ADVANCES IN **SPORT** AND **EXERCISE** SCIENCE SERIES

Nutrition and **Sport**

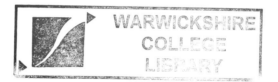

WITHDRAWN

SERIES EDITORS

Neil Spurway MA PhD
Emeritus Professor of Exercise Physiology, University of Glasgow, UK

Don MacLaren BSC MSc PhD CertEd
Professor of Sports Nutrition, School of Sport and Exercise Sciences,
Liverpool John Moores University, Liverpool, UK

For Elsevier:
Commissioning Editor: Dinah Thom
Development Editor: Catherine Jackson
Project Manager: Emma Riley
Designer: Stewart Larking
Illustration Buyer: Bruce Hogarth
Illustrations: David Graham

ADVANCES IN **SPORT** AND **EXERCISE** SCIENCE SERIES

Nutrition and Sport

Edited by

Don MacLaren BSc MSc PhD CertEd

Professor of Sports Nutrition, School of Sport and Exercise Sciences,
Liverpool John Moores University, Liverpool, UK

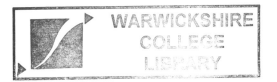

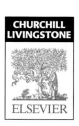

CHURCHILL LIVINGSTONE

ELSEVIER

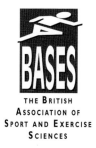

THE BRITISH
ASSOCIATION OF
SPORT AND EXERCISE
SCIENCES

EDINBURGH LONDON NEW YORK OXFORD PHILADELPHIA ST LOUIS SYDNEY TORONTO 2007

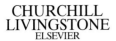

CHURCHILL
LIVINGSTONE
ELSEVIER

First published 2007

ISBN: 978 0 443 10341 4

British Library Cataloguing in Publication Data
A catalogue record for this book is available from the British Library.

Library of Congress Cataloging in Publication Data
A catalog record for this book is available from the Library of Congress.

Notice
Knowledge and best practice in this field are constantly changing. As new research and experience broaden our knowledge, changes in practice, treatment and drug therapy may become necessary or appropriate. Readers are advised to check the most current information provided (i) on procedures featured or (ii) by the manufacturer of each product to be administered, to verify the recommended dose or formula, the method and duration of administration, and contraindications. It is the responsibility of the practitioner, relying on their own experience and knowledge of the patient, to make diagnoses, to determine dosages and the best treatment for each individual patient, and to take all appropriate safety precautions. To the fullest extent of the law, neither the Publisher nor the Editor assumes any liability for any injury and/or damage to persons or property arising out of or related to any use of the material contained in this book.

The Publisher

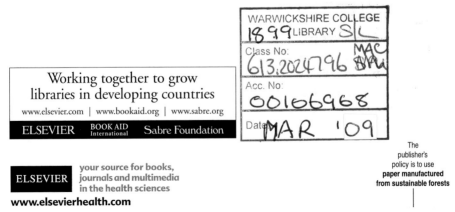

The publisher's policy is to use paper manufactured from sustainable forests

ELSEVIER   your source for books, journals and multimedia in the health sciences

www.elsevierhealth.com

Printed in China

Contents

Contributors

Katherine A Beals PhD RD FACSM
Katherine is an Associate Professor (clinical) in the Division of Nutrition and Department of Family and Preventive Medicine at the University of Utah. She is also the Director of the University of Utah Nutrition Clinic which services university athletes, faculty, staff, students and the greater Salt Lake community. Kathie holds a PhD in Exercise Science and Physical Education from Arizona State University, is a Registered Dietitian, and a Fellow of the American College of Sports Medicine. She has published over a dozen articles on disordered eating and the female athlete triad and recently published a book with Human Kinetics entitled Disordered Eating Among Athletes: A Comprehensive Guide for Health Professionals.

Jo Bowtell BSc PhD
Jo is a Principal Lecturer in Exercise Physiology and Biochemistry at London South Bank University where she is responsible for the nutrition and metabolism modules in the undergraduate and postgraduate programmes. She has published in various areas of nutrition and metabolism as well as on neuromuscular function.

Graeme L Close BSc (Hons) PhD
Graeme is a Senior Research Associate at the University of Liverpool, working in the division of metabolic and cellular medicine. He specializes in free radicals and antioxidants in health and exercise and has published widely in this area. Graeme is a former professional rugby league player and currently works as nutrition and strength/conditioning advisor with several rugby and rowing clubs.

Jeanette Crosland MSc RD
Jeanette is a Registered Dietitian and an accredited Sports Dietitian who has worked in the field of sports nutrition for the last 25 years. She has worked with an extensive range of athletes across many disciplines and has been a consultant to a wide range of squads and organizations such as the British Olympic Association. She is currently the consultant to the British Paralympic Association and lectures at a number of universities as a visiting lecturer in applied sports nutrition. She has written and co-written a number of books about sports nutrition and its practical application.

Allan Hackett BSc MPhil PhD SRD

Allan is a Reader in Community Nutrition at Liverpool John Moores University where he teaches on Community Nutrition, Nutrition and Food & Nutrition programmes. He has published many research papers mainly concerning the dietary habits and nutritional status of children and is particularly interested in dietary survey methodology. He is currently involved in Europe's largest study of the fitness, dietary habits and nutritional status of children of 9–10 years of age which aims to promote physical activity and healthier eating habits. Allan is a member of the Nutrition Society and the British Dietetic Association.

Asker Jeukendrup BSc PhD

Asker is a Professor of Exercise Metabolism at the School of Sport and Exercise Sciences and Director of the Human Performance Laboratory at the University of Birmingham. Asker has published extensively on the links between nutrition, exercise metabolism and performance using stable isotopic techniques and mass spectrometry. He has also written books on Sport Nutrition and High Performance Cycling, is the Editor of the European Journal of Sport Science and member of the editorial board of several other journals. In 2005 he was awarded a Danone Chair in Nutrition at the Free University Brussels in Belgium. Besides this he has worked with many top athletes including track and field athletes of UK Athletics, Chelsea Football Club, and Tour de France cyclists. Asker is also an Ironman triathlete himself.

Francis McArdle BSc (Hons) PhD

Frank is a lecturer working in the division of metabolic and cellular medicine at the University of Liverpool. He specializes in free radical biochemistry and antioxidant nutrition in general, with particular emphasis on selenium biochemistry and nutrition. He has published widely in the fields of both free radical biochemistry and antioxidant nutrition. Frank has recently been appointed to the position of renal lecturer, and hopes to apply his expertise to renal failure.

Don MacLaren CertEd BSc MSc PhD

Don is a Professor of Sports Nutrition at Liverpool John Moores University where he is responsible for the nutrition and metabolism modules in the undergraduate and postgraduate programmes. He has published widely in various areas of nutrition and metabolism as well as on nutritional ergogenic aids. Much of his work is in applied sports nutrition, and he is currently nutrition advisor to a number of professional soccer and rugby union clubs in the UK. In addition, he is a fellow of both the British Association of Sport and Exercise Sciences, and the European College of Sports Sciences.

Melinda M Manore PhD RD

Melinda is a Professor of Nutrition in the Department of Nutrition and Exercise Sciences at Oregon State University where she does research and teaches undergraduate and graduate nutrition/dietetics and nutrition/exercise courses. Her research focuses on the energy and nutrient needs of active individuals, especially active women and the role that poor energy intake plays in menstrual dysfunction, nutritional status and bone health. She also examines the role that nutrition and exercise play in the prevention of disease. Dr Manore is the author of four books and numerous research articles on nutrition and exercise. She is a Fellow of the American College of Sports Medicine (ACSM) and is on the Board of Trustees, an active member of the American Dietetic Association and its Sports and Cardiovascular Practice Group (SCAN) and a member of the American Society of Nutrition.

Ron J Maughan BSc PhD
Ron is currently Professor of Sport and Exercise Nutrition at Loughborough University, England. His research interests are in the physiology, biochemistry and nutrition of exercise performance, with an interest in both the basic science of exercise and the applied aspects that relate to health and to performance in sport. For 10 years, he chaired the Human Physiology Group of the Physiological Society and he now chairs the Nutrition Working Group of the International Olympic Committee.

Susan Shirreffs BSc PhD
Susan is a Senior Lecturer at Loughborough University where she teaches Physiology and Nutrition modules on both undergraduate and postgraduate programmes. She has research interests in sport and exercise physiology and nutrition and publishes particularly in the areas of body water balance, sweat losses and post-exercise rehydration. Susan is a member of The Physiological Society, The Nutrition Society, the British Association of Sport and Exercise Sciences and is a Fellow of the American College of Sports Medicine.

Jim Waterhouse BA (Oxon) DPhil (Oxon) DSc
Jim is a Professor of Biological Rhythms at Liverpool John Moores University where he is responsible for some of the modules on scientific methodology in the postgraduate MRes course. He has published widely in various areas of chronobiology in humans, with particular reference to jet lag, shift work and indirect measurement of the activity of the body clock. He is a Fellow of the Royal Society of Medicine, and co-editor of Biological Rhythm Research.

Klaas R Westerterp PhD
Klaas is Professor of Human Energetics at Maastricht University, where he coordinates the bachelor and master programme Metabolism and Nutrition. Among his present fields of interest in research are energy metabolism and body composition, with special emphasis on observations in daily living conditions using accelerometers and labelled water. He was from 1997 to 2003 a member of the Editorial Board of the British Journal of Nutrition. From 1999 to 2005 he was head of the Department of Human Biology. He is a member of the FAO/WHO/UNU Expert group on Human Energy Requirements.

Clyde Williams BSc MSc PhD
Clyde is a Professor of Sports Science at Loughborough University where he teaches and conducts research on the influences of nutrition on performance during sport and exercise. During his career at Loughborough he has been head of school and pro-vice-chancellor (research). He was the founding chair of BASES and the first

professor of sports science in the UK. He is also a 'special professor' in sports medicine at Nottingham University. He is chair of the Advisory Board for the Professional Register in Sport Nutrition.

Kathleen Woolf PhD RD

Kathleen is an Assistant Professor in the Department of Nutrition at Arizona State University. She is a member of several professional societies including the Academy for Eating Disorders, the American College of Sports Medicine, the American Dietetic Association, the American Society for Nutrition, and the North American Association for the Study of Obesity. As a researcher, her primary area of interest is the identification, prevention and treatment of chronic diseases through nutrition and physical activity modalities. She has also completed sports nutrition research examining the nutritional status of female athletes and efficacy of nutritional ergogenic aids. She currently provides nutrition guidance to recreational and collegiate swimming teams.

Preface

Sport and exercise nutrition has been recognized as a major component of Sports Science/Studies undergraduate and postgraduate programmes over the last 10–15 years. The plethora of review and research articles published in journals has escalated significantly over this time[1]. Originally, the research focused on the importance of carbohydrates, although more recently there has been a significant apportioning of findings in relation to amino acid and protein intake, 'fat loading', and studies on hydration and rehydration. The 'professionalization' of sport, together with the doping regulations of the IOC, has probably led to the significant increase in research (and sales) on nutritional supplements and ergogenic aids. More recently, the importance of micronutrients has also been recognized; not merely for athletes but also for those engaged in exercise. The concept of free radicals and antioxidants continues to occupy not only space in quality journal articles but also reams of coverage in weekly and monthly magazines. Because there is a great deal of money tied up in sport, practical aspects such as the nutritional impact of crossing time zones or of transferring the theory into practice need to be understood.

As a consequence of the magnitude of research publications in this field, undergraduate and postgraduate students (and indeed senior coaches in a variety of sports) constantly explore appropriate texts to furnish themselves with up-to-date information. This textbook addresses the key issues relating to sport and exercise nutrition by employing a critical review perspective, and is aimed at final year undergraduate and Masters students. I have managed to persuade a number of eminent researchers and practitioners into writing chapters on their areas of expertise. The result is what I consider to be an outstanding sports nutrition treatise for students engaged in such modules and for dietitians and nutritionists who wish to deepen their knowledge in the research behind their practice. I find myself in the unenviable position of being author of an excellent book in which I have not contributed a chapter, essentially because I have selected a number of my friends and colleagues

---

[1]MacLaren DPM 1999 The 'rise' of sports nutrition. Journal of Sports Sciences 17:933-935

who happen to be eminent scientists and experts in the subject areas addressed. Consequently the chapters focus on the key areas endemic to any sports nutrition programme.

The first two chapters explore the concept of energy expenditure and energy intake before examining the contribution and importance of the macronutrients. The chapters on energy critically evaluate the methods of assessments of expenditure and intake since such knowledge is crucial when guiding athletes and 'exercisers' in the amount of food they should consume for weight gain or loss. The three chapters on the macronutrients provide sound metabolic background on their requirements before expanding on the plethora of peer-reviewed published papers reporting on the contribution of these energy sources during exercise. The efficacy of ingesting the various macronutrients before, during, and/or after exercise is also assessed. The clear evidence in support of the need for carbohydrates in offsetting fatigue is matched by the fact that dehydration is also a major factor resulting in fatigue. The chapter on dehydration and rehydration examines the influence of exercise and the environment on dehydration and so provides evidence on strategies employed to reduce dehydration and, in the post-exercise period, promote rehydration. The importance of a balanced diet with sufficient amounts of micronutrients and antioxidants are important considerations for the health of athletes and those engaged in exercise programmes. It is unlikely that large doses of either will help improve performance, although lack of sufficient amounts may compromise health. The chapters on micronutrients and antioxidants describe the roles they play in the health and well-being of athletes, and evaluate whether supplementation is necessary. Most athletes trawl the literature to find out the latest on ergogenic aids with a view to improving performance. Only a select group of purported nutritional ergogenic aids possess sufficient sound background support for their use. The chapter on ergogenic aids guides the reader to carefully consider the balanced evidence rather than ingest a substance based solely on theory. The female athlete presents specific considerations with regard to nutritional support, and so the chapter on the female athlete addresses these issues in detail. With the globalization of sport and the demands of playing sport at many different times of day, the athlete needs to consider how and when to eat and drink in order to adjust to these extraneous demands. Furthermore, many individuals who exercise have to do so at varying times of the day dependent on their work and shift patterns. The chapter on chronobiology provides guidelines to such athletes, coaches and 'workers'. The final chapter contains advice on the practicalities of putting the theory into practice, drawing on the sound science from previous chapters.

I believe the resultant is a text which could conceivably be called sports nutrition: from science to practice. I hope you enjoy the nutritional excursion which most certainly provides you with food for thought.

Liverpool 2007   **Don MacLaren**

Chapter 1

Assessment of energy expenditure

Klaas R Westerterp

LEARNING OBJECTIVES

After studying this chapter, you should be able to:

1. Describe the principles, applicability, limitations and differences between direct and indirect calorimetry for the measurement of energy expenditure.
2. Describe the size, determinants and variation of the components of daily energy expenditure.
3. Describe the methodology to compare and normalize energy expenditure for individual differences in body size and body composition.

4. Describe the effects of endurance exercise for energy expenditure, body composition and physical performance.
5. Predict the individual energy expenditure from body size and physical activity.

INTRODUCTION

Life can be regarded as a combustion process. The metabolism of an organism is a process of energy production by the combustion of fuel in the form of carbohydrate, protein, fat or alcohol. In this process oxygen is consumed and carbon dioxide produced. Measuring energy expenditure means measuring heat production or heat loss, which is called direct calorimetry. The measurement of heat production by measuring oxygen consumption and/or carbon dioxide production is called indirect calorimetry.

Total energy expenditure (TEE) consists of three components, i.e. basal metabolic rate (BMR), the thermic effect of food or diet-induced energy expenditure (DEE), and the energy cost of physical activity or activity-induced energy expenditure (AEE).

Here, the current methodology to measure energy expenditure and the separate components is described. Subsequently, methods for the evaluation of energy expenditure data are presented including three aspects: comparisons and normalization of energy expenditure for body size and body composition; limits to energy expenditure; and prediction equations for energy expenditure, based on body size and physical activity. Where appropriate, the theory is illustrated with an application.

METHODOLOGY

DIRECT CALORIMETRY

The early calorimeters for the measurement of energy expenditure were direct calorimeters. At the end of the eighteenth century Lavoisier constructed one of the first calorimeters, measuring energy expenditure in a guinea pig. The animal was placed in a wire cage, which occupied the centre of an apparatus. The surrounding space was filled with chunks of ice. As the ice melted from the animal's body heat, the water, which collected in a container, could be weighed. The ice cavity was surrounded by an outer space packed with snow to maintain a constant temperature. Thus, no heat flowed from the surroundings to the inner ice jacket. Figure 1.1 shows Lavoisier's calorimeter schematically.

Nowadays the heat loss is measured in a calorimeter by removing the heat with a cooling stream of air or water or measuring the heat flow through the wall. In the first case heat conduction through the wall of the calorimeter is prevented and the flow of heat is measured by the product of temperature

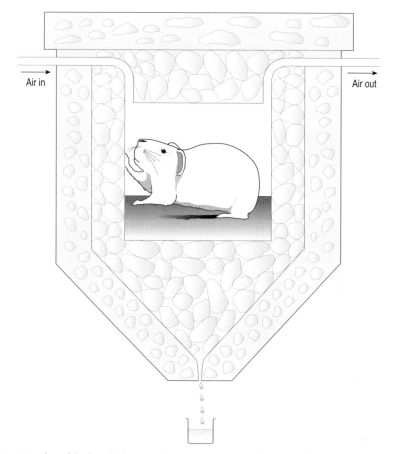

Figure 1.1   Lavoisier's calorimeter. The animal melts the ice in the inner jacket and a mixture of ice and water prevents heat flow to the surrounding container.

difference between inflow and outflow and the rate of flow of the cooling medium. In the latter case instead of preventing heat flow through the wall the rate of this flow is measured from differences in temperature over the wall, so-called gradient layer calorimetry. An example is a suit calorimeter as described below.

INDIRECT CALORIMETRY

In indirect calorimetry heat production is calculated from chemical processes. Knowing for example that 1 mol glucose oxidizes with 6 moles oxygen to 6 moles water and 6 moles carbon dioxide and produces 2.8 MJ heat, we can then calculate heat production from oxygen consumption or carbon dioxide production. The energy equivalent of oxygen and carbon dioxide varies with the nutrient oxidized (Table 1.1).

Brouwer (1957) generated simple formulae for calculating the heat production and the quantities of carbohydrate (C), protein (P) and fat (F) oxidized from oxygen consumption, carbon dioxide production and urine-nitrogen loss. The principle of the calculation consists of three equations with the mentioned three measured variables:

Oxygen consumption	$= 0.829\ C + 0.967\ P + 2.019\ F$
Carbon dioxide production	$= 0.829\ C + 0.775\ P + 1.427\ F$
Heat production	$= 21.1\ C + 18.7\ P + 19.6\ F$

Protein oxidation (g) is calculated as $6.25 \times$ urine-nitrogen (g), and subsequently oxygen consumption and carbon dioxide production can be corrected for protein oxidation to allow calculation of carbohydrate and fat oxidation.

The general formula for the calculation of energy production (E) derived from these figures is:

$$E = 16.20\ \text{oxygen consumption} + 5.00\ \text{carbon dioxide production} - 0.95\ P$$

In this formula the contribution of P to E, the so-called protein correction, is small. In the case of a normal protein oxidation of 10–15% of the daily energy production, the protein correction for the calculation of E is about 1%. Usually one measures only urine nitrogen when information on the contribution of C, P and F to energy production is needed. For calculation of energy production the protein correction is often neglected.

Nowadays, there are many instruments for measuring oxygen consumption and carbon dioxide production, ranging from room-sized respiration chambers to portable devices (Ainsli et al 2003).

Table 1.1 Gaseous exchange and heat production of metabolized nutrients (A) and resulting energy equivalents of oxygen and carbon dioxide (B)

A Nutrient	Oxygen consumption (l/g)	Carbon dioxide production (l/g)	Heat production (kJ/g)
Carbohydrate	0.829	0.829	17.5
Protein	0.967	0.775	18.1
Fat	2.019	1.427	39.6

B Nutrient	Oxygen (kJ/l)	Carbon dioxide (kJ/l)
Carbohydrate	21.1	21.1
Protein	18.7	23.4
Fat	19.6	27.8

Measuring energy expenditure with doubly labelled water

Stable isotopes allow the fully unrestricted measurement of energy expenditure, without the requirement of continuous sampling of respiratory gases. Here, the doubly labelled water method, as the most widespread method, is described in more detail. The doubly labelled water method is a method of indirect calorimetry that was introduced for human use about 20 years ago. The principle of the method is that after a loading dose of water labelled with the stable isotopes of ^2H and ^{18}O, ^2H is eliminated as water, while ^{18}O is eliminated as both water and carbon dioxide. The difference between the two elimination rates is therefore a measure of carbon dioxide production (Fig. 1.2). The deuterium (^2H) equilibrates throughout the body's water pool, and the ^{18}O equilibrates in both the water and the bicarbonate pool. The bicarbonate pool consists largely of dissolved carbon dioxide, which is an end product of metabolism and passes in the bloodstream to the lungs for excretion. The rate constants for the disappearance of the two isotopes from the body are measured by mass spectrometric analysis of samples of a body fluid, blood, saliva or urine.

The method has been developed after the discovery in 1949 that the oxygen atoms in the body water and bicarbonate pools are in equilibration. The method was initially used for studying energy metabolism of small animals in the wild. You capture animals, administer the dose of labelled water, release the animals and then recapture them after an appropriate

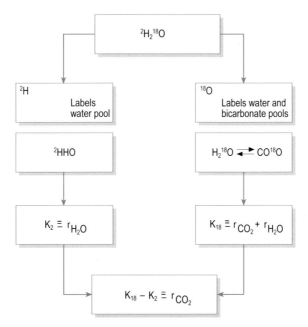

Figure 1.2 Principle of the doubly labelled water method, measuring carbon dioxide production (r_{CO_2}) from the elimination rates of ^{18}O and ^2H after loading with $^2H_2{}^{18}O$.

interval to assess the rate at which the isotopes disappear from their bodies. One of the first such studies involved measuring the energy cost of a 500-kilometre flight by trained racing pigeons. It was not until 1982 that the method was first used in people. The reason is that ^{18}O-water is very expensive and a human being requires a much higher dose than a bird. The isotope is not substantially cheaper now, but isotope ratio mass spectrometers have become so sensitive that the method can now work with much smaller doses of isotope. Presently, the method is frequently used with people in several centres.

The method has been safe to use in humans as the water is labelled with stable isotopes, ^{18}O and ^{2}H, at low abundances. Both ^{18}O and ^{2}H are naturally occurring isotopes, which are present in the body prior to the administration of doubly labelled water. As such, tracer studies depend not on measurement of isotope concentrations, but rather on concentrations in excess of natural abundance or background isotope concentrations. The nominal natural abundances of ^{18}O and ^{2}H are 2000 and 150 ppm, respectively. Typical doses of doubly labelled water only produce excess isotope abundances of 200–300 and 100–150 ppm for ^{18}O and ^{2}H, respectively.

This method can be used to measure carbon dioxide production and hence energy production in free-living subjects for periods of some days to several weeks. The optimal observation period is 1–3 biological half-lives of the isotopes. The biological half-life is a function of the level of the energy expenditure. The optimal observation interval ranges between 3 days for highly active subjects or prematures, respectively, and about 4 weeks in elderly (sedentary) subjects.

An observation starts by collecting a baseline sample. Then, a weighed isotope dose is administered, usually a mixture of 10% ^{18}O and 5% ^{2}H in, for a 70 kg adult, 100–150 cc water. Subsequently the isotopes equilibrate with the body water and the initial sample is collected. The equilibration time is, depending on body size and metabolic rate, for adults 4–8 hours. During equilibration the subject usually does not consume any food or drink. After collecting the initial sample the subject resumes its routines according to the instructions of the experimenter and is asked to collect body water samples (blood, saliva or urine) at regular intervals until the end of the observation period.

Validation studies resulted in an accuracy of 1–3% and a precision of 2–8%, comparing the method with respirometry. The method has now been applied in subjects over a wide range of ages and at different activity levels, from premature infants to elderly and from hospitalized patients to participants in a cycle race. The method needs high precision Isotope Ratio Mass Spectrometry, working at low levels of isotope enrichment for the financial reasons mentioned above (Speakman 1997).

There is still discussion on the ideal sampling protocol, i.e. multi-point versus two-point method. We prefer a combination of both, taking two independent samples at the start, in the midpoint, and at the end of the observation period. Thus an independent comparison can be made within one run, calculating carbon dioxide production from the first samples and the second samples over the first half and the second half of the observation interval.

The doubly labelled water method gives precise and accurate information on carbon dioxide production. Converting carbon dioxide production to energy expenditure needs information on the energy equivalent of CO_2, which can be calculated with additional information on the substrate mixture being oxidized. One option is the calculation of the energy equivalent from the macronutrient composition of the diet. In energy balance, substrate intake and substrate utilization are assumed to be identical. Alternatively substrate utilization can be measured over a representative interval in a respiration chamber (see below). In conclusion, DLW is an excellent method for measuring energy expenditure in unrestrained humans in their normal surroundings over a time period of 1–4 weeks.

DIRECT CALORIMETRY VERSUS INDIRECT CALORIMETRY

Webb et al 1988 performed an experiment where heat loss and metabolic expenditure were measured simultaneously with direct and indirect calorimetry, respectively. Five women and five men were wearing a suit calorimeter while they stayed in a respiration chamber. Observations included rest, walking at different speeds on a motor-driven treadmill, and cycling on an electrically braked cycle ergometer. Heat loss matched metabolic expenditure during rest (Fig. 1.3). During walking, heat loss was lower than metabolic expenditure and the difference was higher at a higher speed. Metabolic

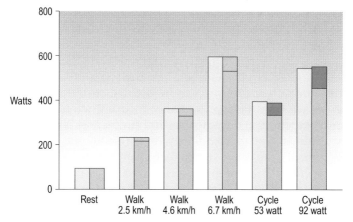

Figure 1.3 Metabolic expenditure (left bar) and heat loss (right-hand bar) as measured simultaneously with direct and indirect calorimetry, respectively, in five women and five men during rest, walking at different speeds on a motor-driven treadmill, and cycling on an electrically braked cycle ergometer. The open part at the top of the right-hand bar during walking is the discrepancy with metabolic expenditure. The dark part at the top of the right-hand bar during cycling is the power produced at the cycle ergometer (adapted from Webb et al 1988).

expenditure matched the sum of heat loss and power produced during cycling, as measured by the ergometer. The results clearly demonstrate the validity of the calorimetric methods, where metabolic expenditure matches the sum of heat loss and power produced, the latter being zero under resting conditions. Thus under resting conditions, the two methods give the same result. During exercise, the discrepancy can be as much as 20%, the ceiling of the efficiency of work-performance by the human body.

COMPONENTS OF DAILY ENERGY EXPENDITURE

BASAL METABOLIC RATE

Basal metabolic rate is the energy expenditure to maintain and preserve the integrity of vital functions. It is defined as the metabolic rate of a subject that is awake, resting, post-absorptive, and in the thermoneutral zone. Thus, basal metabolic rate is commonly measured in the early morning after an overnight fast. Subjects are instructed to refrain from exercise the day before the measurement, including the transport to the laboratory in the morning before the test. A fast of 10–12 hours is the accepted procedure to eliminate the diet-induced energy expenditure. A room temperature of 22–24°C meets the thermoneutral conditions for a normally dressed subject.

An optimal device for the measurement of BMR, under stress-free conditions, is a ventilated hood. The first 10 minutes of a measurement are usually discarded to eliminate habituation to the testing procedure. The following measurement lasts ideally 20 to 30 minutes. Longer intervals increase the risk subjects get restless at the end of the measurement. Thus, the coefficient of variation in BMR is below 5% (Adriaens et al 2003).

DIET-INDUCED ENERGY EXPENDITURE

Diet-induced energy expenditure can be defined as the increase in energy expenditure above basal fasting level after food ingestion. The postprandial rise in energy expenditure lasts for several hours and is often regarded as completely terminated at approximately 10 hours after the last meal but there is still an argument as to when the post-absorptive state is reached.

The experimental design of most studies on DEE is a measurement of resting energy expenditure before and after a test meal, with a ventilated hood system. The observation is started after an overnight fast, where subjects are refrained from eating after the last meal at 20.00 hours at the latest. Thus, with observations starting between 08.00 and 09.00 hours the next morning, the fasting interval is at least 12 hours. Postprandial measurements are made for several hours where subjects have to remain stationary, most often in a supine position, for the duration of the measurements. In some studies, measurements are 30 minutes with 15-minute intervals allowing, e.g., for sanitary activities.

The use of a respiration chamber to measure DEE has the advantage of reproducing more physiological conditions over a longer period of time while regular meals are consumed throughout the day. The DEE, as observed in a respiration chamber over 24 hours, has been evaluated in different ways: (1) as the difference in 24-hour energy expenditure between a day in the fed state and a day in the fasted state; (2) as the difference in daytime energy expenditure adjusted for the variability of spontaneous activity and basal metabolic rate; and (3) as the difference in 24-hour energy expenditure adjusted for the variability of spontaneous activity and basal metabolic rate.

Reported intra-individual variability in DEE, determined with ventilated-hood systems, is 6 to 30%. Reported within-subject variability in DEE, determined with a respiration chamber, is 43 to 48% (Westerterp 2004).

ACTIVITY–INDUCED ENERGY EXPENDITURE

Activity-induced energy expenditure is the most variable component of daily energy expenditure. The doubly labelled water method, in combination with a measurement of BMR by a ventilated hood, has provided truly quantitative estimates of AEE in daily life. Then, AEE is calculated from TEE and BMR with the assumption that DEE is a constant fraction of total energy expenditure in subjects consuming a diet that meets energy requirements. The doubly labelled water method has become the golden standard for the validation of field methods of assessing physical activity. Accelerometers for movement registration are more and more used to objectively assess physical activity including the activity-frequency, -duration and -intensity, and can be used at a larger scale than the more expensive doubly labelled water method.

To test the validity of accelerometers for movement registration, energy expenditure as measured with indirect calorimetry is used as a reference. Thus, many accelerometers have been tested under laboratory conditions during standardized activities, in field settings against portable calorimeters or in the controlled environment of a whole room calorimeter. Most accelerometers show good to very good correlations ($r = 0.74$–0.95) with energy expenditure during walking and running on a treadmill or with other defined activities. An increasing number of accelerometers have also been validated against doubly labelled water under unconfined conditions in daily life. Correlations between accelerometer output and doubly labelled water derived energy expenditure measures, such as AEE or TEE, are often poor and mainly determined by subject's characteristics such as body mass, age, sex and height (Plasqui et al 2005).

Determinants of activity energy expenditure

The main determinants of daily energy expenditure are body size and physical activity. Activity energy expenditure is the most variable component of total energy expenditure. It was assessed whether the physical activity level in confined conditions is an indicator of free-living physical activity (Westerterp & Kester 2003). Activity energy expenditure was measured over one day in the confined environment of a respiration chamber (floor-space 7.0 m²), where activities were restricted to low intensity activities of daily living, and over 2 weeks in the free-living environment with doubly labelled water. Subjects were 16 women and 29 men (31 ± 10 years; 24.2 ± 2.7 kg/m²; means ± SD). Activity energy expenditure in the chamber was 47 ± 13% of the value in daily life, and the two values were correlated (Fig. 1.4, r = 0.50, P <0.001; partial correlation corrected for age, gender and BMI: 0.40, P <0.01). The chamber value explained 25% of the total variance in free-living activity energy expenditure. Thus, the activity level of a subject under sedentary conditions is an indicator for activity energy expenditure in daily life, showing the importance of non-exercise activity for daily energy expenditure. Future studies should indicate whether there is a genetic component in AEE as suggested by a more than twofold variation in AEE between individuals in the same confined environment of a respiration chamber and the significant relation with AEE in free-living conditions. Additionally, behavioural choices could be similar within subjects and different between subjects whether or not they are in a confined living space.

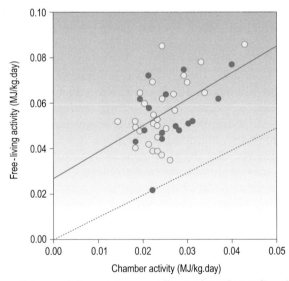

Figure 1.4 Free-living activity energy expenditure plotted as a function of activity energy expenditure in the confined environment of a respiration chamber in 16 women (closed circles) and 29 men (open circles), with the line of identity (dashed) and the linear regression line (continuous).

COMPARISONS AND NORMALIZATION OF ENERGY EXPENDITURE FOR BODY SIZE AND BODY COMPOSITION

BASAL METABOLIC RATE

Basal metabolic rate is usually compared between subjects by standardizing to an estimate of metabolic body size. Fat-free body mass seems to be the best predictor. However, energy expenditure should not be divided by the absolute fat-free mass (FFM) value as the relationship between energy expenditure and FFM has a y and x intercept significantly different from zero. For example, comparing BMR per kg FFM between women and men results in a significantly higher value for women. The smaller the FFM the higher the BMR/FFM ratio and thus the BMR per kg FFM is on average higher in women with on average a lower FFM compared with men. The indicated way of comparing BMR data is by regression analysis. Covariates to be included are FFM, fat mass (FM), age and gender. Then, gender does not come out as a significant contributor to the explained variation. There remains a (theoretical) problem in this approach. The covariates are significantly different for the two groups without much overlap. Ideally one should compare BMR in a group of women and men with comparable body composition. However, then there will be other systematic differences. The women have to be very muscular and lean, i.e. endurance athletes, or the men have to be obese.

Many studies have shown the similarity of BMR of women and men when properly adjusted for differences in body composition as mentioned above. However, some studies showed women to have a higher or a lower BMR compared with men after adjusting for differences in body composition. The differences were largely a function of the menstrual cycle phase that the women were in at the time of measurement. Basal metabolic rate in women is lowest in the late follicular phase and highest in the late luteal phase with an average difference between the two extremes of 5–10%.

In conclusion, BMR is comparable for women and men when properly adjusted for body composition. There are indications that post-ovulation women have the same or slightly higher values and pre-ovulation and post-menopausal women have the same or slightly lower values than men.

Basal metabolic rate and endurance exercise

The main determinant of BMR is the fat-free mass. Energy balance is an extrinsic factor known to influence BMR as well. Below are two examples of the relation between fat-free mass and energy balance and BMR as observed in novice athletes and elite athletes (Westerterp 2001).

In novice athletes, an increase in fat-free mass was induced of 49.5 ± 7.3 to 52.2 ± 7.6 kg (means $\pm$ SD, N = 23, P <0.001) with a 44-week training programme to run a half-marathon. Sleeping metabolic rate, as a proxy of BMR, did not increase; in fact, the opposite occurred: sleeping metabolic rate decreased by 0.3 ± 0.5 MJ/day (means $\pm$ SD, N = 23, P <0.05). Sleeping metabolic rate as a function of FFM was lower after 40 weeks of exercise training than before training (Fig. 1.5A). The decrease in sleeping metabolic rate was related to a decrease in body mass (r = 0.62, P <0.01), possibly as a defence mechanism by the body to maintain energy balance. The results contrast with findings for elite athletes. The BMR of elite athletes from the Swedish national cross-country ski team was compared with that of sedentary non-athletic controls matched for sex and fat-free mass (Fig. 1.5B). Comparisons with theoretical calculations of BMR were also made. The athletes had a 13% higher (P <0.001) BMR than controls if related to fat-free mass and a 16% higher (P = 0.001) BMR if related to both fat-free mass and fat mass. Possible explanations included an increased substrate flux in the athletes, even during the non-exercise phase, for recovery and in anticipation of exercise.

Summarizing, in elite endurance athletes, BMR is increased for two reasons: fat-free mass is higher and BMR adjusted for fat-free mass is also higher. It is suggested that an increased substrate flux is a determinant of the increased BMR in elite athletes. This was confirmed by the value of BMR in an athlete with a previous history of anorexia nervosa. She had a much lower BMR (by 16%) than those of the other female athletes but matched the sedentary controls as well as theoretical calculations. The effect of exercise on BMR was not observed in the intervention study in which (sedentary) subjects were trained over 44 weeks to run a half-marathon. Possibly the interval was too short to induce increases in metabolically active body components like organ tissue. Additionally, the daily energy turnover in the elite athletes was more than twice the highest values reached in the novice athletes after training and most of the novice athletes did not maintain energy balance as reflected in body weight loss over the training interval.

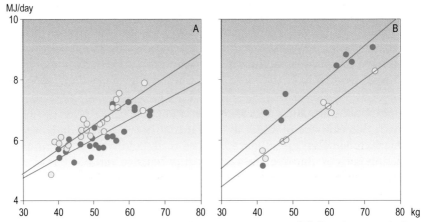

Figure 1.5 Metabolic rate as a function of fat-free mass. (A) Sleeping metabolic rate in novice athletes (n = 23) before (open symbols) and after (filled symbols) 40 weeks of exercise training. (B) Basal metabolic rate in elite athletes (closed symbols) and sedentary control subjects (open symbols).

DIET-INDUCED ENERGY EXPENDITURE

The main determinant of DEE is the energy content of the food, followed by the protein fraction of the food. The thermic effect of alcohol is similar to the thermic effect of protein. Diet-induced thermogenesis is related to the stimulation of energy-requiring processes during the post prandial period; the intestinal absorption of nutrients, the initial steps of their metabolism and the storage of the absorbed but not immediately oxidized nutrients. As such, the amount of food ingested quantified as the energy content of the food is a determinant of DEE. The most common way to express DEE is derived from this phenomenon, the difference between energy expenditure after food consumption and BMR, divided by the rate of nutrient energy administration.

Theoretically, based on the amount of ATP required for the initial steps of metabolism and storage, the DEE is different for each nutrient. Reported DEE values for separate nutrients are 0 to 3% for fat, 5 to 10% for carbohydrate, 20 to 30% for protein, and 10 to 30% for alcohol. In healthy subjects with a mixed diet, DEE represents about 10% of the total amount of energy ingested over 24 hours.

In conclusion, when a subject is in energy balance, where intake equals expenditure, DEE is 10% of total energy expenditure.

Diet composition and diet-induced energy expenditure

To study the effect of diet composition on diet-induced thermogenesis, energy expenditure was measured at two diets with a different macronutrient composition (Westerterp et al 1999). Subjects were eight healthy female volunteers (age 27 ± 3 years; BMI 23 ± 3 kg/m^2). Diets were a high protein and carbohydrate (HP/C) (60:10:30; E% carbohydrate, fat and protein) and high fat (HF) (30:60:10) diet, both isoenergetic, isovolumetric, composed of normal food items and matched for organoleptic properties (taste, smell, appearance). Subjects each spent two 36-hour periods in a respiration chamber consuming both test diets in random order. Components of 24-hour energy expenditure: sleeping metabolic rate, DEE and activity-induced energy expenditure were measured. Figure 1.6 shows the mean pattern of DEE throughout the day, calculated by plotting the residual of the individual relationship between energy expenditure and physical activity in time, as measured over 30-minute intervals from a 24-hour observation in the respiration chamber. Resting metabolic rate did not return to basal metabolic rate before lunch at 4 hours after breakfast, or before dinner at 5 hours after lunch. Overnight, basal metabolic rate was reached at 8 hours after dinner consumption. DEE was higher in all subjects while on the HP/C diet (1295 vs 931 kJ/d; 14.6 vs 10.5% of energy intake; P <0.02). There was no significant difference in other components or TEE, though there was a trend towards higher TEE on the HP/C diet. In conclusion, a high protein and carbohydrate diet induces a greater thermic response in healthy individuals when compared to a high-fat diet.

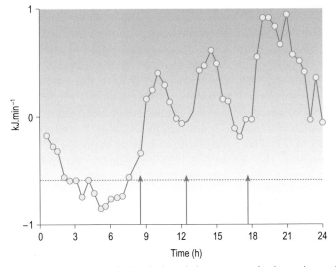

Figure 1.6 The mean pattern of diet-induced thermogenesis throughout the day, calculated by plotting the residual of the individual relationship between energy expenditure and physical activity in time, as measured over 30-minute intervals from a 24-hour observation in a respiration chamber: ––– = level of basal metabolic rate; arrows = meal times.

ACTIVITY-INDUCED ENERGY EXPENDITURE

Activity-induced energy expenditure is the most variable component of total energy expenditure. There is no consensus on the way to normalize AEE for differences in body size. A frequently used method to quantify physical activity is by expressing TEE as a multiple of BMR, the physical activity index:

$$PAI = \frac{TEE}{BMR}$$

It assumes that the variation in total energy expenditure is due to body size and physical activity. The effect of body size on total energy expenditure is corrected for by expressing TEE as a multiple of BMR. Sometimes it is stated that the expression of total energy expenditure as a multiple of BMR for comparison between subjects is precluded by the fact that the nature of the relation between total energy expenditure and BMR is highly variable between studies and often has a non-zero intercept. Subsequently, it proposed to adjust total energy expenditure for BMR to correct for the effect of body size in a linear regression analysis. A third alternative method many studies have used to adjust AEE for differences in body size is by expressing AEE per kg body mass, assuming that energy expenditure associated with physical activity is weight dependent.

Recently, it was shown that PAI does not fully adjust for differences in body size. In children, the increase in AEE and PAI during growth does not equate to a higher level of physical activity expressed as body movement. An increase in AEE and PAI was more likely due to an increase in body size or body weight, and therefore these estimates were not the best indicators of the total amount of physical activity in comparisons between groups who differ in body size. Similarly, the obese have higher energy expenditure for an activity than non-obese subjects, especially for weight bearing activities. Obese and normal-weight subjects who differed in body weight by more than 40 kg did not differ in activity counts obtained during the performance of a standard activity, i.e., walking at 4 km/h, but AEE during this standard activity was significantly higher in the obese group. Additionally, physical activity assessed by accelerometry was significantly lower in the obese group, whereas there was no difference between the obese and normal-weight in AEE under free-living conditions. AEE per kilogram body mass has to be similar to allow the same body movement in an obese as in a non-obese subject.

In conclusion, activity-induced energy expenditure can be compared between individuals with the physical activity index, i.e. total energy expenditure as a multiple of basal metabolic rate, by adjustment of total energy expenditure for basal metabolic to correct for the effect of body size in a linear regression analysis, and by expressing activity-induced energy expenditure per kg body mass.

LIMITS TO ENERGY EXPENDITURE

Activity-induced energy expenditure sets the limits of TEE, where diet-induced energy expenditure can be assumed to be a constant fraction of 10% of TEE and BMR is determined by body size. Interestingly, there is a narrow distribution of the PAI of subjects. Already, Black et al (1996) suggested that there are boundaries for activity levels within the general population. They suggested a PAI range of 1.2–2.5 for 'sustainable lifestyles'. At PAI values around 2.5 subjects indeed have problems to maintain energy balance. Only in exceptional groups like endurance athletes, higher PAI values are reached while body weight is maintained. Training studies of sedentary subjects also give confirmation for the upper limit of PAI in the general population at a value of 2.5.

Training does not have the expected effect on energy expenditure when food intake is not ad libitum. A clear example is that the addition of exercise to an energy -restricted diet results in little further weight loss. Weight loss is not different for groups undergoing dietary restriction and dietary restriction plus exercise. The latter implicates that the direct cost of the exercise training is compensated by a reduction of activity-associated energy expenditure outside the training sessions. Evidence for the fact that energy restriction negatively affects physical activity also comes from studies of energy restriction per se on physical activity.

Physical activity declines with age. Black et al (1996) concluded from an analysis of 574 doubly labelled water measurements that the physical activity index is fairly constant between 18 and 65 years. There seems to be a gradual decline with age, starting at about age 65 and getting more pronounced after age 80. On average, subjects of 65 years and over have a PAI below 1.65, i.e. spent less than 30% of daily energy expenditure on physical activity. Subjects of over 80 generally have an extremely low physical activity index, well below the level of 1.5 as defined for sedentary adults. It is intriguing to observe that the physical activity level of younger subjects was modified with exercise training while exercise training had no effect in older subjects.

EXERCISE TRAINING AND LIMITS TO ENERGY EXPENDITURE

There are a limited number of well-controlled exercise intervention studies measuring the effect on energy expenditure. The size of the change in energy expenditure associated with physical activity is generally higher than the energy cost of the training intervention. The discrepancy between the expected increase and the measured increase in TEE is a function of the training time. This is most clearly illustrated in the study of Westerterp et al (1992) where seven subjects were measured at the start and 8, 20 and 40 weeks after the start of the training. Figure 1.7 shows how the training volume doubled from 25 to 50 km running per week without any change in PAI. Apparently the effect of an exercise intervention on daily energy turnover decreases in time, i.e. novice runners increase the efficiency of the exercise as

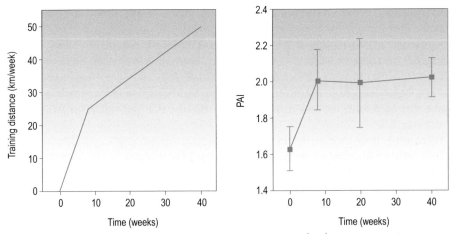

Figure 1.7 Training distance and physical activity index (PAI) in seven novice athletes (three women and four men) at baseline and 8, 20 and 40 weeks after the start of a training period in preparation for the half-marathon.

a result of the training. Another interesting aspect is the value of the PAI, already reached at the first observation point, 8 weeks after the start of the training period.

At the start of the training period, the seven subjects had a mean PAI of 1.63 ± 0.12, a value for a sedentary lifestyle. The value PAI reached after the start of the training corresponds with the upper limit, as defined above, where at PAI values around 2.5 subjects have problems to maintain energy balance. Indeed, individual values did not exceed this value, resulting in a mean PAI value around 2.0.

PREDICTION EQUATIONS FOR ENERGY EXPENDITURE, BASED ON BODY SIZE AND PHYSICAL ACTIVITY

In many situations, information on energy expenditure is required while no real measurement can be performed. Then, energy expenditure can be predicted from body size and a measure of physical activity. Body size determines BMR, the largest component of TEE. Physical activity determines additional variation as reflected in AEE. The third component, DEE, is 10% of total energy expenditure when a subject consumes a mixed diet and is in energy balance. Thus, energy expenditure can be expressed as multiples of BMR, i.e., the PAI.

There are several equations for the prediction of BMR from body size. The FAO/WHO/UNU Expert Committee on Human Energy Requirements reported on the use and validity. The determinants in the equation are body composition or weight, age, height and gender. In the latter type of equations, based on weight, age, height and gender, ethnicity should be taken into account as well. The difference between ethnic groups disappears when BMR is predicted from body composition.

The complex nature of physical activity makes it difficult to accurately measure all its aspects and assess the impact on energy expenditure. Different measuring techniques available can be grouped into four categories: behavioural observation, self-report (questionnaires and activity diaries), physiological markers (heart rate, body temperature, and ventilation), and motion sensors (pedometers and accelerometers). Ideally, physical activity should be assessed during daily life, over periods long enough to be representative for the habitual activity level and with minimal discomfort to the subject. Self-report (questionnaires and activity diaries), physiological markers (heart rate), and motion sensors (pedometers and accelerometers) are applied most frequently. Accelerometers are the most promising tool for the objective assessment of physical activity in daily life.

The tri-axial accelerometer for movement registration, as developed in our laboratory, showed correlations between PAI and activity counts of 0.79, 0.73 and 0.78 in children, in healthy young adults, and in the elderly, respectively. The total explained variation in TEE of 83%, based only on subjects' characteristics, age, body mass, and height, and Tracmor counts, is the highest reported so far.

DISCUSSION

Energy expenditure can be measured with direct or indirect calorimetry. The result is a function of body size, food intake and physical activity. In daily life conditions, the minimum value is basal metabolic rate. Depending on body size and physical fitness, a five- to twentyfold increase of metabolic rate can be sustained for a few minutes, while a healthy young adult can, if necessary, develop five to eight times the BMR over an 8-hour working day. In the general population, the PAI ranges between 1.2 and 2.2–2.5 over intervals of 1 week or longer. In proportion of TEE, AEE varies from 5% in a subject with a minimum PAI of 1.2 to 45–50% in a subject with a PAI of 2.2–2.5. At a PAI value of 1.75, close to the average reported for the general population, AEE is one-third of total energy expenditure.

Energy expenditure data are the basis for the estimation of energy requirements. With the introduction of the doubly labelled water for human use, the FAO/WHO/UNU formulated this as a principle, instead of reported energy intake. Doubly labelled water studies have shown there is not yet a method for the accurate determination of dietary intake. All methods rely on self-report and the reporting bias can be as high as 50%, depending on physical and psychological characteristics of study. Additionally, the degree of mis-reporting increases with repeated dietary assessment in the same subjects, confounding the results of intervention studies.

Judging the effect of changes in food intake or physical activity on energy balance one might evaluate the effect from a change in body composition. Body composition can reflect the cumulative effect of a non-detectable difference between energy intake and energy expenditure. The precision of body composition estimates is in the order of magnitude of minimally 1.5 kg fat mass and fat-free mass. A combination of independent measurements can reduce this measurement bias. In a three-compartment model, based on the measurement of body mass, body volume and total body water, the claimed precision is 1.0 kg for fat mass and 0.7 kg for fat-free mass. A further slight improvement is reached in a four compartment model for body composition, subdividing fat-free mass in: total body water, protein mass and bone or mineral mass. The four compartment model nowadays is the 'gold standard' for body composition, measuring four variables: body mass, body volume and total body water with the 'traditional' methods, and mineral mass with dual energy X-ray absorptiometry. The precision will never reach the level of 0.001 kg for body mass with integrating electronic balances. On the other hand the precision of an average household bathroom scale for the measurement of body mass usually is not better than 1.0 kg. Putting the scale in another corner of the room often results in a difference of 0.5–1.0 kg. Everybody is familiar with discrepancies of body weight measurements between different scales. Thus the essential starting point of the measurement of body composition and changes in body composition is an accurate measurement of body mass. For comparative studies subjects should be measured with minimal clothing, minimal gut contents (post-absorptive) and with an empty bladder.

WHAT HAVE WE LEARNED FROM THE DOUBLY LABELLED WATER TECHNIQUE?

The doubly labelled water technique allows measurement of energy expenditure under free-ranging conditions, not interfering with food intake and physical activity. Thus, energy intake recommendations are nowadays based on energy requirements as measured with doubly labelled water. Total energy expenditure increases with body size, as we know since the application of the doubly labelled water technique in humans. Earlier observations of energy intake showed the opposite, a lower reported food intake in obese than in non-obese subjects. Similarly, studies on exercise training showed under-reporting of food intake, with an increasing discrepancy between reported intake and measured energy expenditure when observations were repeated in the same subjects (Westerterp et al 1992).

Another major finding since the application of doubly labelled water technique is the limit of total energy expenditure. The physical activity index in the general population, calculated as doubly labelled water total energy expenditure as a multiple of basal metabolic rate has an upper limit of 2.2 to 2.5. The upper limit of sustainable metabolism is about twice as high in endurance athletes, mainly because of long-term exercise training with simultaneous consumption of carbohydrate rich food during exercise. Endurance athletes have an increased fat-free mass and can maintain energy balance at a physical activity index value of 4.0 to 5.0 (Westerterp 2001).

KEY POINTS

1. Total energy expenditure is a function of body size and body composition, thermic effect of food, physical activity, thermoregulation and energy expended in synthesizing new tissues or in producing milk. For an adult human subject in the non-reproductive phase, the latter two components can be neglected and total energy expenditure depends on sex and varies primarily as a function of body size and physical activity.
2. Nowadays, there are many instruments to measure oxygen consumption and carbon dioxide production from room-sized respiration chambers to portable devices.
3. The most applied method for the measurement of energy expenditure is indirect calorimetry.
4. The doubly labelled water technique is typical application of indirect calorimetry to measure energy expenditure in unrestrained subjects over a time period of 1–4 weeks.

References

Adriaens MPE, Schoffelen PFM, Westerterp KR 2003 Intra-individual variation of basal metabolic rate and the influence of physical activity before testing. British Journal of Nutrition 90:419–423

Ainslie PN, Reilly T, Westerterp KR 2003 Estimating human energy expenditure: a review of techniques with particular reference to doubly-labelled water. Sports Medicine 33:683–698

Black AE, Coward WA, Cole TJ, Prentice AM 1996 Human energy expenditure in affluent societies: an analysis of 574 doubly-labelled water measurements. European Journal of Clinical Nutrition 50:72–92

Brouwer E 1957 On simple formulae for calculating the heat expenditure and the quantities of carbohydrate and fat oxidized in metabolism of men and animals from gaseous exchange (oxygen intake and carbonic acid output) and urine-N. Acta Physiologica Neerlandica 6:795–802

Plasqui G, Joosen AMCP, Kester AD et al 2005 Measuring free-living energy expenditure and physical activity with tri-axial accelerometry. Obesity Research 13:1363–1369

Speakman JR 1997 Doubly labelled water, theory and practice. Chapman & Hall, London

Webb P, Saris WHM, Schoffelen PFM et al 1988 The work of walking: a calorimetric study. Medical Science in Sports Exercise 20:331–337

Westerterp KR 2001 Limits to sustainable human metabolic rate. Journal of Experimental Biology 204:3183–3187

Westerterp KR 2004 Diet induced thermogenesis. Nutrition & Metabolism 1:1–5

Westerterp KR, Kester ADM 2003 Physical activity in confined conditions as an indicator of free-living physical activity. Obesity Research 11:865–868

Westerterp KR, Meijer GAL, Janssen EME et al 1992 Long term effect of physical activity on energy balance and body composition. British Journal of Nutrition 68:21–30

Westerterp KR, Wilson SAJ, Rolland A 1999 Diet-induced thermogenesis measured over 24h in a respiration chamber: effect of diet composition. International Journal of Obesity 23:287–292

Chapter 2

Dietary survey methods

Allan Hackett

LEARNING OBJECTIVES

After studying this chapter, you should be able to:

1. Discuss the range of methods available for measuring food intake and their advantages and disadvantages.
2. Distinguish between estimating nutrient intake and intake of foods, and their advantages and disadvantages.
3. Discuss the concept of validity as applied to dietary surveys and in particular the role of biomarkers in assessing validity.
4. Discuss the concept of reliability as applied to estimates of habitual intake (dietary exposure) and some strategies for improving reliability.
5. Appreciate the value of collecting dietary data in order to motivate change in eating habits.

INTRODUCTION

The measurement of food intake has been described as the most difficult of physiological measurements. The methods available tend to be time consuming and problematic and many poor quality dietary surveys are conducted (and some are still published). Why bother? It is axiomatic that the food we eat has a profound influence on our metabolism and hence health, both in the short and long terms. Indeed, the food eaten by us as children (and by our mothers during pregnancy) may have serious consequences for us after we retire. Our growth, development and performance (intellectual and physical) are also affected. It is essential therefore to have information on what we eat, and why, both to understand the relationship between food and our bodies and to give effective dietary advice. During the twentieth century nutrition science has moved away from the study of deficiencies, through the study of the effects of excess intake (so-called diseases of affluence) to consider how dietary intake can be optimized. Most recently, nutrient/gene interactions are being probed which may account for the very varied responses to dietary intake and eventually enable dietary advice to be truly personalized.

Nutritional epidemiology has gained increasing recognition. Some very large-scale studies of the relationship between diet and disease are in progress and the rigour expected of dietary survey methods has increased dramatically. However, fundamental problems remain with the estimation of food intake and these will be discussed. One major problem to address is akin to Heisenberg's principle of uncertainty; the more precise the method used to estimate intake the greater the likelihood that the intake will be distorted by the method used. The extent and nature of the distortion is also likely to change.

Dietary counselling requires high level skills. It must be understood that food choice is intimately and inextricably related to all other aspects of lifestyle, for example social class, income, physical activity, education, occupation, gender, age, ethnicity .... the list is a very long one and includes very personal behaviours, relationships and emotional make-up. Dietary counselling is not to be undertaken lightly therefore and talking about food intake can often reveal deep-seated problems. Apparently simple changes in food choice may require a major change in attitude and significant changes to lifestyle and relationships.

THE METHODS

There are a variety of methods for conducting dietary surveys but there is no best method (or 'gold standard'). The method chosen must be appropriate to the reason for which the data are being collected. Dietary data are normally required from individuals, but data collected on the whole population (per capita) or on families or groups can be useful to describe trends over time such as responses to interventions. There are two reasons for collecting dietary data from individuals. The first is for 'research' including epidemiological and experimental studies which vary in scale from a handful of volunteers put through taxing programmes of manipulation and measurement, for example to probe metabolic responses, to studies of tens of thousands of individuals to try to understand the aetiology of disease. In the latter type of study data on individuals are usually pooled to enable sophisticated statistical techniques to be applied, hence the quality and value of the data depend upon the group, not any individual. This will be discussed further in the sections on validity and reliability. The second reason is to facilitate dietary advice, but it should be borne in mind that ultimately, with few exceptions, dietary advice, can only be given in terms of foods, not nutrients. This explains why there is no best method; a point well worth repeating.

Several fundamental decisions have to be taken before choosing a dietary survey method:

- To what use will the information be put (what information is needed)?
- How will amounts of food eaten be estimated (is this necessary)?
- Do estimates of food intake need to be converted into estimates of nutrient intake? If so, how will this be done? Are particular nutrients (dietary components) of interest?
- What degree of statistical power is required? This will be a function of precision of the method chosen, sample size and reliability of the method.
- Is an estimate of concurrent food intake required?
- Is a retrospective estimate of food intake required? If so, for what period?
- Is an estimate of 'normal' intake required?
- How many and which days need to be surveyed?

NATIONAL SURVEYS

Per capita

These data are based on records of the production, import and export of food commodities making allowances for waste and crops fed to animals. This method forms the basis of many international comparisons and can yield useful trends and help define the nation's diet.

The expenditure and food survey

Formerly, but incorrectly, known as the 'National Food Survey', this survey has a long pedigree dating back to the 1940s when it began as a study of expenditure. Its protocol has been modified several times to allow it to estimate food and nutrient intake. Unusually the estimates are based on family or household units. Thus there are estimates of intake (per head), for example for families of two adults and two children, but not for adults or children. The method is based on an inventory of all food in the house, food purchases during 1 week and a second inventory at the end of the week. Allowances are

then made for food consumed outside the home (which affects such important items as confectionery and alcoholic drinks). It is conducted quarterly and
an annual report produced (quarterly data are available).

SURVEYS OF INDIVIDUALS

The national diet and nutrition survey (NDNS) is a rolling programme of
surveys of different population groups (e.g. children, adults, elderly) conducted by the Office of Population Censuses and Surveys (OPCS) for the
Department of Health (DH) and the Food Standards Agency (FSA). Thus any
one group is periodically surveyed, typically at 10-year intervals, but not
necessarily at any given interval. To date, the NDNS invariably uses the
weighed inventory method.

Duplicate portions
This involves each subject collecting a duplicate of everything that he or she
eats for a period of time (often only 24 hours). Thus twice as much food as
normal must be purchased, prepared and two exactly similar portions weighed
out. The food is later analysed for its chemical composition; typically trace
elements, vitamins or contaminants.

Advantages.   The ONLY method which can give precise estimates of intake
of some dietary components, e.g. trace elements, vitamins, pesticides etc. See
section on tables of food composition.

Disadvantages.   Very expensive, very time consuming, very demanding.
Likely to distort intake greatly. Normally only very well educated and
motivated people can complete such studies, otherwise the study has to be
completed in a closed 'metabolic unit'.

Weighed inventory method
Until quite recently this method was regarded by many, apparently for no
particularly good reason, as the 'gold standard' method. The subject weighs
each portion of food served to him or her just before eating. He or she later
weighs any left-over food. Electronic balances which are now very light, portable and precise have enhanced this method. Most often a record for seven
consecutive days is attempted.

Advantages.   If carried out according to instructions, by subjects willing
and able to behave exactly as 'normal', it should give as good a quantitative
record of intake, in the field, as it is possible to get.

Disadvantages.   Only literate subjects can take part and only very well
motivated subjects will follow all the instructions precisely. A biased sample
is almost inevitable. Not all food *will* be weighed, and not all food *can* be
weighed, for example food eaten outside the home in restaurants, and snack
foods are perhaps most likely not to be weighed or ignored. The subjects
often become very conscious not only of what they eat, but also, of how

much; possibly for the first time. Validity is likely to be compromised. Food composition tables are still needed.

Food diaries

These involve keeping a written record of everything consumed over a set period, usually 7, 5 or 3 consecutive days. Sometimes diaries are sent out and returned by post. I find it very difficult to interpret much of the information recorded without interviewing the subject individually (usually for about 20 minutes). Even the best records usually require some clarification (spelling and writing), such as, what kind of milk was used (skimmed, semi-skimmed or whole milk)? It is also very common to need to add foods which have been 'forgotten', for example the custard consumed with apple pie. These details should not be taken for granted. Some investigators use interviews by phone but this precludes using various methods of estimating portion size.

Advantages.   Much less onerous than the weighed inventory method and it can be used in all circumstances (eating out). Relatively cheap but logistically difficult; the subjects have to be instructed how to complete the diaries and then interviewed the day after the diary has been completed. A good level of motivation is required but it is a very flexible method and can generate motivation for change in suitable subjects. An excellent prelude to dietary counselling and for many people the only prompt needed to make useful changes to their eating habits.

Disadvantages.   Only literate well motivated subjects will follow the instructions (a high level of illiteracy can be compensated for by the interview). Estimating portion sizes is problematical. Needs a well trained interviewer familiar with eating habits of target group. Food composition tables are still needed.

Diet histories

These are based entirely on interviews and can only give retrospective information. There are two varieties of diet history.

1. Usual consumption.   The only method which was specifically designed to measure usual or normal intake. There are many variants on Bertha Burke's original protocol. Perhaps the commonest protocol is as follows: the subject is interviewed and asked to describe his or her intake for a typical week. Each day is systematically worked through, for example what do you normally eat first thing in the morning on a Monday? (N.B. I try to avoid the term breakfast which is value laden and some people do eat before breakfast – tea and biscuits in bed.) This record is then cross-checked against an inventory of food purchases recalled for a typical week.

Advantages.   Fast (perhaps 1 hour per subject) and therefore relatively cheap.

Disadvantages.   Does a normal or usual intake exist? Some people do eat the same foods on particular days of the week, others have very erratic eating habits. Needs a well trained interviewer familiar with eating habits of target group. Estimating portion sizes is problematical. Food composition tables are still needed.

2. Dietary recall.   This is a one-to-one interview normally conducted face-to-face but occasionally by telephone. The subject is normally asked to recall all foods and drinks consumed during the previous 24 hours – although the previous day is more usually recalled (very occasionally longer periods). The interviewer asks about each time of day from waking up until going to sleep. It is vital to take nothing for granted nor to suggest 'acceptable' answers, for example asking 'What did you have for breakfast?' implies that eating breakfast is desirable. The interviewer should also record the other activities for the period which can often serve as a memory aid, for example if the subject went to the cinema on the previous day it is possible that they ate some snack food there (e.g. pop-corn). A high level of detail is required and information on brand names, cooking methods, recipes, waste and accompaniments is necessary.

Advantages.   Very quick (perhaps 20 minutes per subject) hence relatively cheap.

Disadvantages.   Needs a well trained interviewer familiar with eating habits of target group. Estimating portion sizes is problematical. Food composition tables are still needed. Memory is known to be a significant problem and whole meals can be 'forgotten'. Very susceptible to effects of the day, for example if the previous day was the subject's birthday or they were ill the intake could be very abnormal. Some subjects are much more aware of their eating habits than others; men are notoriously vague. Interviews can include other family members to good effect but this can pose the problem of who to believe if conflicting information is given (when interviewing children I almost invariably believe children rather than parents in such cases).

Food frequency questionnaires
A check list of foods is provided with a stem question such as: 'How often do you eat ... ?'. A restricted list of alternatives is offered, for example: 'daily', once or twice per week', 'monthly' etc. Many versions have been used.

Advantages.   Self-completed and can be delivered and returned by post. Can be used on very large samples and data inputting can be automated (but this can be problematic).

Disadvantages.   Are the questions meaningful? It assumes rather stable eating habits; how often do you eat fish? Estimation of portion size can be very crude (choose: small, medium or large) or more usually, may depend on averages or centiles based on surveys probably several years old and data collected in populations which may differ from the target population. Food composition tables are still needed but coding can be especially problematical (may assume everyone who ate apple pie ate same type).

Food intake questionnaires

A check list of foods with a stem question such as: 'Did you, at any time yesterday, eat any amount of .... ?' A restricted list of alternatives is offered, for example: 'sweets', 'fruit', 'chips' etc. May or may not attempt to estimate amount of each food consumed.

Advantages. Self-completed and can be delivered and returned by post. Can be used on very large samples and data inputting can be automated.

Disadvantages. Not designed to estimate nutrient intakes. Of very limited use if working with individuals.

Establishing portion size

It would seem axiomatic that in order to estimate the amount of food consumed measurements must be taken. This is the basis of the weighed inventory method but experience has revealed that this is associated with three major problems: (i) distortion of intake, (ii) increasingly, situations when weighing food is impossible, and (iii) careful studies (using bio-markers) have shown that the data obtained are not necessarily more precise than those obtained from non-weighed methods. Many foods are consumed in standard portion sizes (confectionery, beer, tins, packets etc.) which greatly facilitates estimating consumption. Furthermore, some people have a very keen appreciation of the amount of food purchased and used in recipes. Thus estimating portion size may not be as crude as it may initially appear to be, especially with an experienced interviewer and some training for the subjects. It should be understood that most dietary survey methods work only at the level of ranking the sample; sorting out the 'big eaters' from the 'small eaters', which is sufficient for many purposes when absolute estimates are of less importance than relative amounts.

1. Verbal descriptions only. The interviewer asks the subject to describe the amount of food consumed as well as he or she can and forms an estimate of the amount based on judgement.

Advantages. Rapid.

Disadvantages. Interviewer needs extensive experience of portion sizes. Interviewers are unlikely to fully agree. At worst little more than (educated) guesswork at the mercy of the prejudices of the interviewer.

2. Photographic food atlas. Several attempts have been made to use photographs to help subjects describe the amount of food they have eaten. The most commonly used atlas (Nelson et al 1997) contains colour pictures of 76 foods, one page per food, with eight pictures per page arranged from smallest portion to largest. The portion sizes were chosen ranging from the 5th to 95th centiles for portion sizes taken from the National Diet and Nutritional Survey for adults (Gregory et al 1990). Photographs also represent the amount of butter on bread, a further 13 food groups (e.g. tins and some fruits) are represented by 'guide' photographs, and a range of utensils is shown. The subject is then asked to pick out the portion which corresponds most closely to that consumed. Computer programs are now being developed to allow the subject to choose and define portion sizes.

Advantages.   Can help inarticulate subjects express themselves. Can differentiate extremes. Photographs can be mailed and interviews conducted by trained non-specialists. Should diminish inter-interviewer bias.

Disadvantages.   The interview can be a very slow process. Portion size is effectively delimited by the NDNS used. It is debatable whether the atlas is appropriate for subjects dissimilar to those in the NDNS survey, e.g. children. Pictures of all foods cannot be provided.

3. Food models/household measures.   The subjects are asked to record their intake in terms of household measures. Sophisticated plastic models of common foods can be purchased but few are available in several portion sizes. The subjects can then point at the appropriate model and interpolate from it, for example 'about half of that slice of bread'.

Less sophisticated three-dimensional shapes (in polystyrene) have been used with calibrated utensils; cups, spoons, bowls and glasses. These enable the subject to select what he or she feels is the best representation of each portion from whatever is available.

Advantages.   Helps focus the interview and foods are easily recognized.

Disadvantages.   The models are very expensive and relatively few foods have been modelled and fewer still in different portion sizes. Lack of choice is likely to lead to spurious agreement that the portion presented was appropriate. The portion sizes modelled seem to be arbitrary. One study has shown poor performance of such models when compared with photographs.

4. Average portions.   Some surveys, especially food frequency questionnaires and those conducted by post/telephone, simply assume an average or typical portion size was consumed.

Advantages.   Very simple and fast. Can be automated.

Disadvantages.   Results are entirely dependent on assumptions based on a prior survey/data for estimating mean portion size. In effect it becomes a survey of frequency only.

Food composition tables: computer programs

Most dietary surveys rely on 'food tables' to convert estimates of food consumption into estimates of nutrient intake. Food tables are simply a catalogue of the chemical composition of foods. Those used in the UK are in McCance & Widdowson's *The Composition of Foods*, now in its 6th edition (FSA 2002), named in honour those who began the process in the 1940s. Currently the tables are compiled by the Royal Society of Chemistry, the Food Standards Agency and the Institute of Food Research. Over 1200 foods are included and some 46 nutrients are listed (however, there are some woeful gaps and the data for many nutrients are so incomplete as to be of very little value). Many new foods are marketed each year and the tables are not able to include many new products and then only in infrequent supplements/revisions. Thus nutritional analyses are not available for many foods, which weakens the accuracy of estimates of intake. Values are listed for macronutrients, minerals and vitamins, fatty acids, amino acids and a variety of other components. Using the food tables accurately requires a great deal of technical knowledge concerning the way they are organized (coding), the methods used for analysis and how to handle missing data. THEY ARE NOT TO BE CONSIDERED ANALOGOUS TO TABLES OF ATOMIC WEIGHTS (Widdowson & McCance 1943).

Clearly only a very limited number of samples of each food can be analysed and only one mean figure is given. The components and composition of many foods are very variable. Consider apple pie, was it commercially or home produced? How much apple and what variety was used? How much sugar (which sugars)? How much pastry (top and bottom?) – and what kind of fat and flour? Was the pie dusted with sugar? How was it cooked? Finally, the leftovers may not be comparable to the initial product, for example the individual who does not eat the thickest parts of the pastry crust. All these will affect its final nutritional value. There are many limitations in using the tables and they should not be used without a thorough understanding of these. The introductions to the hard copy text are essential reading (I recommend reading the introductions from all three of the last editions of the tables: 4th, 5th and 6th) but these are not available in the computer programs.

In order to use the tables a computer program is highly desirable and many are available which do not infringe copyright but they are expensive (typically £500 for a single copy). Such programs are powerful but potentially very dangerous because they enable the tables to be used with minimal understanding. It is very unwise to use food tables developed for use in other countries to the one in which the survey was conducted.

VALIDITY

Perhaps the question asked most frequently of anyone who has conducted a dietary survey is 'How do you know the subjects were telling the truth?'. A study is valid if it measures what you set out to measure. When trying to record and measure behaviour, except in very rare cases, the individual will report his or her own intake. This provides an opportunity for each subject to 'filter' his or her report, either consciously or subconsciously, to describe an intake either different to that actually consumed (an untruth), or to change intake for the duration of the study. The net result is the same; an invalid record is produced. Dietary records, however, are unlikely to be either 'valid' or 'invalid' but may differ from 'reality' to a greater or lesser extent. A further complication is that the mis-reporting of, or actual change in, eating habits may be very specific to certain food items and may also differ between subjects in quality and extent. Those items most likely to be affected are those regarded as most sensitive, such as alcohol, confectionery and snack foods.

There are other reasons why an invalid description of intake may be obtained; items may be forgotten, or badly described or miscoded, especially by nonspecialists. A further problem occurs in studies where data are being collected by more than one person. Inter-observer variability must be assessed and eliminated as far as possible (by adequate training even, perhaps especially, for experienced observers). In large-scale studies there may also be 'observer drift', that is, a tendency for estimates to change either systematically (getting larger or smaller) or randomly (increased or decreased variance) as time passes. These are issues of quality control vital to any survey.

It is now regarded as imperative that any dietary survey is conducted with some evaluation of its validity and some of the methods for doing this are indicated below. There is, however, no one single method which can 'validate' a dietary survey or enable 'calibration' to be carried out (the adjustment of figures produced to allow for inaccuracies in the data). At best, perhaps, they allow the limitations of the method used to be appreciated.

BIOMARKERS

A biomarker is some physical, physiological or biochemical parameter which varies quickly and quantitatively with a specific measurable aspect of food intake. For example the nitrogen content of the urine would be expected to reflect protein intake and its sodium content, sodium intake. In fact measuring sodium excretion is probably the only way to estimate sodium intake with any useful degree of precision (although, to give effective dietary advice some indication of the sources of the sodium based on records of dietary intake is essential).

Energy expenditure

If weight is stable energy intake must equal energy expenditure but the situation is rather more complex than it might appear. Energy balance is dynamic and only achieved over a period of time (which is unknown and is probably variable both between and within subjects) – it is certainly not normally achieved on a day-by-day basis and even 7 days need not reflect 'balance'. Body weight does indeed fluctuate from day to day (± 1 kg is not unusual) and from week to week. Thus if an estimate of intake does not match expenditure this is not proof of under- or over-reporting.

Energy expenditure (EE) can be measured with precision using doubly labelled water but this method is far too expensive for general use. Several key studies using it have strongly suggested systematic under-reporting of energy intake especially by overweight/obese subjects.

Dr Gail Goldberg and colleagues calculated cut-offs for 'valid' estimates of energy intake based on comparisons between calculated basal metabolic rate (BMR), derived from the Schofield equations, and energy intake (EI). A ratio of EE to BMR of 1.4 is generally considered to represent a sedentary individual; their energy expenditure is only 1.4 times their basal metabolic rate. This probably applies to most of the population. Thus a ratio of EI:BMR of less than 1.4 may represent under-reporting; however, since energy intake varies so much it must occasionally and naturally dip below the amount necessary to maintain weight (at other times it will be above). Thus Goldberg et al's cut-offs make statistically derived allowances (based on the day-to-day variation in intake, the number of days information available and whether BMR was calculated or measured) and the cut-offs used are lower. Typically, an EI:BMR below 1.2 or 1.3 is often used to indicate under-reporting has occurred.

The use of the 'Goldberg' equations is complex and the reader is urged to refer to the original papers as only the principles have been described here. Their use has become the most frequently used means of assessing the likelihood of under-reporting. Curiously, over-reporting is not usually investigated. A draw-back of the Goldberg equations is that they do not allow for physical activity and attempts to estimate activity, to add to the estimate of BMR, have been problematic. Motion sensors (pedometers and accelerometers) provide an objective, if partial, measure of activity and have been used with some success.

Urine nitrogen excretion

Protein cannot be stored and so nitrogen intake is rapidly reflected by nitrogen excretion. Most, but not all, nitrogen is lost in the urine (mainly as urea); the non-urine nitrogen losses, however, are quite constant from day to day and in adults amount to about 2 g per day. Thus measuring urine nitrogen can lead to estimates of protein intake independent of the dietary records and so can validate the ranking of protein intakes based on the dietary survey. The problem is that collecting valid and reliable urine samples is almost as problematic as collecting dietary data. The completeness of urine collections, normally for 24 hours, can be verified using markers (para amino benzoic acid – PABA) but nitrogen excretion fluctuates and it has been estimated that an 8-day collection is needed to get an acceptably reliable estimation of usual mean nitrogen excretion. This will be totally unacceptable to most people.

Other biomarkers: serum parameters and body fat composition

A variety of other markers have been used, including:

- blood: carotenoids, white blood cell vitamin C levels, iron levels*
- urine: sodium, potassium, creatinine, sugars (sucrose and fructose)

---

*Blood haemoglobin levels have not always been shown to relate to estimates of iron intake, even after taking into account a range of factors which affect iron availability. Transferrin and ferritin are regarded as much better indicators of iron status but neither appears to be a sensitive enough indicator of dietary intake for use as a biomarker.

- adipose tissue: fatty acid composition of body fat (from biopsy), change in body weight before/after survey†
- hair and nails: zinc and other trace metals. Samples are very easily contaminated, for example by shampoo.

Ideally the marker should be selected to reflect the nutrient of paramount interest (bear in mind that malnutrition cannot be diagnosed from dietary data, only from physical/biochemical measurements). Blood tests are only useful if a simple relationship exists between intake and blood level. For example there is no point measuring blood calcium level since it is so tightly regulated and there are very large stores and so only the most abnormal pathological conditions would be detected.

There is no consensus on how information from biomarkers should be used. Suspect records might be excluded, more data could be collected or different methods used. Calibration does not seem to be possible at present. At the least their use will give a better understanding of the quality of the data and hence how it can be used, in particular the strength of any conclusions drawn.

RELIABILITY

In order to give dietary advice an estimate of true intake is required but in research it is often most important to be able to put the subjects in the correct rank order; that is, to separate the 'big eaters' from the 'small eaters'. Unless this is possible relationships with disease or responses to programmes of intervention (clinical trials) cannot be determined. If this process of ranking is unreliable then incorrect conclusions may be drawn. The crucial question in dietary study design is: How many and which days to survey?

HOW MANY AND WHICH DAYS?

This is partly a problem of validity and partly of reliability. Reliability improves as the amount of information collected increases; the estimate of the mean is closer to the 'true' mean (crudely, the high and low intakes begin to balance out). This assumes that this variation is random, which is acceptable only up to a point since dietary intake might also vary systematically. For example week days tend to be different to weekend days, summer from winter and intake changes with age (quite quickly during puberty) and in response to training programmes.

This variability may be evident from the foods consumed; ice cream consumption is still higher in the summer (although not as markedly so as in

---

†It is interesting to note that many people lose weight when asked to record their food intakes for a few days. This clearly suggests under-reporting of usual intake.

the past) but the effect on nutrient intake is less evident. The intake of many nutrients simply follows energy intake, which suggests that more or less food of all sorts is being eaten (it also suggests that, when comparing intakes, energy intake must be taken into account, perhaps by comparing proportion of energy supplied by the nutrient or by calculating intake of nutrient per MJ energy). The intake of some nutrients can be very stable but not others. For example protein is found in almost all foods and its intake tends to be remarkably constant. In fact it is a characteristic of the wider population since it is determined largely by very general social factors. Iron, however, is found in appreciable amounts in relatively few foods and so if a dietary survey happened to include a day when liver was consumed iron intake would be well above the true mean on that occasion. The only solution to this problem is to collect information over a longer time period but this will reduce volunteer and completion rates and so a compromise has to be reached.

To estimate the true usual intake of an individual may require a lengthy survey which includes all days of the week perhaps on more than one occasion. It should also include the different seasons and other events such as holidays and work days. Surveys of groups should ensure that all these are covered within the group although not perhaps by every individual, which might limit the use to which the data can be put. It has been suggested that a continuous survey lasting for 3 months might be required to identify all the foods regularly eaten by an individual.

INTER–INDIVIDUAL VARIATION

Intake varies greatly from one person to another even after allowing for sex, age and weight. The relationship between physical activity levels and intake is complex and in practice estimates of energy expenditure do not correlate strongly with estimates of intake in the short term. This variation is partly systematic (as discussed above) but there is also a large apparently random element. Typical coefficients of variation for inter-individual variation in energy intake are 25% (values for other nutrients are invariably higher and some very much so). A sufficient number of days must be surveyed to deliver the degree of reliability required to meet the needs of the survey. One estimate of the sources of variance in the estimation of energy intake of children found that 28% was attributable to differences between subjects, the rest was within-subject variation; 18% due to differences between surveys but 54% was due to day-to-day variation in intake (Hackett et al 1983).

INTRA–INDIVIDUAL VARIATION

Intake therefore varies greatly from day to day in the same person; feasts and famines. The coefficient of variation for an individual is also of the order of 20–25% and fourfold differences in energy intake over the period of a few days are not uncommon. A short survey therefore could reflect a high day or a low day purely by chance, which could completely upset a rank order.

This matter is further complicated since the variability is itself variable both between and within people. It is suggested that the intake of some sectors of the population is very stable (elderly people) but in others is very erratic (young adults). For these groups as a whole this is probably a reasonable generalization but it could be very misleading for any individual (some young adults eat very monotonous diets). More information would be needed from those with erratic habits compared with those with stable eating habits to achieve the same level for reliability but in practice this is never done.

There are different approaches to estimating reliability; the estimation of reliability coefficients (Hackett et al 1983) or calculating the number of people misclassified into, for example, tertiles of distribution or calculating the number of days information required to estimate intake of a nutrient to within a specified degree of precision.

Estimates of the number of days required to estimate intake of different nutrients to a given degree of precision are shown in Table 2.1. This shows very clearly that the intake of some nutrients is far more variable than that for others. Thus 5 days' intake may be enough to estimate energy intake but 36 days' data are required for vitamin C.

The reliability of different study designs (in this example for estimating sugars intake of children, the figures for estimating energy intake are very similar) is shown in Table 2.2. A reliability coefficient of 1.0 is perfect – the order of ranking individuals in relation to their sugars intake is perfect (it says nothing about the absolute estimates). Clearly a huge amount of data is required to give estimates approaching 1.0. The compromise decided upon will depend upon the purpose of the study. The table shows that reliability improves more rapidly with increases in the number of surveys rather than with increases in the duration of each survey. This is because the information

Table 2.1 Effect of day-to-day variation in intake on the precision of estimates of mean nutrient intake (after Bingham 1987)

	Estimate of within-person variation (%)	Number of days intake required to be ± 10% of true mean intake
Energy	23	5
Carbohydrate	25	6
Protein	27	7
Fat	31	10
Fibre	31	10
Calcium	32	10
Iron	35	12
Cholesterol	52	27
Vitamin C	60	36

Table 2.2 Reliability of estimating sugars intake according to different combinations of length of study (days) and numbers of studies conducted (after Hackett et al 1983)

Number of days per survey	Number of surveys					
	1	2	4	5	10	15
1	26	41	59	64	78	84
2	37	54	70	74	85	90
3	42	59	74	78	88	92
5	48	65	79	82	90	93
7	51	68	81	84	91	94
14	56	71	83	86	93	95

collected at one time is likely to be linked whereas that collected at different times (from more surveys) is more likely to be independent and hence represent true intake more effectively. In practice, however, very few studies involve more than one estimate of intake (except longitudinal studies which pose special problems not discussed here) for logistical reasons. Note that increasing the duration of the survey from 3 to 5 days makes little difference to reliability and even extending the survey to 7 days (which many people find onerous) does not represent a substantial improvement.

The ability to discriminate between groups/individuals is facilitated if intra-individual variation is low but inter-individual variation is high. The sample size to deliver sufficient power to discriminate will reflect this (Table 2.3). This table shows that both increasing the number of days and the number of

Table 2.3 Schematic table to illustrate the notional relationship between power to discriminate between mean intake of groups of subjects and the study design (number of subjects and number of days surveyed)

Reliability*	Number of subjects	Differences in intake which can be detected Small <==================================> Large
Low	Small	
High	Large	

*As explained above, this is a combination between number of surveys conducted and the duration of each survey in days.

subjects contribute to the power to discriminate between groups. A decision will have to be taken about the power required (magnitude of difference thought to be important) and how to achieve this; by increasing sample size, by improving the reliability of individual estimates of intake (number of days) or by using both of these approaches. Inevitably resource implications play a part in this decision, which usually results in a compromise. The level of compromise which is acceptable requires very fine subjective judgement. It is usual to maximize sample size rather than overloading the volunteers by requesting more extensive information.

The number of subjects required to discriminate between groups with different intakes can be calculated by use of a simple formula (Hall 1983). It requires estimates of the mean and standard deviations of the intake of the two groups, a subjective decision about the magnitude of the difference which would be considered important and the setting of the ability to rule out the probability of achieving the result by chance.

$$n = 2. \left[\frac{(z_\alpha - z_\beta)\sigma}{\delta} \right]^2$$

Where n = sample size in each group (i.e. study size = 2n)

$Z\alpha$ = probability false positive
$Z\beta$ = probability false negative
σ = standard deviation of variable
δ = difference in population means thought to be important.

If a 5% chance of achieving a false-positive result or false-negative result is considered acceptable and if the mean intakes are about 2200 kcal and SD 525, then Table 2.4 shows the sample sizes required.

Do remember that small differences in intake can be important. For example consuming 100 kcal per day less than the amount of energy expended over 6 months, if real, could result in a weight loss of 3.65 kg.

Table 2.4 Sample size required to discriminate between the mean energy intake of two groups of subjects

Difference in mean energy intakes considered important (kcal)	Sample size in each group (n)	Total sample size (n)
50	2401	4802
100	600	1200
200	150	300
400	38	76
600	17	34

CONCLUSIONS

Dietary surveys cannot diagnose malnutrition. They can identify poor eating habits and related problems and suggest useful changes which could be made. They have also made useful contributions to epidemiology and clinical trials (treatment). They are vital for a comprehensive understanding of cause and effect. Eating habits are in a constant state of flux (new products come onto the market, fads are embraced and ideas change) and need constant review so that advice can be tailored to current habits.

RECORDS OF INTAKE AS A BASIS FOR DIETARY ADVICE

Keeping a record of intake is an excellent basis for giving dietary advice to an individual or group, for example the basis of discussions in schools. It is vital that the individual appreciates the need for an unbiased record of 'normal' intake. If the record is biased it is useless. An interview will be needed to help establish to what extent the record is a true representation of normal intake; especially to record infrequent or erratic habits (for example alcohol intake and meals out) which may be crucial. For well motivated individuals who are seeking advice a 7-day record is a reasonable request. For reluctant subjects a much shorter period, or interview only, is more appropriate. Dietary advice can, and indeed must, be given in terms of foods which can remove some of the problems.

A study of New Zealand jockeys (Leydon & Wall 2002) used the 7-day weighed inventory method to estimate intake. Energy and nutrient intakes were low and 5 of the 20 jockeys showed signs of disordered eating. Delayed menarche was noted in some of the women and 44% were classified as osteopenic associated with low calcium intake. Thus detailed dietary information helped to identify the problems of individuals which required urgent action which was thought could compromise their sporting performance and their short- and long-term health.

RECORDS OF INTAKE AS A BASIS FOR RESEARCH AND POLICY

Research needs are usually related to estimating the intake of groups or establishing a rank order of intake within a group. Dietary surveys are beset with pitfalls. They are labour intensive (and specialist knowledge is required) and hence expensive and yet the information is often of low reliability and questionable validity. Sample size needs to be 'large' to compensate for the high variability in intake (within people especially) and the large errors (uncertainty) associated with every method. All surveys must address these twin problems. There are some key questions to ask:

- What information is (really) needed?
- Why is the information needed (what will be done with it)?

- Are sufficient resources (expertise) available to support the collection of the information (badly collected data are worse than useless)?

The value of dietary data to general advice for athletes is shown by the study of van Erp-Baart et al (1989) who recorded the eating habits of elite athletes in the Netherlands using dietary diaries. They identified that low intakes (<10 MJ/d) were associated with low intakes of iron and calcium and that high energy intakes (>20 MJ/d) were associated with very high refined carbohydrate intakes and a lower nutrient density for thiamine. As a result they suggested that supplements must be considered. In addition they found that body builders and cyclists took very high doses of vitamins. This study therefore identified a range of issues previously unsuspected which sports coaches need to be aware of.

It is sometimes argued that surveys of nutrient intake (especially micronutrients) are worthless. Although problematic, I believe dietary data can be useful – the key to their use lies in selecting an appropriate method in the first place, understanding the method's weaknesses (and assessing these whenever possible) and, crucially, interpreting the findings in the light of this knowledge.

KEY POINTS

1. The measurement of food intake is problematic because of problems associated with validity and reliability.
2. There is no 'best method' (gold standard); the method chosen must fit the purpose of the study and its limitations acknowledged.
3. Food records are an excellent basis for dietary advice and for motivating change.

References

Bingham S 1987 The dietary assessment of individuals; methods, accuracy, new techniques and recommendations. Nutrition Abstracts and Reviews (Series A) 57:705–742

Black AE, Bingham SA, Johansson G, Coward WA 1997 Validation of dietary intakes of protein and energy against 24 hour urine N and DLW energy expenditure in middle aged women, retired men and post-obese subjects: comparisons with validation against presumed energy requirements. European Journal of Clinical Nutrition 51:405–413

Cameron ME, van Staveren WA 1988 Manual on methodology for food consumption studies. Oxford University Press, Oxford

FSA (Food Standards Agency) 2002 McCance and Widdowson's The composition of foods, 6th edn. Royal Society Chemistry, Cambridge (Ten supplements to the 5th edn were published)

Goldberg G, Black AE, Jebb SA et al 1991 Critical evaluation of energy intake data using fundamental principles of energy physiology: 1. Derivation of cut-off limits to identify under-recording. European Journal of Clinical Nutrition 45:569–581

Gregory J, Foster K, Tyler H, Wiseman M 1990 The dietary and nutritional survey of British adults. HMSO, London

Hackett AF, Rugg-Gun AJ, Appleton DR 1983 Use of a diary and interview to estimate the food intake of children. Human Nutrition: Applied Nutrition 37A:293–300

Hall JC 1983 A method for the rapid assessment of sample size in dietary studies. American Journal of Clinical Nutrition 37:473–477 (note letter in following issue)

International Journal of Epidemiology 1997 (supplement 1) (this whole issue is devoted to assessing dietary intake in the context of the EPIC study)

Leydon MA, Wall C 2002 New Zealand jockeys' dietary habits and their potential impact on health. International Journal of Sport Nutrition and Exercise Metabolism 12:220–237

Macdiarmid J, Blundell J 1998 Assessing dietary intake: who, what and why of under-reporting. Nutrition Research Reviews 11:231–253

MAFF (1940–2000) Household food consumption and expenditure. Annual Report of the National Food Survey Committee. Stationery Office, London

ONS/DEFRA (2001) The expenditure and food survey. Stationery Office, London

Margetts B, Nelson M (eds) 1997 Design concepts in nutritional epidemiology, 2nd edn. Oxford University Press, Oxford

Marr JW 1971 Individual dietary surveys: purposes and methods. World Review of Nutrition and Dietetics 13:105

NDNS (various authors) ONS (various dates) National nutrition surveys published rolling programme of different population groups: infants, children & adolescents, adults, elderly, low income

Nelson M, Atkinson M, Meyer J 1997 Food portion sizes – a photographic atlas. FSA, London

van Erp-Baart AMJ, Saris WMH, Binkhorst RA, Elvers JWH 1989 Nationwide survey on nutritional habits of elite athletes. Part 11: mineral and vitamin intake. International Journal of Sports Medicine 10:S11–S16

Web site

European Food Consumption Survey Method. Final Report 2001

http://europa.eu.int/comm/health/ph_projects/1999/monitoring/fp_monitoring_1999_frep_10_en.pdf

Chapter 3

Carbohydrate as an energy source for sport and exercise

Clyde Williams

LEARNING OBJECTIVES

After studying this chapter, you should be able to:

1. Describe the storage of carbohydrates.
2. Describe in broad terms the degradation of muscle glycogen, i.e. glycogenolysis.
3. Describe the relationship between carbohydrate and fat metabolism during exercise.

4. Describe the relationship between aerobic and anaerobic ATP production.
5. Describe the mechanisms underlying glycogen resynthesis.
6. Describe the methods of increasing the rate of muscle glycogen resynthesis.
7. Describe the relationship between muscle glycogen and blood glucose.
8. Describe the classical studies that show the links between pre-exercise carbohydrate feeding and exercise performance.
9. Describe the relationship between carbohydrate feeding during exercise and performance.
10. Describe the studies that show the impact of carbohydrate nutrition on recovery of exercise performance.

INTRODUCTION

Carbohydrates are a mixture of starches and sugars. Sugars (monosaccharides) are the simplest form of carbohydrates, e.g. glucose and fructose. Combining these simple sugars produces disaccharides, trisaccharides and so on to more complex polymers called polysaccharides, i.e. starches. The largest polysaccharides can contain a million or more glucose molecules. These polymers of glucose can form in two ways: one is as linear chains of glucose and this polymer is called amylose; the other is amylopectin, which has many branched chains of glucose molecules and this form is called amylopectin. For example, the starch in potato is composed of 20% amylose and 80% amylopectin: in wheat the amylose content is 25% and the amylopectin content is 75%. These starches are the main edible forms of carbohydrate found in plants and are used to manufacture the carbohydrate foods that form an essential part of our diet. The carbohydrate content of animal tissue is a relatively insignificant dietary source of carbohydrate. The 'starch' in animal tissues, such as skeletal muscle, is also glucose polymer but called glycogen.

TYPES OF CARBOHYDRATE

Bread, potatoes, pasta, rice, vegetables and sugars are examples of carbo-hydrate containing foods. The classification of carbohydrate foods as simple and complex was largely based on their fibre content. High-fibre carbohydrates were classified as complex whereas foods with low content that contain a significant proportion of simple sugars such as glucose and fructose were described as simple carbohydrates.

The common assumption was that after consuming simple, rather than complex, carbohydrates there is a rapid rise in blood glucose. However, this is not the case with all simple carbohydrates or, indeed, all complex carbohydrates.

A more informative way of describing carbohydrates is one that describes the degree to which they raise blood glucose concentrations. Carbohydrates which produce a large increase in blood glucose concentration are classified as having a high glycaemic index. A glycaemic index is given to a carbohydrate by comparing the area under a glucose-time curve following the ingestion of 50 g of the food. The reference value of 100 is assigned to the changes in blood glucose concentration following the ingestion of 50 g of glucose. Carbohydrates which have a high glycaemic index are glucose, white bread, rice, sweet corn and potatoes, whereas low glycaemic index carbohydrates are apples, dates, peaches, fructose and milk ice-cream. Fructose is a simple sugar but has a glycaemic index of less than 60. There is a clear difference between the blood glucose concentrations following the consumption of the same amount of high and low glycaemic index individual carbohydrate foods (Fig. 3.1). However, this difference is not so marked when HGI and LGI carbohydrates are part of mixed meals.

The glycaemic index provides additional information about a carbohydrate, which is particularly useful when designing diets to deliver glucose to working muscles rapidly or to optimize metabolism.

CARBOHYDRATE STORES

MUSCLE GLYCOGEN

Carbohydrate is stored as a polymer of glucose called glycogen. The largest glycogen stores are in the liver and skeletal muscles but there are also

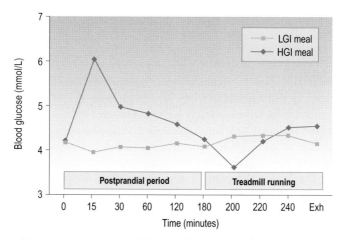

Figure 3.1   Glycaemic response to high and low glycaemic index carbohydrate pre-exercise meals followed by a run to exhaustion at 70% $\dot{V}O_2$max (adapted from Wee et al 1999).

glycogen stores in adipose tissue, kidneys, cardiac muscle and in the brain. Glycogen is described in terms of the number of 'glucose or glucosyl units' it contains and in skeletal muscle the normal concentration is within the range 60 to 150 mmol glucosyl units/kg body mass, wet weight (ww) or 250 to 650 mmol glucosyl units/kg body mass, dry weight (dw). Bearing in mind that muscle makes up about 40% of the body mass of an adult then the total glycogen concentration is equivalent to about 550 g. (Many studies report glycogen and glycolytic intermediates as dry weight rather than wet weight values because they freeze dry their muscle samples before analysis. Freeze dried muscle samples are easier to handle and analyse than fresh samples. On the basis that the water content of human muscle is approximately 77%, wet weight concentrations can be converted to dry weight values by using a conversion factor of 4.3.)

LIVER GLYCOGEN

The size of the store of glycogen in the liver depends on the nutritional state of the individual. For example, in the fed state the adult liver weighing about 1.8 kg contains approximately 550 mmol glucosyl units (90 g) whereas after an overnight fast the concentration of glycogen falls to about 200 mmol glucosyl units. After a number of days on a high carbohydrate diet the liver glycogen concentration can increase to about 1000 mmol glucosyl units. Whereas an overnight fast severely reduces liver glycogen stores it has no such effect on muscle glycogen stores.

Prolonged fasting reduces the liver glycogen stores which may compromise the function of the brain by failing to maintain an adequate supply of blood glucose for cerebral metabolism. In an attempt to maintain the supply of glucose the liver is able to manufacture glucose from the breakdown products of carbohydrate, fat and protein metabolism. This process is called glyconeo-genesis and uses metabolites such as lactate, glycerol and amino acids such as alanine to produce glycogen in the liver.

BLOOD GLUCOSE

Liver glycogen is the reservoir from which glucose is released to maintain normal concentrations within a fairly narrow range of values of 4 to 5 mmol/L. Therefore, there is about 4 to 5 g of glucose within the systemic circulation. It is under the control of the hormone glucagon that is released from the alpha cells of the Islets of Langerhans in the pancreas when blood glucose concentrations fall. The brain, the central nervous system, blood cells and kidneys use about 75% of the available blood glucose in resting individuals. The brain and central nervous system use about 120 g of glucose a day and so a fall in blood glucose concentrations to values below 3 mmol/L, i.e. hypoglycaemia, may cause lack of motivation, headaches and even dizziness.

The passage of glucose into the liver, as a result of the digestion and absorption of carbohydrate foods, is not under hormonal control as is the entry of glucose into muscle cells and adipose tissue. Insulin is released from the beta cells of the Islets of Langerhans when there is an increase in the concentration of blood glucose. Insulin controls the uptake of glucose into adipose tissue and into muscle cells mainly during the postprandial period that follows a meal. During exercise the release of insulin is suppressed by an increase in the concentrations of noradrenaline and adrenaline. Even during low intensity exercise there is an increase in noradrenaline as a result of an outflow of this neurotransmitter from the sympathetic nerve endings whereas adrenaline release from the adrenal medulla occurs at higher exercise intensities. The inhibition of insulin secretion during exercise may be regarded as a safety mechanism to protect us from a life threatening hypoglycaemia. For example, during prolonged submaximal exercise carbohydrate metabolism can be sustained at a rate of 2.5–3 g/minute to the point where glycogen concentrations fall to very low values and exercise intensity cannot be maintained. If skeletal muscle had free access to blood glucose under these conditions then there would be a rapid onset of hypoglycaemia as muscle 'soaked up' the relatively small amount of circulating glucose. One of the many metabolic adaptations to endurance training is a reduction in the contribution of blood glucose to muscle metabolism during submaximal exercise.

FUELS FOR EXERCISE

The relative contributions of carbohydrate and fat to energy production changes with exercise intensity and duration. For example, when going from walking to running, the fuel for energy production shifts from the oxidation of fatty acids and a minor contribution from blood glucose to a large contribution from muscle glycogen and a smaller amount from fatty acids (Romijn et al 1973, van Loon et al 2001). The recruitment of glycogen to energy production during moderate to high intensity exercise is necessary because glycogen can be degraded rapidly to maintain high rates of ATP production necessary to support the activity. Although there is an abundant store of fat in the body, fatty acids cannot be oxidized rapidly enough to support ATP production during heavy exercise. Nevertheless, during prolonged moderate to heavy exercise muscle glycogen is degraded relatively quickly and the rate of fatty acid oxidation is increased in an attempt to cover the loss of glycogen to ATP production. However, this up-regulation of fat metabolism is generally inadequate to cover the required high rate of ATP production. The contribution of blood glucose to muscle metabolism increases but is also inadequate even when high concentrations are maintained throughout exercise by glucose infusion (Claassen et al 2005). As a consequence of a decreased rate of ATP production the contractile activity of working muscles cannot be maintained and so the athlete slows down. The loss of muscle glycogen during prolonged constant pace running occurs most rapidly in the type 1 fibres (slow contracting, slow fatiguing) than in the type 2 fibres (fast contracting, fast fatiguing). However, at the point of fatigue the concentrations of muscle glycogen are very low in both fibre populations (Tsintzas et al 1996a).

Sprinting recruits both fibre populations in order to generate enough power to develop high speeds. During prolonged intermittent high intensity running it appears that glycogen is reduced most rapidly in the type 2 fibres (Nicholas et al 1999). These changes in muscle metabolism during prolonged exercise may not be the only determinants of the onset of fatigue during prolonged exercise. Changes in brain metabolism of glucose may also contribute a 'central' element to the onset of fatigue (Nybo et al 2003). This may be part of what has been termed a central 'glucostat' that might have an influence on muscle fibre recruitment and in turn on the decrease in pace towards the end of prolonged exercise (Rauch et al 2005).

GLYCOGEN METABOLISM

Glycogen is degraded in a stepwise process that leads to the production of the useable form of cellular energy, i.e. ATP. Glycogen degradation is called glycogenolysis and the speed of the process is facilitated by the presence of enzymes at key points in the process. Some of these enzymes are critical to the process because their activity can be influenced by the presence of end products of metabolism resulting in a more rapid or less rapid rate of glycogenolysis.

The metabolic intermediates in glycogenolysis are shown in Figure 3.2 together with the points in the pathway that contain the enzymes that are critical to the control of the process. The first step in the degradation of glycogen is the activation of an inactive form of the enzyme phosphorylase b to the active form of the enzyme phosphorylase a. This conversion to an active enzyme is stimulated by the release of calcium (Ca^{++}) ions into the sarcoplasm (cytosol) of the muscle cells from their storage site, namely the sarcoplasmic reticulum. Calcium ions released into the sarcoplasm then combine with a regulatory protein called troponin that is situated at intervals along the length of the tropomyosin/actin complex, all of which are part of the myofibrillar structure in skeletal muscles. The attachment of the Ca^{++} ions to the active sites on the troponin leads to a series of changes in the configuration of the tropomyosin such that the active sites on actin become exposed to the heads of the myosin protein resulting in cross-bridge formation. Repeated making and breaking of the cross-bridges between actin and myosin results in the shortening of the muscle fibres that is the basis of the contractile activity of skeletal muscles. The energy required for the breaking of the cross-bridges is ATP; however, there is only enough ATP available for a few contractions. Therefore to continue the contractile activity of the muscle ATP has to be resynthesized rapidly. This is achieved by the immediate degradation of a high energy phosphate compound called phosphocreatine (PCr). The following reactions provide immediate replenishment of the ATP used in contractile activity and produce bi-products that continue to play a role in energy production, i.e. ADP (adenosine

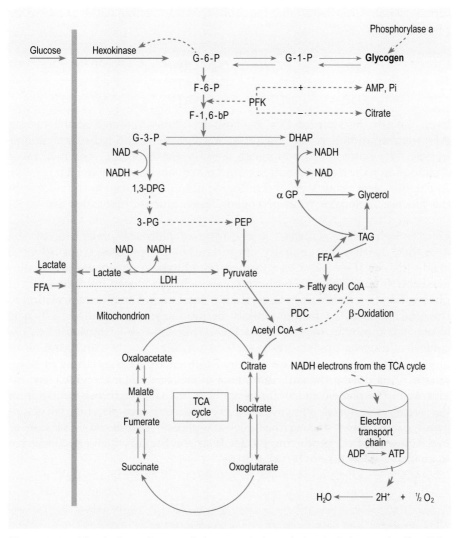

Figure 3.2 Metabolic pathways of glycogenolysis and glycolysis in muscle. G-6-P is glucose-6-phosphate. G-1-P is glucose-1-phosphate. F-6-P is fructose-1-phosphate. F-1,6-bP is fructose-1,6-bisphosphate. G-3-P is glyceraldehyde-3-phosphate. 3-PG is 3-phosphoglycerate. PEP is phosphoenolpyruvate. DHAP is dihydroxacetonephosphate. α GP is alpha glycerolphosphate. NAD is nicotinamide-adenine-dinucleotide. NADH is nicotinamide-adenine-dinucleotide (reduced form). LDH is lactate dehydrogenase. PDC is pyruvate dehydrogenase complex. PFK is phosphofructokinase. FFA is free fatty acids. TAG is triacylglycerides.

diphosphate), AMP (adenosine monophosphate), creatine (Cr) and inorganic phosphate (Pi).

$$
\begin{array}{llll}
& \text{Contraction} & & \\
\text{ATP} & \xrightarrow{\hspace{2cm}} & \text{ADP} + \text{Pi} \\
\text{ADP} + \text{PCr} & \xrightarrow{\hspace{1.5cm}} & \text{ATP} + \text{Cr} \\
\text{ADP} + \text{ADP} & \xrightarrow{\hspace{1.5cm}} & \text{ATP} + \text{AMP}
\end{array}
$$

Even though the store of PCr is about five times the size of the resting ATP concentration it is not enough to support the continued contraction of muscle. Therefore, in order to match the resynthesis of ATP with the rate of degradation requires contributions from other substrates (Table 3.1).

The first step major step in the degradation of glycogen is the release of the glucose molecules from glycogen. These glucose molecules are phosphorylated to first become glucose-1-phosphate and then are converted to glucose-6-phosphate. Glucose in the form of glucose-6-phosphate can be degraded further but equally importantly, the process traps glucose inside the cell (Fig. 3.2). Once formed the glucose-6-phosphate is indistinguishable from the glucose-6-phosphate which is produced from the entry of glucose into the muscle from the systemic circulation. The phosphorylation of this glucose is aided by the activity of the enzyme hexokinase which is located on the inner membrane of the sarcolemma and contributes to the control of glucose uptake into muscle. An increase in the concentration of glucose-6-phosphate exerts an inhibitory influence over the activity of hexokinase. Thus during the early moments of exercise when the glycogen and glucose-6-phosphate concentrations are high, the rate of glucose uptake from the blood is reduced. However, as exercise continues the rate of glycogenolysis decreases and so the glucose-6-phosphate-induced inhibition of hexokinase is lifted, producing intracellular conditions which are conducive to an increased uptake of blood glucose.

Table 3.1 ATP yield from aerobic and anaerobic metabolism

		ATP per mol of substrate	Respiratory Exchange Ratio (RER)
Glycogen	Lactate	3	–
Glycogen	CO_2, H_2O	37	1.00
Glucose	Lactate	2	–
Glucose	CO_2, H_2O	36	1.00
Fatty acids	CO_2, H_2O	138	0.70
Acetoacetate	CO_2, H_2O	23	1.00
Hydroxybutyrate	CO_2, H_2O	26	0.80

AEROBIC METABOLISM

The end product of glycolysis is the formation of pyruvate which has several potential fates. Most of the pyruvate enters the mitochondria where it is converted into acetyl CoA by a process that is largely regulated by the enzyme pyruvate dehydrogenase complex (PDC). The acetyl CoA undergoes stepwise degradation by the process known as the 'Krebs Cycle' or more correctly the 'tricarboxylic acid cycle (TCA)' resulting in the production of carbon dioxide, water and ATP. The TCA cycle in conjunction with the 'electron transport chain (ETC)' is the process that converts ADP to ATP and the overall process is called 'oxidative phosphorylation'. It is oxidative in a number of ways, not least because when the intermediates of the TCA cycle are degraded to simpler molecules, hydrogen ions are released and eventually combine with oxygen to form water and carbon dioxide via the 'electron transport chain' (Fig. 3.2). The oxygen molecules become the terminal acceptors of the electrons released from the TCA cycle and without which the whole process would stall completely.

Fatty acids are transformed into fatty acyl CoA molecules when they first enter the muscle and then after transport into the mitochondria they are converted to acetyl CoA via beta oxidation before being oxidized via the TCA cycle (Fig. 3.2). An increase in the activity of the TCA cycle produces an increase in citrate which is one of the few intermediates that can leave the mitochondria. An accumulation of citrate has been shown to have an inhibitory influence on the glycolytic enzyme phosphofructokinase (PFK) and so has the potential to reduce the rate of glycolysis in skeletal muscle. This is one of the mechanisms that have been suggested as an explanation for the decrease in glycogenolysis in the presence of an increased fatty acid oxidation. The 'glucose-fatty-acid cycle' has been shown to operate in animal muscle and may occur in humans at rest but the evidence of its operation in human skeletal muscle during exercise has yet to be confirmed.

ANAEROBIC METABOLISM

When the rate of pyruvate formation exceeds the capacity of the mitochondria to accept and oxidize this glycolytic intermediate then it is converted mainly into lactate and to a lesser extent alanine. The glycogen to pyruvate part of the pathway or more correctly the Embden–Meyerhof pathway normally has a greater capacity for pyruvate formation than has muscle mitochondria to oxidize the pyruvate formed. The Embden–Meyerhof pathway does not require oxygen for the stepwise degradation of glycogen (and glucose-6-phosphate) to pyruvate and so it is often called 'anaerobic metabolism'. However, the term 'anaerobic metabolism' has often caused confusion because it has been misused in describing the energy production of muscles during exercise. An increased production of pyruvate and lactate is a reflection of an increased rate of glycogenolysis, i.e. activity of the anaerobic pathway, but it does not mean that all the energy production supporting active muscles is taking place in an oxygen-free or hypoxic environment.

The important role of lactate formation is often overlooked because it has traditionally been associated with fatigue. In the glycolytic pathway the conversion of the intermediate G-3-P to 1,3-DPG (Fig. 3.2) occurs because NAD is converted to NADH (via electron transfer). This important step in glycolysis can only continue as long as there is sufficient NAD to support the reaction. In the formation of lactate NAD is regenerated from NADH that has been produced further up the glycolytic pathway. Therefore without lactate formation the rate of glycolysis would be significantly slower.

During glycolysis, glucose-6-phosphate, which is a six carbon atom molecule, is converted into two three carbon atom molecules. So during glycolysis the six carbon atom molecule glucose-6-phosphate produces two three atom molecules of pyruvate. This increased glycolytic activity during exercise increases the number of molecules and as such changes the osmotic balance within the cell. However, there are 3 to 4 g of water stored with every gram of glycogen and so the degradation of glycogen may not, therefore, cause a disruptive osmotic change in muscle during exercise.

The flux of glycolytic intermediates down the glycogenolytic pathway is controlled largely by increasing or decreasing the activity of the enzymes that are located at key points in the pathway. For example, the three main enzymes that control glycogenolysis in skeletal muscles are (i) 'phosphorylase a', (ii) phosphofructokinase (PFK) and (iii) pyruvate dehydrogenase complex (PDC). The active form of phosphorylase, i.e. phosphorylase a or b, initiates glycogen degradation: PFK is the enzyme that controls flux of intermediates down the glycolytic pathway whereas the conversion of pyruvate to acetyl CoA is controlled by the pyruvate dehydrogenase complex (PDC). Metabolic signals from other parts of the glycogenolytic pathway influence the activity of the enzymes. For example when muscles are working hard the match between ATP used and the amount resynthesized may be less than optimal and so some ADP is degraded to AMP. An increase in AMP concentration is a strong metabolic signal that additional ATP is needed. The accumulation of AMP and inorganic phosphate (Pi) activates PFK so that a more rapid flux of glycolytic intermediates down the pathway occurs to produce pyruvate. An increase in pyruvate concentration activates PDC, so facilitating the conversion of pyruvate to acetyl Co A in the mitochondria, resulting in an increased rate of ATP production.

A high rate of fatty acid oxidation (i.e. fatty acyl CoA) will lead to an accumulation of acetyl CoA within the mitochondria. An excess accumulation of acetyl CoA will inhibit the activity of PDC and so there is a decrease in the uptake of pyruvate into mitochondria. Similarly when there is an accumulation of the TCA intermediate citrate in resting, but possibly not during exercise, it leaks out of the mitochondrion and has a negative influence on PFK. Thus a high rate of fat oxidation will lead to a decrease in glycogenolysis and so have a glycogen sparing effect. Endurance training increases the mitochondrial density in skeletal muscles and so the capacity for fatty acid oxidation is increased. An increase in fatty acid oxidation and a decrease in carbohydrate metabolism during submaximal exercise is one of the most important adaptations to endurance training.

GLYCOGEN RESYNTHESIS

MECHANISMS

The process of glycogen resynthesis begins immediately after exercise and is most rapid during the first 5 to 6 hours of recovery (Fig. 3.3) (Goforth et al 2003, Piehl 1974). The uptake of glucose by the formerly active muscle fibres is accelerated by the appearance at the muscle membrane of specific glucose transporter proteins (GLUT-4). The GLUT-4 proteins are released from storage vesicles in the sarcoplasm of the muscle fibres as a consequence of the contractile activity and the reduction in glycogen concentration (Ivy & Kuo 1998, Jentjens & Jeukendrupt 2003) (Fig. 3.4). They remain in an active state during the immediate post-exercise period. The enzyme that speeds up glycogen resynthesis is glycogen synthase which is activated mainly as a consequence of a reduction in glycogen stores. Thus the GLUT-4 transporter proteins and enzyme glycogen synthase are probably the two most important components in the glycogen resynthesis process (Fisher et al 2002). The size of the subsequent glycogen store also appears to limit further resynthesis, i.e. evidence of autoregulation (Laurent et al 2000). In addition to the fundamental influence of muscle contraction per se on glucose transport and glycogen resynthesis, the presence of insulin also makes a significant contribution to this process. Insulin contributes to glycogen resynthesis by either extending the time that GLUT-4 transporters are active or may even stimulate the

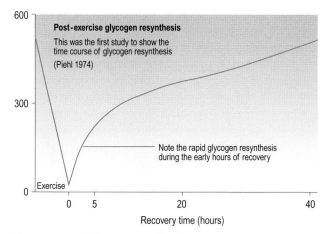

Figure 3.3   Time course of glycogen synthesis.

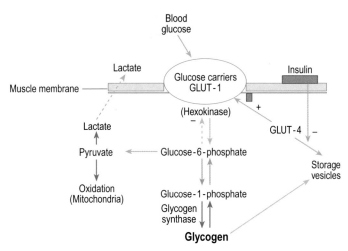

Figure 3.4 Summary of mechanisms for glycogen resynthesis in skeletal muscles.

release of more transporters from a different storage site (Jentjens & Jeukendrupt 2003). Thus the glycogen resynthesis process occurs in two parts: first there is the non-insulin resynthesis period that lasts for about an hour and is the result of muscle contractions per se; the second part is a consequence of the action of insulin and this period of glycogen resynthesis can last many hours into the recovery period. The activities of the GLUT-4 transporters and glycogen synthase are increased with endurance training and decrease during a period of inactivity (Greiwe et al 1999).

NUTRITION

The early studies on post-exercise glycogen resynthesis recommended that the optimum amount of carbohydrate is about 1 to 1.5 g/kg body mass, consumed immediately after exercise and at 2-hour intervals until the next meal (for review see Ivy 1991). Consuming carbohydrate at a rate of 1.2 g.kg^{-1} h^{-1} every 30 minutes during a 4-hour recovery period results in a maximum rate of glycogen resynthesis of approximately 45 mmol.kg^{-1} h^{-1} (van Loon et al 2000b). However, smaller amounts might be advisable because athletes may experience intolerable abdominal discomfort during subsequent exercise.

Elevated post-exercise insulin concentrations play an essential role in promoting high rates of glycogen resynthesis. Adding protein and some amino acids to carbohydrate generally results in an increase in insulin concentrations to values that are higher than those achieved with an equal amount of carbohydrate (van Loon et al 2000a, Zawadzki et al 1992). Ivy and colleagues were among the first to report that consuming a carbohydrate-protein mixture immediately after exercise increased the rate of post-exercise muscle glycogen resynthesis beyond that which occurs with carbohydrate alone (Ivy et al 2002, Zawadzki et al 1992). However, not all authors report a greater increase in glycogen resynthesis following the ingestion of carbohydrate-protein mixtures immediately after exercise (Carrithers et al 2000, Jentjens et al 2001, van Hall et al 2000, van Loon et al 2000b).

Another mixture that has been shown to be effective in increasing the rate of glycogen resynthesis after exercise is carbohydrate and creatine mono-hydrate (Nelson et al 2001, Roberts et al 2004, Robinson et al 1999). The proposed mechanism for the greater increase in glycogen storage is an increase in cell volume (Robinson et al 1999) rather than an increase in post-exercise insulin concentration (Roberts et al 2004).

CARBOHYDRATE LOADING – A PRACTICAL APPROACH

It is well established that if the diet after prolonged heavy exercise is rich in carbohydrate then supra-normal muscle glycogen stores may be achieved (Bergstrom & Hultman 1966). Therefore, nutritional strategies have been developed to take advantage of this super-compensatory response of glycogen-depleted muscle to carbohydrate intake. The traditional method of increasing muscle and liver glycogen stores after prolonged cycling to exhaustion is to eat a diet low in carbohydrate for the first 3 days of recovery and then switch to a high carbohydrate diet for the next 3 days (Astrand 1967, Bergstrom et al 1967). The classic study by Bergstrom and colleagues was one of the first to show the links between increased muscle glycogen concentration following carbohydrate loading and improvement in exercise capacity. They reported that when their subjects exercised to exhaustion on a cycle ergometer at an intensity equivalent to 65–70% $\dot{V}O_2$max after their normal mixed diet they fatigued after 58 minutes. Thereafter they ate a low carbohydrate diet for 3 days and then cycled to exhaustion again before consuming a high carbohydrate diet for 3 days. At the end of the period on the high carbohydrate diet they again cycled for just over 3 hours before the onset of fatigue (Bergstrom et al 1967).

The original carbohydrate loading method for increasing muscle glycogen concentration has also been shown to be an effective preparation for endurance races. Karlsson & Saltin (1971) reported that when a group of runners undertook carbohydrate loading in preparation for a 30 km cross-country race they increased their glycogen stores and improved their performance time by 8 minutes compared with their performance after consuming a mixed diet before the race.

Although this carbohydrate loading method is effective, athletes generally find that even light training during the low carbohydrate phase is unpleasant and so alternative ways of restocking glycogen stores were developed. Among the most successful was the 'taper method' shown by Sherman et al (1981) and colleagues to be as effective for runners as the traditional method of carbohydrate loading. Runners tapered their training intensity and volume during the week leading up to competition and increased the carbohydrate content of their diet to 9 to 10 g/kg^{-1} body mass during the last 3 to 4 days before the event. This was an important study because it was one of the first to show that carbohydrate loading could produce high muscle glycogen concentrations after running as after cycling.

Athletes are eager to continue training while carbohydrate loading but are concerned that this might delay the restoration of muscle glycogen stores. There does appear to be some slowing of glycogen resynthesis during the first hour of recovery even while performing low intensity exercise (40–50% $\dot{V}O_2$max) compared with passive recovery (Choi et al 1994). However, more recent research suggests that daily 20-minute sessions of light exercise (~65% $\dot{V}O_2$max) do not limit the supercompensation process (Goforth et al 2003). Furthermore, having achieved high muscle glycogen concentrations they persist for 3 to 4 days after the 3 day carbohydrate-loading phase on a diet that consists of a lower carbohydrate intake (60% energy intake) (Goforth et al 1997, 2003).

Most studies on restoring glycogen concentrations after exercise have used men as subjects. Earlier studies on carbohydrate loading in women suggested that, unlike in men, 'glycogen supercompensation' does not occur (Tarnopolsky et al 1990) or at least not to the same extent (Walker et al 2000). However, when the carbohydrate intake of men and women are matched then it is clear that women can increase their glycogen stores to supra-normal values (James et al 2001). Even so it appears that some female endurance cyclists can maintain a high daily training mileage on a very low carbohydrate diet (e.g. 3 g/kg body mass per day) (Dolins et al 2003).

CARBOHYDRATE INTAKE AND PERFORMANCE

Most of the studies on exercise performance fall into two broad categories whether the mode of exercise is cycling or running. Those exercise tests that require their subjects to complete a fixed amount of work as quickly as possible or do as much work as possible in a set time, usually during cycling, may be regarded as assessing 'exercise performance'. Those exercise tests that require subjects to exercise as long as possible at a fixed power output (cycling) or at set pace (running) may be regarded as assessing 'endurance capacity'.

PRE-EXERCISE CARBOHYDRATE INTAKE

In one of the early endurance performance studies, subjects ate a breakfast consisting of bread, cereal, milk and fruit juice (200 g carbohydrate) 4 hours before cycling to exhaustion (Neufer et al 1987). This meal increased pre-exercise muscle glycogen concentration by about 15% (though this was not statistically significant). The performance test required the subjects to cycle for 45 minutes at 77% $\dot{V}O_2$max and then to cycle as fast as possible for 15 minutes. The total work accomplished during the last 15 minutes of the test was greater (22%) after the pre-exercise meal than it was following the no-meal trial. However, not all performance studies have found such marked improvements in performance following the ingestion of a high carbohydrate pre-exercise meal. One such cycling study reported by Whitley et al (1998) found no differences in time trial performances when they provided their subjects with a meal containing 215 g of carbohydrate, or no meal, 4 hours before a 10 km time trial. Their cyclists completed 90 minutes at 70% $\dot{V}O_2$max and then the 10 km as fast as possible, but the 10 km times for the fed (878 s) and the fasted (874 s) trials were almost identical.

These two examples of exercise performance studies are typical of those reported in the early literature and as a generalization the benefits of eating a high carbohydrate meal before an exercise performance test are not as clear as are the results from those studies that assess endurance capacity.

In one such endurance capacity study, Schabort et al (1999) gave their subjects a commercially available breakfast cereal (100 g CHO) and milk 3 hours before they cycled to exhaustion at 70% $\dot{V}O_2$max. They also obtained muscle biopsy samples from their subjects before each trial and then again at the end of exercise to assess the use of muscle glycogen. Endurance capacity was significantly greater after the carbohydrate breakfast than when their subjects exercised to exhaustion after an overnight fast (136 minutes vs 109 minutes). There were no differences in the muscle glycogen concentrations at the end of exercise in the two trials, but a direct comparison of the respective rates of glycogenolysis cannot be undertaken because the final biopsy samples were obtained at different times.

Of course, the amount of carbohydrate ingested in a pre-exercise meal is also an important consideration. For example, Sherman et al (1989) showed that although small amounts of carbohydrate (46 g and 156 g) consumed 4 hours before intermittent cycling improved endurance capacity, a larger amount of carbohydrate (312 g) was even more effective. After this larger amount of carbohydrate the exercise capacity was 15% greater (56 minutes) than after the water placebo (48 minutes) trial.

Two related studies examined the benefits of pre-exercise meals on subsequent endurance running capacity. The studies found that the longest run time to fatigue was the result of a high carbohydrate breakfast (2 g/kg body mass), consumed 3 hours earlier, and the ingestion of a carbohydrate-electrolyte solution throughout the treadmill run. The next most effective treatment was the high carbohydrate breakfast and the ingestion of water throughout the endurance run. The third most effective treatment was when the runners fasted but ingested a carbohydrate-electrolyte solution throughout the endurance run. The poorest performance followed an overnight fast and the ingestion of only water during the endurance run. The pre-exercise carbohydrate meal and the carbohydrate-electrolyte solution increased running time by 9% (125 minutes) more than when only the meal was consumed (115 minutes) but 21% more (103 minutes) than when the runners completed the test without breakfast and had fasted overnight (Chryssanthopoulos & Williams 1997, Chryssanthopoulos et al 2002). Thus, the weight of available evidence supports the recommendation that a high carbohydrate meal before exercise is of greater benefit to performance than undertaking exercise in the fasting state.

CARBOHYDRATE COMPOSITION OF PRE-EXERCISE MEALS

Accepting that a high carbohydrate pre-exercise meal is of benefit to performance, the next question is whether there is an advantage in selecting one type of carbohydrate over another. The ingestion of carbohydrates with different glycaemic indices (GI) will produce markedly different changes in plasma glucose and insulin concentrations. A pre-exercise meal containing low (LGI) carbohydrates results in higher rates of fat oxidation during 60 minutes of submaximal treadmill running 3 hours later than after a high (HGI) meal (Wu et al 2003). The greater rate of fat oxidation and lower rate of carbohydrate oxidation are conditions that result in an improvement in endurance running capacity. Whether or not the improved endurance capacity is a consequence of sparing the limited glycogen stores both in the liver and in skeletal muscle or simply in skeletal muscles has yet to be established. A LGI carbohydrate pre-exercise meal results in a greater rate of fat oxidation because the insulin-suppressed mobilization of fatty acids is not as great as after a HGI carbohydrate meal. Therefore the benefits of LGI carbohydrate pre-exercise meals are probably more evident during prolonged low intensity exercise than during high intensity exercise. This may explain why some studies have reported benefits on endurance capacity and other studies have found no benefits on time-trial performance. Furthermore, the majority of studies report that their subjects were fed only an hour or so before exercise (Febbraio & Stewart 1996). Even when a HGI meal is consumed 3 hours before exercise it seems that not all the carbohydrate has been digested and absorbed. For example, the muscle glycogen concentrations of a group of runners were determined before and 3 hours after HGI and LGI carbohydrate meals (2–2.5 g/kg body mass). There was an increase in resting muscle glycogen concentration of only 11–15% after the HGI meal (Chryssanthopoulos et al 2004, Walker et al 2000) but no significant increase after the LGI carbohydrate pre-exercise meal (Wee et al 2005). These are modest changes in muscle glycogen concentrations and suggest that performing exercise 3 hours after a large carbohydrate meal may be insufficient time for complete digestion and absorption. Of course, some of the carbohydrate will have been stored in the liver and so may contribute to muscle metabolism during exercise but even so 3 hours is insufficient time for the complete dispersal of ingested carbohydrate to the liver and skeletal muscles.

CARBOHYDRATE INTAKE WITHIN THE HOUR BEFORE EXERCISE

Earlier studies on the influence of ingesting carbohydrate within the hour before exercise suggested that this practice would have a detrimental influence on performance (Costill et al 1977, Foster et al 1979). These studies showed that there was a greater rate of glycogen degradation during exercise after ingesting a concentrated carbohydrate solution (25% w/v) (Costill et al 1977) and fatigue occurred sooner (19%) during cycling to exhaustion at 80% $\dot{V}O_2$max (Foster et al 1979). However, this highly publicized recommendation has not been supported by subsequent studies (Burke et al 1998, Chryssanthopoulos et al 1994).

These early studies also showed a sharp peak in blood glucose concentrations following the ingestion of the concentrated glucose solution and then a rapid fall at the onset of exercise. For most people the transient fall in blood glucose concentrations during the first few minutes of exercise appears to go unnoticed and has little influence on subsequent exercise capacity (Chryssanthopoulos et al 1994).

CARBOHYDRATE INTAKE DURING EXERCISE

Submaximal exercise

The influence of drinking carbohydrate solutions during exercise on subsequent performance has been extensively studied (for reviews see Coyle 2004, Maughan & Murray 2000). Although most of the studies on carbohydrate intake and endurance capacity have used cycling, there are relatively fewer studies on running. Some running studies have used constant pace treadmill running to exhaustion (Tsintzas et al 1996b) to assess the benefits of drinking carbohydrate solutions during exercise and others have simulated races both on treadmills (Millard-Stafford et al 1997, Tsintzas et al 1995) and on the open road (Tsintzas et al 1993). Most have shown improvements in treadmill run times to exhaustion and improvements in road race finishing times following the ingestion of carbohydrate solutions than after ingesting taste and colour matched placebo solutions.

The mechanisms responsible for the improved performance following the ingestion of carbohydrate solutions during exercise have been the focus of several recent studies. Depletion of muscle glycogen is largely responsible for the onset of fatigue during prolonged exercise as has been demonstrated in many studies. For example, when a group of runners ingested a carbohydrate-electrolyte solution or taste matched placebo immediately before and throughout a constant pace treadmill run to exhaustion (70% $\dot{V}O_2$max) their run time was 104 minutes during the placebo trial and 132 minutes during the carbohydrate trial. The placebo trial was completed first so that changes in muscle glycogen could be assessed at the point of fatigue under both conditions. Muscle biopsies were obtained before and at the point of fatigue in the placebo trial whereas in the carbohydrate trial an additional biopsy sample was obtained at the time of fatigue in the placebo trial (104 minutes). Glycogen concentration in the vastus lateralis muscle was very low at the point of fatigue in the placebo trial. However, at the same time point in the carbohydrate trial the glycogen concentration was significantly higher than in the placebo trial and then reached the same low values at the point of fatigue. When the muscle samples were analysed for glycogen in the type 1 and type 2 fibre populations it was clear that there was a reduction in glycogen in both fibre types at the end of exercise. The glycogen sparing seemed to occur in both type 1 and type 2 fibres (Tsintzas & Williams 1998).

Following the ingestion of a carbohydrate there is a steady increase in the rate of carbohydrate oxidation during the first 80 minutes of exercise and then it levels off at about 1.1 g/minute (Jeukendrup & Jentjens 2000). The ingestion of ever greater quantities of carbohydrate will not lead to a proportional increase in carbohydrate oxidation during exercise. The limitation may not be gastric emptying of the ingested carbohydrate but the absorption across the intestinal wall of the gut. Therefore, the optimal amount of exogenous carbohydrate that will achieve the maximum oxidation rate is about 70 g/hour. Accompanying the increased rate of oxidation of the exogenous carbohydrate is an almost complete shut down in hepatic glucose output (Jeukendrup et al 1999). Thus the ingestion of carbohydrate during exercise has a glycogen sparing effect on the liver. Late in exercise when muscle glycogen concentrations are low the uptake of blood glucose into muscle contributes to the high rates of carbohydrate oxidation. However, this contribution cannot cover the loss of muscle glycogen for very long. Nevertheless, the contribution of blood glucose does make a significant contribution to extending exercise time to fatigue. Therefore, an adequate liver glycogen store that is able to continue to maintain normal blood glucose concentrations for cerebral as well as muscle metabolism makes a significant contribution to endurance capacity during prolonged exercise.

Multiple-sprint exercise
Even during brief periods of maximal exercise muscle glycogen makes a significant contribution to ATP production. For example, during a 6-second maximal sprint muscle glycogen contributes about 50% to ATP turnover, 48% is derived from phosphocreatine and about 2% from the muscle's ATP store (Boobis 1987). During repeated periods of brief high intensity exercise muscle glycogen stores are gradually depleted and so carbohydrate loading prior to exercise helps delay the onset of fatigue (Balsom et al 1999).

Some studies have also examined the benefit of ingesting carbohydrate-electrolyte solutions during prolonged intermittent high intensity running in an attempt to assess the applicability to sports such as football, rugby and hockey. Nicholas and colleagues designed a shuttle running test (LIST) that requires participants to repeatedly run, walk, jog and sprint between two lines 20 metres apart in 15-minute blocks of activity with 3 minutes recovery between each block. When continued for the full 90 minutes the participants cover about 12 km during which they perform 66 maximum sprints and expend in total about 1300 kcal (Nicholas et al 2000). These distances covered and energy expended are similar to those reported for mid-field players in professional football (Bangsbo et al 2006).

In one study a group of recreational football players completed 5 blocks of the LIST before undertaking an endurance test. This test required the subjects to continue sprinting and jogging back and forth over the 20 m course to the point of fatigue. They found that the distance covered was 33% greater when the football players drank a carbohydrate-electrolyte solution (6.5%) than when they drank a flavoured placebo solution (Nicholas et al

1995). A subsequent study examined the amount of glycogen used during the completion of 6 blocks of the LIST (90 minutes) and reported that less glycogen was used when their subjects consumed the carbohydrate-electrolyte solution than when they consumed flavoured water placebo (Nicholas et al 1999). Welsh and colleagues used a similar protocol but gave their subjects greater amounts of carbohydrate and found even greater improvements in endurance capacity (50%) than when their subjects drank a placebo solution during the test (Welsh et al 2002).

Drinking a carbohydrate-electrolyte solution also appears to improve endurance capacity during intermittent exercise even when players have high pre-exercise muscle glycogen stores. Foskett et al (2004) studied the influence of drinking a carbohydrate-electrolyte solution on endurance capacity during intermittent shuttle running after the subjects had increased their pre-exercise muscle glycogen concentrations by carbohydrate loading for the previous 48 hours. Six male recreational footballers were required to continue running repeated 15-minute blocks of the LIST to the point of fatigue. On one occasion they drank a flavoured placebo and on another they drank a 6.4% carbohydrate-electrolyte solution throughout the exercise test. Muscle biopsy samples were obtained from subjects after an overnight fast, i.e. before exercise, after 90 minutes of the LIST and then again at fatigue. All six subjects ran for longer when they drank the carbohydrate-electrolyte solution (158 minutes) than when they drank the flavoured placebo solution (131 minutes). However, there were no differences in the muscle glycogen concentrations after 90 minutes of running during the two trials, endorsing the important role of blood glucose during the later stages of prolonged exercise (Claassen et al 2005, Coggan & Coyle 1989, Coyle et al 1983, 1986).

Carbohydrate intake during recovery of performance

It is essential that athletes who train hard and compete regularly recover quickly from training and competition. Recovery from exercise depends on the nature of the exercise, its intensity, duration and the time between training sessions. Successful recovery involves the completion of several essential physiological and metabolic processes that act in concert to prepare the athlete for the next bout of exercise. Assuming that the athlete has not suffered injury or severe muscle soreness then the key components of recovery are resynthesis of the body's carbohydrate stores, rehydration and rest.

CARBOHYDRATE AND RECOVERY

RECOVERY OVER SEVERAL DAYS OF CONSTANT PACE FIXED TIME EXERCISE

Several studies have explored what the optimum amount of carbohydrate should be for athletes who undertake daily training. Kirwan and colleagues changed the training demands and the daily carbohydrate intake of ten highly trained endurance athletes. The athletes completed 5 days of increased training (20 km/day ~80% $\dot{V}O_2$max): on one occasion they had a low carbohydrate intake and on another they had a high carbohydrate intake. The high carbohydrate diet was calculated to match the demands of the runners' daily energy expenditure (~530 g or 8 gm/kg body mass) and the low carbohydrate diet (240 g or 3.8 g/kg BM) was calculated to cover only 50% of the runner's estimated daily expenditure (Kirwan et al 1988). Each runner completed 5 days of training at an intensity equivalent to 80% $\dot{V}O_2$max and a duration equivalent to 1.5 times the distance normally covered in training. They found that even during the high carbohydrate trial there was a significant decrease in muscle glycogen at the end of the 5 days of training. When the runners completed a treadmill run to assess their running economy they all found it harder when they had consumed the low carbohydrate recovery diet. Similar results have been reported for 3 and 7 consecutive days of training when the subjects either cycled or ran on a treadmill at exercise intensities equivalent to approximately 75% $\dot{V}O_2$max. In these studies there is a clear trend for glycogen concentrations to be lower after cycling than after running. Even though muscle glycogen concentrations were significantly lower after 3 and 7 days on a moderate carbohydrate diet the subjects were able to cope with each day's training (Pascoe et al 1990, Sherman et al 1993). Nevertheless, performance after several weeks of training appears to be better after high rather than moderate carbohydrate diets (Achten et bal 2004, Simonsen et al 1991).

RECOVERY OF PERFORMANCE AFTER 24 HOURS: PROLONGED EXERCISE

Consuming a high carbohydrate diet during the 24 hours after prolonged heavy exercise (Goforth et al 2003, Keizer et al 1987) or even without heavy exercise (Bussau et al 2002, Goforth et al 2003) restores muscle glycogen concentrations to normal pre-exercise values. Keizer and colleagues (1987) noted that when a sub-group of their subjects were allowed to eat ad libitum during their 22-hour dietary recovery study they failed to restore their muscle glycogen concentrations. Therefore, it is essential that the amount of carbohydrate that athletes consume during the recovery period is prescribed for them if they wish to recover in 24 hours. One of the key questions is whether eating a high carbohydrate diet that restores muscle glycogen will also recover performance? Unfortunately, there are only a few studies that have addressed this question. In one such study successful recovery of endurance running capacity 22 hours after prolonged exercise was reported by Fallowfield & Williams (1997). They found that when their subjects ran for 90 minutes or to fatigue (whichever occurred first) on treadmill at 70% $\dot{V}O_2$max and were then fed either a high carbohydrate (9 g/kg BM, CHO) or isocaloric mixed diet (6 g/kg BM, CHO) during a 22-hour recovery only those runners on the high carbohydrate diet were able to match their previous day's run time of 90 minutes. Those runners who consumed the mixed diet could only manage to complete 78% of their previous day's exercise even though their recovery diet contained their normal carbohydrate intake.

The type of carbohydrate consumed during recovery may also have an influence on the rate of muscle glycogen resynthesis and subsequent performance. Burke and colleagues (1993) reported that muscle glycogen resynthesis after a 24-hour recovery from prolonged exercise was greater when their subjects consumed a high (HGI) rather than a low (LGI) glycaemic index carbohydrate recovery diet; although they did not assess the exercise capacity of their subjects after the 24-hour recovery on the two different carbohydrate diets it is reasonable to assume that a greater endurance capacity would have been achieved after the HGI diet. This hypothesis was examined by Stevenson et al (2005) who found that the treadmill run time to exhaustion was 12 minutes longer and fat oxidation higher after the LGI rather than the HGI recovery diet. It is reasonable to assume that the greater rate of fat oxidation during the run to exhaustion would have compensated for the lower pre-exercise glycogen stores after the LGI recovery diet. It is also interesting to note that the runners reported that they never felt hungry on the LGI diet even after the overnight fast prior to the run to exhaustion on the second day of the trial. This was not the case when they consumed the HGI recovery diet that was matched for energy and macronutrient composition with the LGI recovery diet. Therefore, it may be more effective to consume HGI carbohydrates for the first few hours after exercise and then consume LGI carbohydrate meals for the remainder of the recovery period. In this way the HGI carbohydrate will contribute quickly absorbed substrate during the most rapid period of glycogen resynthesis and the LGI carbohydrates will provide high satiety.

RECOVERY OF PERFORMANCE IN 24 HOURS: INTERMITTENT HIGH INTENSITY EXERCISE

Although the numbers of participants in sports that include endurance running and cycling are large they are much less than those who participate in multiple-sprint or 'stop-go' sports such as football, soccer, field and ice hockey, rugby, tennis and basketball. The prolonged intermittent high intensity exercise that is part of these sports reduces muscle glycogen stores and impairs performance, as is the case in constant pace exercise (Balsom et al 1999). For example, the muscle glycogen concentrations of professional soccer players are severely reduced after 90 minutes of match play (Jacobs et al 1982, Saltin 1973). It is well established that those players who begin match play with modest or low glycogen concentrations cannot fully engage in the game because of the early onset of fatigue (Saltin 1973).

In a study on nutrition and soccer specific fitness, Bangsbo et al (1992) and colleagues showed that when players consumed a high carbohydrate diet for 48 hours before a series of soccer specific tests their endurance capacity during prolonged intermittent high intensity treadmill running was significantly better than when a normal mixed diet was the nutritional preparation for the tests.

Using prolonged intermittent high intensity shuttle running as an exercise protocol that mimics the activity patterns common in soccer, Nicholas and colleagues examined the influence of different nutritional strategies on exercise capacity during the last 15 minutes of the 90 minutes of the test (Nicholas et al 2000). The 90-minute intermittent shuttle running test severely reduced the glycogen concentrations in both the type 1 and 2 fibre populations in the vastus lateralis muscles of the participants (Nicholas et al 1999). Nicholas and colleagues also showed that recovery of intermittent high intensity shuttle running capacity was restored 22 hours later when the subjects consumed a recovery diet that provided a carbohydrate intake of 10 g/kg body mass (Nicholas et al 1997). However, when the subjects consumed their normal amount of carbohydrate with additional protein and fat to match the energy intake of the carbohydrate recovery diet they failed to match their previous day's running capacity.

PERFORMANCE FOLLOWING SHORT RECOVERY PERIODS

It is quite common for athletes to train twice a day with as little as 4 to 5 hours recovery between training sessions. In some sports athletes also have to compete more than once a day and so optimal recovery is even more important than recovery between training sessions. After training or competition there will be a real need to rehydrate and to begin to replace some of the carbohydrate stores before the next session. Consuming carbohydrate beverages immediately after exercise has been shown to accelerate muscle glycogen resynthesis during a recovery as short as 4 hours. However, even though there is solid evidence to support benefits of drinking a carbohydrate solution immediately after exercise there is relatively little information on the impact of this recommendation on subsequent exercise performance. In one study Fallowfield & Williams (1993) examined the endurance capacity runners who followed the recommendations that have emerged from the studies on glycogen resynthesis. Their subjects ran on a treadmill at 70% $\dot{V}O_2max$ for 90 minutes or to fatigue (whichever occurred first) and then they were allocated to either the placebo or the carbohydrate group. The carbohydrate group ingested a carbohydrate solution that provided the equivalent of 1 g.kg^{-1} BM of carbohydrate immediately after exercise and then again 2 hours later. The placebo group drank the same volume of flavoured coloured water at the same times as the carbohydrate group. After the 4 hours' recovery both groups ran to exhaustion at the same treadmill speeds as on the first occasion. The group that ingested the sports beverage were able to run for 20 minutes longer than the group who ingested the flavoured placebo solution. Even following the simple recommendation to consume about 50 g of carbohydrate immediately after exercise (Coyle 1991) results in greater endurance capacity during subsequent exercise than consuming only water during a 4-hour recovery period (Wong et al 2000).

However, ingesting a greater amount of carbohydrate immediately after exercise may not result in the expected further improvements in endurance capacity during subsequent exercise. Wong et al (2000) gave a group of runners 50 g of carbohydrate from a 6.5% carbohydrate-electrolyte beverage immediately after 90 minutes of treadmill running (70% $\dot{V}O_2$max) and then rehydrated them by providing either water or the carbohydrate beverage in sufficient quantity to cover 150% of the body mass lost during the initial run. Surprisingly there was no difference in running time to exhaustion when the runners had consumed 175 g of carbohydrate or 50 g during the 4-hour recovery. In a subsequent study that used exactly the same recovery rehydration solutions and experimental design muscle biopsy samples were obtained to examine the changes in glycogen concentration after the 4-hour recovery. Analyses of the muscle samples showed that there was a significant increase in muscle glycogen concentration during the 4-hour recovery when the runners ingested the larger amount of carbohydrate (Tsintzas et al 2003).

The results of this study confirmed those of an early study that used exactly the same exercise and recovery protocols but provided runners with either low (1 g.kg^{-1} BM) or high (3 g.kg^{-1} BM) amounts of carbohydrate from a 6.5% carbohydrate solution during the 4-hour recovery (Fallowfield & Williams 1997). There were not only no differences between run times to fatigue after the 4-hour recovery but several runners fell asleep after the ingesting the larger amount of carbohydrate, i.e. 3 g.kg^{-1} BM, and had to be woken in order to obtain blood samples and to complete the second run.

These results are paradoxical because it would be reasonable to expect an improved exercise capacity following short term recovery during which more carbohydrate was consumed. Possible explanation(s) include a rate limited uptake of glucose during the recovery period and an insulin-induced reduction in the availability and oxidation of fatty acids. The consumption of carbohydrate may have been sufficient to depress fat oxidation but insufficient to make up the deficit in substrate provision and so overall there is no net gain in endurance capacity.

Consuming a carbohydrate-protein mixture (4:1 CHO-protein) after prolonged exercise has been shown to be more effective in replenishing muscle glycogen stores 4 hours later than consuming carbohydrate alone (Zawadski et al 1992). Ivy and colleagues have also explored the influences of ingesting a carbohydrate-protein mixture during recovery on subsequent endurance capacity. In their initial study their subjects performed prolonged cycling to deplete muscle glycogen concentration and then ingested either the carbohydrate-protein mixture or a carbohydrate solution (6% CHO) immediately after exercise and again 2 hours later. After a recovery of 4 hours their subjects cycled to exhaustion at an intensity equivalent to 85% $\dot{V}O_2$max. The time to exhaustion following the ingestion of the CHO-protein mixture was 55% greater than following the ingestion of the commercially available sports beverage (Williams et al 2003). Unfortunately the study is difficult to interpret because it did not compare like with like: the carbohydrate-protein mixture provided far more carbohydrate than was available in the sports beverage during the recovery period therefore it might not be surprising that there were differences in exercise capacity.

In a similar study using running rather than cycling Betts and colleagues examined the influences of a carbohydrate-protein mixture and a matched amount of carbohydrate on endurance running capacity at 85% $\dot{V}O_2$max 4 hours after a 90-minute treadmill run at 70% $\dot{V}O_2$max (Betts et al 2005). A 9.3% carbohydrate solution and the same solution containing 1.5% protein was used to provide carbohydrate equivalent to 1.2 g.kg^{-1} BM.h^{-1} for one trial and the same amount of carbohydrate plus protein for the other trial. The runners ingested the solutions immediately after the 90-minute run and then at 30-minute intervals during the 4-hour recovery. Although the solutions ingested were matched for carbohydrate the carbohydrate-protein mixture contained 17% more energy. There was a large variation in run times to fatigue in both trials but there were no overall differences in endurance capacity (CHO: 14.5 minutes vs CHO-protein: 18 minutes). In this study several of the subjects complained of abdominal discomfort which was probably the consequence of the large amounts of carbohydrate ingested during the recovery period. Therefore a second study was undertaken using exactly the same exercise and recovery protocol with the same carbohydrate plus protein mixture but on this occasion the runners ingested smaller amounts (0.8 g.kg^{-1} BM.h^{-1}) during the 4-hour recovery. Again there were no differences in the run times to fatigue in the two trials (CHO: 18 minutes vs CHO-protein: 19.5 minutes) (Betts et al 2005).

In a more recent study Betts et al (2004) repeated their earlier studies with exactly the same exercise, the same type of carbohydrate-protein mixture and feeding schedule but the run to exhaustion after the 4-hour recovery was at 70% $\dot{V}O_2$max. The exercise intensity was reduced from 85% to 70% $\dot{V}O_2$max because it would allow longer run times and so offer a greater challenge to the runner's carbohydrate stores. Six runners completed three trials: in one trial they ingested a carbohydrate-protein mixture (0.8 g.kg^{-1}.h^{-1} plus 0.3 g.kg^{-1}.h^{-1} of whey protein isolate), in another they ingested the same amount of carbohydrate as in the carbohydrate-protein trial (8 g.kg^{-1}.h^{-1}) and in the third trial they ingested the carbohydrate equivalent to the energy content of the carbohydrate-protein mixture (1.1 g.kg^{-1}.h^{-1}). After the 4-hour recovery the run times to fatigue at 70% $\dot{V}O_2$max were significantly longer in the carbohydrate-protein and the energy matched carbohydrate trials than in the carbohydrate only trial, i.e. 91 minutes, 99.9 minutes vs 83.7 minutes. There were no significant differences between the run times to fatigue between the carbohydrate-protein and energy match carbohydrate trials (Betts et al 2004). These studies show no differences in muscle glycogen resynthesis rates after ingesting the carbohydrate-protein mixture and the energy matched carbohydrate solution or any differences in performance. However, some studies report that the degree of muscle soreness experienced by their subjects is generally less after ingesting a carbohydrate-protein solution than after ingesting carbohydrate alone (Millard-Stafford et al 2005, Saunders et al 2004). Again it is difficult to offer a rational explanation for these observations in the absence of further information.

In summary the daily carbohydrate intake should be adjusted according to the intensity and duration of the training programme and the time available for recovery. For example, a daily carbohydrate intake of 5 to 7 g/kg body mass is recommended for male athletes undertaking daily training of moderate intensity that lasts about an hour. For male endurance athletes who train for between 1 and 3 hours daily the recommendation is a daily carbohydrate intake of 7 to 10 g/kg body mass (Burke et al 2001). However, female athletes may not require such large amounts of carbohydrate to support their daily training programmes but this has yet to be confirmed by further research (Dolins et al 2003).

KEY POINTS

1. Carbohydrate is stored as polymers of glucose in plants as starch and in animal tissue as glycogen.
2. Carbohydrates are classified according to their glycaemic responses, i.e. high (HGI) and low (LGI) glycaemic carbohydrates.
3. High glycaemic carbohydrates are characterized by a rapid large rise in blood glucose after ingestion whereas low glycaemic carbohydrates are characterized by a low and even slow rise in blood glucose concentration after ingestion.
4. The degradation of muscle glycogen, i.e. glycogenolysis, occurs along two major biochemical pathways, i.e. anaerobic which occurs on the surface of the mitochondria and aerobic metabolism that occurs inside the mitochondria via the tricarboxylic acid cycle (TCA).
5. Carbohydrate is stored mainly in the liver and in skeletal muscles but in limited amounts when compared with the fat stores of the body.
6. Fatigue during prolonged exercise is associated with the depletion of muscle glycogen stores.
7. Dietary carbohydrate loading in the days before prolonged exercise increases muscle glycogen concentrations and generally results in an increase in endurance capacity.
8. Muscle glycogen resynthesis can be accelerated by consuming a carbohydrate-rich diet immediately after exercise.
9. Post-exercise glycogen resynthesis begins immediately after exercise following a contraction-induced activation of glucose transport proteins (GLUT-4) from their storage vesicles within the sarcoplasm of muscle and the activation of the enzyme glycogen synthase.
10. Post-exercise muscle glycogen resynthesis is also accelerated in the presence of insulin which indirectly results in the GLUT-4 transporter proteins remaining active in glucose transport for longer than in the absence of insulin.
11. Muscle glycogen stores can be replenished within 24 hours when the carbohydrate intake is equivalent to approximately 10 g/kg body mass.

References

Achten J, Halson S, Moseley L et al 2004 Higher dietary carbohydrate content during intensified running training results in better maintenance of performance and mood state. Journal of Applied Physiology 96:1331–1340

Astrand P-O 1967 Diet and athletic performance. Federation Proceedings 26:1772–1777

Balsom P, Gaitanos G, Soderlund K, Ekblom B 1999 High intensity exercise and muscle glycogen availability in humans. Acta Physiologica Scandinavica 165:337–345

Bangsbo J, Norregaard L, Thorsoe F 1992 The effect of carbohydrate diet on intermittent exercise performance. International Journal of Sports Medicine 13:152–157

Bangsbo J, Mohr M, Krustrup P 2006 Physical and metabolic demands of training and match play in the elite player. Journal of Sports Sciences 24:665–674

Bergstrom J, Hultman E 1966 Muscle glycogen synthesis after exercise: an enhancing factor localized to the muscle cell in man. Nature 20:309–310

Bergstrom J, Hermansen L, Hultman E, Saltin B 1967 Diet, muscle glycogen and physical performance. Acta Physiologica Scandinavica 71:140–150

Betts J, Williams C, Grey E, Griffin J 2004 Carbohydrate-protein mixtures on recovery of endurance capacity. Medicine and Science in Sports and Exercise 36:S42

Betts J, Stevenson E, Williams C et al 2005 Recovery of endurance running capacity: effect of carbohydrate-protein mixtures. International Journal of Sport, Nutrition and Exercise Metabolism 15:590–609

Boobis LH 1987 Metabolic aspects of fatigue during sprinting. In: Macleod D et al (eds) Exercise, benefits, limitations and adaptations. E & FN Spon, p 116–140

Burke L, Collier G, Hargreaves M 1993 Muscle glycogen storage after prolonged exercise: effect of the glycaemic index of carbohydrate feedings. Journal of Applied Physiology 75:1019–1023

Burke L, Claassen A, Hawley J, Noakes T 1998 Carbohydrate intake during prolonged cycling minimises effect of glycemic index of preexerise meal. Journal of Applied Physiology 85:2220–2226

Burke L, Cox G, Cummings N, Dresbrow B 2001 Guidelines for daily carbohydrate intake. Sports Medicine 31:267–299

Bussau V, Fairchild T, Rao A et al 2002 Carbohydrate loading in human muscle: an improved 1 day protocol. European Journal of Applied Physiology 87:290–295

Carrithers J, Williamson D, Gallagher P et al 2000 Effects of postexercise carbohydrate-protein feedings on muscle glycogen restoration. Journal of Applied Physiology 88:1876–1982

Choi D, Cole K, Goodpaster B et al 1994 Effect of passive and active recovery on the resynthesis of muscle glycogen. Medicine and Science in Sports and Exercise 26:992–996

Chryssanthopoulos C, Hennessy L, Williams C 1994 The influence of pre-exercise glucose ingestion on endurance running capacity. British Journal of Sports Medicine 28:105–109

Chryssanthopoulos C, Williams C 1997 Pre-exercise carbohydrate meal and endurance running capacity when carbohydrates are ingested during exercise. International Journal of Sports Medicine 18:543–548

Chryssanthopoulos C, Williams C, Novitz C et al 2002 The effect of a high carbohydrate meal on endurance running capacity. International Journal of Sport, Nutrition and Exercise Metabolism 12:157–171

Chryssanthopoulos C, Williams C, Nowitz A, Bogdanis G 2004 Skeletal muscle glycogen concentration and metabolic responses following a high glycaemic carbohydrate breakfast. Acta Physiologica Scandinavica 22:1065–1071

Claassen A, Lambert E, Bosch A et al 2005 Variability in exercise capacity and metabolic response during endurance exercise after a low carbohydrate diet. International Journal of Sport, Nutrition and Exercise Metabolism 15:97–116

Coggan A, Coyle E 1989 Metabolism and performance following carbohydrate ingestion late in exercise. Medicine and Science in Sports and Exercise 21:59–65

Costill D, Coyle E, Dalsky G et al 1977 Effects of elevated plasma FFA and insulin on muscle glycogen usage during exercise. Journal of Applied Physiology 43:695–699

Coyle E 1991 Timing and method of increased carbohydrate intake to cope with heavy training, competition and recovery. Journal of Sports Sciences 9:S29–S52

Coyle E 2004 Fluid and fuel intake during exercise. Acta Physiologica Scandinavica 22:39—59

Coyle E, Hagberg J, Hurley B et al 1983 Carbohydrate feeding during prolonged strenuous exercise can delay fatigue. Journal of Applied Physiology 55:230–235

Coyle EF, Coggan AR, Hemmert MK, Ivy JL 1986 Muscle glycogen utilization during prolonged strenuous exercise when fed carbohydrate. Journal of Applied Physiology 61:165–172

Dolins KR, Boozer C, Stoler F 2003 Effect of variable carbohydrate intake on exercise performance in female endurance cyclists. International Journal of Sport, Nutrition and Exercise Metabolism 13:422–435

Fallowfield J, Williams C 1993 Carbohydrate intake and recovery from prolonged exercise. International Journal of Sports Nutrition 3:150–164

Fallowfield J, Williams C 1997 The influence of a high carbohydrate intake during recovery from prolonged constant pace running. International Journal of Sports Nutrition 7:10–25

Febbraio M, Stewart K 1996 CHO feeding before prolonged exercise: effect of glycemic index on muscle glycogenolysis and exercise performance. Journal of Applied Physiology 82:1115–1120

Fisher J, Nolte L, Kawanaka K et al 2002 Glucose transport rate and glycogen synthase activity both limit skeletal muscle glycogen accumulation. American Journal of Physiology, Endocrinology and Metabolism 282:1214–1221

Foskett A, Tsintzas K, Williams C, Boobis L 2004 The effects of carbohydrate ingestion on muscle glycogen utilisation during exhaustive high-intensity intermittent running. Journal of Physiology 555P:C63

Foster C, Costill D, Fink W 1979 Effects of pre-exercise feedings on endurance performance. Medicine and Science in Sports and Exercise 11:1–5

Goforth H Jr, Arnall D, Bennett B, Law P 1997 Persistence of supercompensated muscle glycogen in trained subjects after carbohydrate loading. Journal of Applied Physiology 82:342–347

Goforth H Jr, Laurent D, Prusaczyk W et al 2003 Effects of depletion exercise and light training on muscle glycogen supercompensation in men. American Journal of Physiology, Endocrinology and Metabolism 285:E1304–E1311

Greiwe J, Hickner R, Hansen P 1999 Effects of endurance exercise training on muscle glycogen accumulation in humans. Journal of Applied Physiology 87:222–226

Ivy J, Goforth H Jr, Damon B, McCauley T, Parsons E 2002 Early post-exercise muscle glycogen recovery is enhanced with a carbohydrate-protein supplement. Journal of Applied Physiology 93:1337–1344

Ivy JL 1991 Muscle glycogen synthesis before and after exercise. Sports Medicine 11:6–19

Ivy JL, Kuo C-H 1998 Regulation of GLUT-4 protein and glycogen synthase during muscle glycogen synthesis after exercise. Acta Physiologica Scandinavica 162:293–304

Jacobs I, Westlin N, Karlsson J et al 1982 Muscle glycogen and diet in elite soccer players. European Journal of Applied Physiology 48:297–302

James A, Cullen L, Goodman C et al 2001 Muscle glycogen supercompensation: absence of a gender-related difference. European Journal of Applied Physiology 85:533–538

Jentjens R, Jeukendrup A 2003 Determinants of post-exercise glycogen resynthesis during short term recovery. Sports Medicine 33:117–144

Jentjens R, van Loon L, Mann C et al 2001 Addition of protein and amino acids to carbohydrates does not enhance postexercise muscle glycogen synthesis. Journal of Applied Physiology 91:839–846

Jeukendrup A, Jentjens R 2000 Oxidation of carbohydrate feedings during prolonged exercise: Current thoughts, guidelines and directions for future research. Sports Medicine 29:407–424

Jeukendrup A, Wagenmakers A, Stegen J et al 1999 Carbohydrate ingestion can completely suppress endogenous glucose production during exercise. American Journal of Physiology, Endocrinology and Metabolism 276:E672–E683

Karlsson J, Saltin B 1971 Diet, muscle glycogen and endurance performance. Journal of Applied Physiology 31:203–206

Keizer H, Kuipers H, van Kranenburg G 1987 Influence of liquid and solid meals on muscle glycogen resynthesis, plasma fuel hormone response, and maximal physical working capacity. International Journal of Sports Medicine 8:99–104

Kirwan J, Costill D, Mitchell J et al 1988 Carbohydrate balance in competitive runners during successive days of intense training. Journal of Applied Physiology 65: 2601–2606

Laurent D, Hundal R, Dresner A et al 2000 Mechanism of glycogen autoregulation in human muscle. American Journal of Physiology, Endocrinology and Metabolism 278:E663–E668

Maughan R, Murray R 2000 Sports drinks: basic science and practical aspects. CRC Press, London

Millard-Stafford M, Rosskopf L, Snow T, Hinson B 1997 Water versus carbohydrate-electrolyte ingestion before and during a 15 km run in the heat. International Journal of Sports Nutrition 7:26–38

Millard-Stafford M, Warren G, Thomas L et al 2005 Recovery from run training: efficacy of a carbohydrate-protein beverage. International Journal of Sport, Nutrition and Exercise Metabolism 15:610–624

Nelson A, Arnall D, Kokkonen J et al 2001 Muscle glycogen supercompensation is enhanced by prior creatine supplementation. Medicine and Science in Sports and Exercise 33:1096–1100

Neufer PD, Costill DL, Flynn MG et al 1987 Improvements in exercise performance: effects of carbohydrate feedings and diet. Journal of Applied Physiology 62:983–988

Nicholas C, Williams C, Lakomy H et al 1995 Influence of ingesting a carbohydrate-electrolyte solution on endurance capacity during intermittent, high-intensity shuttle running. Journal of Sports Sciences 13:283–290

Nicholas C, Green P, Hawkins R, Williams C 1997 Carbohydrate intake and recovery of intermittent running capacity. International Journal of Sports Nutrition 7:251–260

Nicholas C, Williams C, Boobis L, Little N 1999 Effect of ingesting a carbohydrate-electrolyte beverage on muscle glycogen utilisation during high intensity, intermittent shuttle running. Medicine and Science in Sports and Exercise 31:1280–1286

Nicholas C, Nuttall F, Williams C 2000 The Loughborough intermittent shuttle test: a field test that simulates the activity pattern of soccer. Journal of Sports Sciences 18:97–104

Nybo L, Moller K, Pedersen B et al 2003 Association between fatigue and failure to preserve cerebral energy turnover during prolonged exercise. Acta Physiologica Scandinavica 179:67–74

Pascoe D, Costill D, Robergs R et al 1990 Effects of exercise mode on muscle glycogen restorage during repeated days of exercise. Medicine and Science in Sports and Exercise 22:593–598

Piehl K 1974 Time course of refilling of glycogen stores in human muscle fibres following exercise-induced glycogen repletion. Acta Physiologica Scandinavica 90:297–302

Rauch H, Gibson A, Lambert E, Noakes T 2005 A signalling role for muscle glycogen in regulation of pace during prolonged exercise. British Journal of Sports Medicine 39:34–38

Roberts P, Fox J, Jones S et al 2004 The time-course of creatine mediated augmentation of skeletal muscle glycogen storage following exhaustive exercise in man. Journal of Physiology 555P:C59

Robinson T, Swell D, Hultman E, Greenhaff P 1999 Role of submaximal exercise in promoting creatine and glycogen accumulation in human skeletal muscle. Journal of Applied Physiology 87:598–604

Romijn J, Coyle E, Sidossis L et al 1993 Regulation of endogenous fat and carbohydrate metabolism in relation to exercise intensity and duration. American Journal of Physiology 265:E380–E391

Saltin B 1973 Metabolic fundamentals of exercise. Medicine and Science in Sports and Exercise 15:366–369

Saunders M, Kane M, Todd M 2004 Effects of a carbohydrate-protein beverage on cycling performance and muscle damage. Medicine and Science in Sports and Exercise 36:1233–1238

Schabort E, Bosch A, Weltan S, Noakes T 1999 The effect of a preexercise meal on time to fatigue during prolonged cycling exercise. Medicine and Science in Sports and Exercise 31:464–471

Sherman W, Costill D, Fink W, Miller J 1981 Effect of exercise-diet manipulation on muscle glycogen and its subsequent utilization during performance. International Journal of Sports Medicine 2:114–118

Sherman W, Brodowicz G, Wright D et al 1989 Effects of 4h preexercise carbohydrate feedings on cycling performance. Medicine and Science in Sports and Exercise 21:598–604

Sherman M, Doyle J, Lamb D, Stauss R 1993 Dietary carbohydrate, muscle glycogen and exercise performance during 7d of training. American Journal of Clinical Nutrition 57:27–31

Simonsen JC, Sherman WM, Lamb DR et al 1991 Dietary carbohydrate, muscle glycogen, and power output during rowing training. Journal of Applied Physiology 70:1500–1505

Stevenson E, Williams C, McComb G, Oram C 2005 Improved recovery from prolonged exercise following the consumption of Low Glycemic Index Carbohydrate Meals. International Journal of Sport, Nutrition and Exercise Metabolism 15:333–349

Tarnopolsky LJ, MacDougall JD, Atkinson SA et al 1990 Gender differences in substrate for endurance exercise. Journal of Applied Physiology 68:302–307

Tsintzas K, Williams C 1998 Human muscle glycogen metabolism during exercise: effect of carbohydrate supplementation. Sports Medicine 25:7–23

Tsintzas K, Liu R, Williams C et al 1993 The effect of carbohydrate ingestion on performance during a 30-km race. International Journal of Sports Nutrition 3:127–139

Tsintzas O, Williams C, Singh R et al 1995 Influence of carbohydrate-electrolyte drinks on marathon running performance. European Journal of Applied Physiology 70:154–160

Tsintzas O, Williams C, Boobis L, Greenhaff P 1996a Carbohydrate ingestion and single muscle fiber glycogen metabolism during prolonged running in men. Journal of Applied Physiology 81:801–809

Tsintzas O, Williams C, Wilson W, Burrin J 1996b Influence of carbohydrate supplementation early in exercise on endurance running capacity. Medicine and Science in Sports and Exercise 28:1373–1379

Tsintzas K, Williams C, Boobis L et al 2003 Effect of carbohydrate feeding during recovery from prolonged running on muscle glycogen metabolism during subsequent exercise. International Journal of Sports Medicine 24:452–458

van Hall G, Shirreffs S, Calbet J 2000 Muscle glycogen resynthesis during recovery from cycle exercise: no effect of additional protein ingestion. Journal of Applied Physiology 88:1631–1636

van Loon L, Kruijshoop M, Verhagen H et al 2000a Ingestion of protein hydrolysate and amino acid-carbohydrate mixtures increases postexercise plasma insulin responses in men. Journal of Nutrition 130:2508–2513

van Loon L, Saris W, Kruijshoop M, Wagenmakers A 2000b Maximizing postexercise muscle glycogen synthesis: carbohydrate supplementation and the application of amino acid or protein hydrolysate mixtures. American Journal of Clinical Nutrition 72:106–111

van Loon L, Greenhaff P, Constantin-Teodosiu D et al 2001 The effects of increasing exercise intensity on muscle fuel utilisation in humans. Journal of Physiology 536:295–304

Walker L, Heigenhauser G, Hultman E, Spriet L 2000 Dietary carbohydrate, muscle glycogen content, and endurance performance in well trained women. Journal of Applied Physiology 88:2151–2158

Wee S-L, Williams C, Gray S, Horabin J 1999 Influence of high and low glycemic index meals on endurance running capacity. Medicine and Science in Sports and Exercise 31:393–399

Wee S, Williams C, Tsintzas K, Boobis L 2005 Ingestion of a high-glycemic index meal increases muscle glycogen storage at rest but augments its utilization during subsequent exercise. Journal of Applied Physiology 99:707–714

Welsh R, Davis M, Burke J, Williams H 2002 Carbohydrates and physical/mental performance during intermittent exercise to fatigue. Medicine and Science in Sports and Exercise 34:723–731

Whitley H, Humphries S, Campbell I et al 1998 Metabolic and performance relationship during endurance exercise after high fat and high carbohydrate meals. Journal of Applied Physiology 85:418–424

Williams M, Raven P, Fogt D, Ivy J 2003 Effects of recovery beverages on glycogen restoration and endurance exercise performance. Journal of Strength & Condition Research 17:12–19

Wong S, Williams C, Adams N 2000 Effects of ingesting a large volume of carbohydrate-electrolyte solution on rehydration during recovery and subsequent exercise capacity. International Journal of Sport, Nutrition and Exercise Metabolism 10:375–393

Wu C-L, Nicholas C, Williams C et al 2003 The influence of high-carbohydrate meals with different glycaemic indices on substrate utilisation during subsequent exercise. British Journal of Nutrition 90:1049–1056

Zawadzki K, Yaspelkis III B, Ivy J 1992 Carbohydrate-protein complex increases the rate of muscle glycogen storage after exercise. Journal of Applied Physiology 72:1854–1859

Chapter 4

The role of fats as an energy source

Asker Jeukendrup

LEARNING OBJECTIVES

After reading this chapter, you should be able to:

1. Have an understanding of the regulation of carbohydrate and fat metabolism during exercise.
2. Critically discuss the factors that influence substrate utilization during exercise.
3. Have an understanding of the ways to increase fat oxidation.
4. Distinguish between facts and fallacies as far as nutrition supplements are concerned.

5. Appreciate the importance of fat oxidation in health and disease (in particular with endurance training and metabolic diseases such as diabetes).

INTRODUCTION

Carbohydrate and fat are the main sources of energy for muscle contraction during exercise. Both fuels are stored within the body but the fat stores are very large in comparison with carbohydrate stores. The total amount of energy stored as glycogen (the form in which carbohydrate is stored) in the muscle and liver has been estimated to be 500 g or 8000 kJ (2000 kcal), although this may depend on diet and muscle mass. The carbohydrate stores are so small that they can become performance limiting. In some forms of exercise (e.g. prolonged cycling or running), carbohydrate depletion has been associated with fatigue and carbohydrate depletion can occur within 1 hour to 2 hours of strenuous exercise (see Chapter 3). Fat stores can contain more than 50 times the amount of energy in carbohydrate stores. A person with a body mass of 80 kg and 15% body fat has 12 kg of fat. Most of this fat is stored in subcutaneous adipose tissue, but some fat can also be found in muscle as intramuscular triacylglycerol. In theory, the fat stores could provide sufficient energy for a runner to run at least 1300 km.

Ideally, athletes like to tap into their fat stores as much as possible and save the carbohydrate for later in a competition. Researchers, coaches and athletes have therefore tried to devise strategies to enhance fat metabolism, spare carbohydrate stores, and, hence, improve endurance performance. Understanding the effects of various nutritional strategies requires an understanding of fat metabolism and the factors that regulate fat oxidation during exercise. The aim of this chapter, therefore, is to provide an understanding of the regulation of fat metabolism during exercise and to give an overview of ways in which researchers and athletes have tried to enhance fat metabolism by nutritional manipulation and training.

FAT METABOLISM DURING EXERCISE

In order to provide energy for muscle contraction, fatty acids must be broken down to acetyl CoA which can then enter the tricarboxylic acid (TCA) cycle resulting in adenosine triphosphate (ATP) production. This high energy phosphate will then enable muscle contraction. Fatty acids are broken down to acetyl CoA in the mitochondria and therefore all fats have to be transported to the muscle and into the mitochondria in order to provide energy (Fig. 4.1).

Fatty acids that are oxidized in the mitochondria of skeletal muscle during exercise are derived from various sources. The main two body stores of fat are adipose tissue and muscle triacylglycerols (Fig. 4.1). A third fuel, plasma triacylglycerol, may also be utilized, but the importance of this

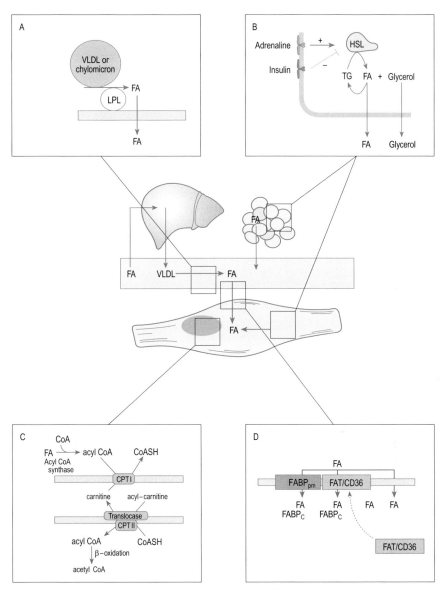

Figure 4.1   Schematic illustrating various stages of lipid mobilization and transport. (A) Transport form of lipids in blood before hydrolysis by LPL (lipoprotein lipase) to fatty acids near muscle cells. (B) Activation and hydrolysis of stored TGs in adipose tissue and muscle via HSL (hormone-sensitive lipase) to fatty acids and glycerol. (C) Transport of fatty acids across the mitochondrial membrane. (D) Methods of transport across a plasma membrane.

fuel is subject to debate (Fig. 4.1A). The mobilization and utilization of these fuels will be discussed below as well as the regulation of the processes involved.

ADIPOSE TISSUE

The vast majority of fat is stored in adipose tissue as triacylglycerols and this energy source is mobilized by splitting triacylglycerols into fatty acids and glycerol, a process called lipolysis (Fig. 4.1B). This process is initiated when the enzyme hormone-sensitive lipase (HSL) is activated. As the name of this enzyme suggests, the regulation of the activity of the enzyme is dependent on hormonal concentrations, mainly adrenaline and insulin. Adrenaline is a potent stimulant of HSL, whereas insulin is a strong inhibitor. HSL is also activated by the sympathetic nervous system. When HSL is activated, triacylglycerol moieties are cleaved into fatty acids and glycerol. When exercise is started increased adrenergic stimulation will increase HSL activity and increase the mobilization of fatty acids. The fatty acids that are released have to be transported out of the adipocyte to become available and adipose tissue blood flow plays an important role in the removal of fatty acids from the adipose tissue. During exercise, a proportion of fatty acids is not released into the circulation but is used to form new triacylglycerols within the adipose tissue, a process called re-esterification. Because fatty acids are not soluble in water, they are usually bound to proteins in the body. In cells they are bound to so-called fatty-acid-binding proteins (FABPs) and in the blood they are bound to albumin. Albumin is a large protein with three high-affinity binding sites for fatty acids. The removal rate of fatty acids from adipose tissue is dependent, not only on blood flow, but also on the transport capacity of the blood (i.e. the albumin concentration and the saturation of albumin with fatty acids). The fatty acids that are released into the circulation are transported to other tissues and taken up by skeletal muscle during exercise. Glycerol is also released into the circulation and transported to the liver, where it serves as a gluconeogenic substrate for the synthesis of new glucose.

PLASMA TRIACYLGLYCEROLS

Circulating triacylglycerols (for example in very-low-density lipoprotein (VLDL) can also serve as a fuel although its importance is subject to debate. Plasma triacylglycerols can temporarily bind to lipoprotein lipase (LPL) which is present in the walls of the vascular bed (Fig. 4.1A). The enzyme hydrolyzes (breaks down) some of the triacylglycerols in circulating lipoproteins passing through the capillary bed. As a result, fatty acids are released that the muscle can take up and use for oxidation. However, it has been suggested that the fatty acid uptake from plasma lipoprotein triacylglycerols occurs slowly and accounts for fewer than 3% of the energy expenditure during prolonged exercise. Therefore, it is generally believed that plasma triacylglycerols contribute only minimally to energy production during exercise. However, some interesting observations may indicate that the role of plasma triacylglycerol has been underestimated in the past. For instance, LPL activity is significantly increased after training and after a high-fat diet; in both situations, fat oxidation is markedly increased. In addition, acute exercise also stimulates LPL activity. Nevertheless, arteriovenous balance studies suggest that the contribution of plasma triacylglycerols to energy provision is small.

Fatty acids derived from adipose tissue triacylglycerol and circulating plasma triacylglycerol have to be transported across the muscle membrane. For a long time, the transport of fatty acids into the muscle cell was believed to be a passive process. This belief was based on early observations that fatty acid uptake increased linearly with fatty acid concentration. However, recently, specific carrier proteins have been identified which are likely to be responsible for the transport of most fatty acids across the sarcolemma (Fig. 4.1D). Probably the most important protein is FAT/CD36 which can translocate from intracellular vesicles to the cell membrane in a similar manner as the GLUT-4 protein. Muscle contraction increases the amount of membrane bound FAT/CD36 and increases the transport of fatty acids into the muscle.

MUSCLE TRIACYLGLYCEROL

A third source of fat resides inside the muscle in the form of intramuscular triacylglycerol. These triacylglycerols can be seen under a microscope as little lipid droplets usually located adjacent to the mitochondria and have been recognized as an important energy source during exercise. Studies in which muscle samples were investigated under a microscope revealed that the size of these lipid droplets decrease during exercise. Intramuscular triacylglycerols are hydrolyzed by a muscle-specific hormone-sensitive lipase (HSL), and fatty acids are transported into the mitochondria for oxidation in the same way fatty acids from plasma and plasma triacylglycerol are utilized.

Similar to HSL in adipose tissue, muscle HSL is activated by beta-adrenergic stimulation and inhibited by insulin (Fig. 4.1B). Fatty acids derived from the breakdown of intramuscular triacylglycerols may be released into the blood, re-esterified, or oxidized within the muscle. Because, at least in trained muscle, the lipid droplets are located close to the mitochondria, most of the fatty acids released after lipolysis are assumed to be oxidized.

Once fatty acids have entered the muscle cell they have to be transported across the mitochondrial membrane (Fig. 4.1C). Fatty acids in the sarcoplasm will be activated by the enzyme acyl CoA synthetase or thiokinase to form an acyl CoA complex (often referred to as an activated fatty acid). This acyl CoA complex is used for the synthesis of intramuscular triacylglycerols, or it is bound to carnitine under the influence of the enzyme carnitine palmitoyl transferase I (CPT I), which is located at the outside of the outer mitochondrial membrane.

The bonding between carnitine and the activated fatty acid is the first step in the transport of the fatty acids into the mitochondria. As carnitine binds to the fatty acid, free CoA is released. The fatty acyl-carnitine complex is transported with a translocase and reconverted into fatty acyl CoA at the matrix side of the inner mitochondrial membrane by the enzyme carnitine palmytoyl transferase II (CPT II). The carnitine that is released diffuses back across the mitochondrial membrane into the cytoplasm and thus becomes available again for the transport of other fatty acids. Fatty acyl-carnitine crosses the inner membrane in a 1:1 exchange with a molecule of free carnitine. Although short-chain fatty acids (SC fatty acids) and medium-chain fatty acids (MC fatty acids) are believed to diffuse freely into the mitochondrial matrix, carrier proteins with a specific maximum affinity for short-chain or medium-chain acyl CoA transport at least some of the fatty acids.

Once in the mitochondrial matrix, the fatty acyl CoA is subjected to β-oxidation, a series of reactions that splits a 2-carbon acetyl CoA molecule of the multiple carbon fatty acid chain. The β-oxidation pathway uses oxygen and generates some ATP through substrate-level phosphorylation. The acetyl CoA is then oxidized in the tricarboxylic acid (TCA) cycle. The complete oxidation of fatty acids in the mitochondria depends on several factors, including the activity of enzymes of the β-oxidation pathway, the concentration of TCA-cycle intermediates and activity of enzymes in the TCA cycle (these factors determine the total TCA-cycle activity), and the presence of oxygen.

REGULATION OF FAT METABOLISM

A common misconception is that fuel selection will switch from carbohydrate to fat once the carbohydrate stores become depleted. In reality, carbohydrate and fat are always oxidized simultaneously, and whether carbohydrate or fat is the predominant fuel depends on a variety of factors, including the intensity and duration of exercise, the level of aerobic fitness, diet, and carbohydrate intake before or during exercise. Below the changes in fat metabolism that occur in the transition from rest to exercise will be discussed as well as the various factors that influence fat mobilization and oxidation.

After an overnight fast, most of the energy requirement is derived from the oxidation of fatty acids from adipose tissue. Lipolysis in adipose tissue depends on the hormonal milieu (adrenaline will stimulate lipolysis and insulin will inhibit lipolysis). After a meal when blood insulin concentrations are high lipolysis will be suppressed and fat oxidation will be reduced. At rest, most of the fatty acids liberated after lipolysis are re-esterified within the adipocyte. Some fatty acids enter the bloodstream, but only about half of these fatty acids are oxidized. Resting plasma FA concentrations are typically between 0.2 mmol/L and 0.4 mmol/L.

When exercise is initiated, the rate of lipolysis and the rate of fatty acid release from adipose tissue are increased. During moderate-intensity exercise, lipolysis increases approximately threefold, mainly because of an increased beta-adrenergic stimulation (by catecholamines). In addition, during moderate-intensity exercise, the blood flow to adipose tissue is doubled and the rate of re-esterification is halved. Blood flow in skeletal muscle is increased dramatically, and, therefore, the delivery of fatty acids to the muscle is increased manyfold.

During the first 15 minutes of exercise, plasma fatty acid concentrations usually decrease because the rate of fatty acid uptake by the muscle exceeds the rate of fatty acid appearance from lipolysis. Thereafter, the rate of appearance is in excess of the utilization by muscle, and plasma fatty acid concentrations increase. The rise in fatty acid depends on the exercise intensity. During moderate-intensity exercise, fatty acid concentrations may reach 1 mmol/L within 60 minutes of exercise, but at higher exercise intensities, the rise in plasma fatty acids is very small or may even be absent. Plasma fatty acid concentrations do not normally exceed 2 mmol/L as this would be close to the maximum binding capacity of albumin. A further increase in fatty acid appearance in the circulation would result in an increase in the unbound fraction (normally <0.1% of the fatty acids is unbound) and this could have detrimental effects since unbound fatty acids are toxic. The body seems to have protective mechanisms to prevent rises above 2 mmol/L. One of these mechanisms could be increased incorporation of fatty acids into plasma triacylglycerol. During every pass through the liver, a fraction of the fatty acids is extracted from the circulation and incorporated into VLDL particles.

In all situations, carbohydrate and fat together constitute most, if not all, of the energy provision. The percentage contribution of these two fuels, however, varies depending on the factors discussed previously. The rate of carbohydrate utilization during prolonged strenuous exercise is closely related to the energy needs of the working muscle. In contrast, fat utilization during exercise is not tightly regulated. No mechanisms closely match the metabolism of fatty acids to energy expenditure. Fat oxidation is therefore mainly influenced by fat availability and the rate of carbohydrate utilization.

There is evidence to suggest that an increase in plasma fatty acid concentration can cause a decrease in the rate of muscle glycogen breakdown. This action could theoretically be beneficial, because muscle glycogen depletion is one of the prime causes of fatigue. Researchers have artificially elevated plasma fatty acid concentrations by raising plasma triacylglycerol concentrations by means of a fat meal or intravenous infusion of triacylglycerol (Intralipid), followed by a heparin injection. This method has repeatedly shown that an increase in plasma fatty acid concentration can reduce carbohydrate dependence.

In a study by Costill et al (1977), Intralipid was infused and heparin was injected during exercise at 70% $\dot{V}O_2$max. After 60 minutes, a muscle biopsy was taken and muscle glycogen was measured before and after the exercise bout. Muscle glycogen breakdown was reduced with the elevated plasma fatty acid concentrations. The classical glucose–fatty acid cycle or Randle cycle was originally thought to explain this interaction between carbohydrate and fat metabolism. This theory states that with an increase in plasma fatty acid concentration, uptake of fatty acids increases and these fatty acids undergo β-oxidation in the mitochondria, in which they are broken down to acetyl CoA. An increasing concentration of acetyl CoA (or increased acetyl CoA/CoA ratio) inhibits the pyruvate dehydrogenase (PDH) complex that breaks down pyruvate to acetyl CoA. Also, increased formation of acetyl CoA from fatty acids increases muscle citrate levels, and after diffusing into the sarcoplasm, could inhibit phosphofructokinase (PFK), the rate-limiting enzyme in glycolysis. The effect of increased acetyl CoA and citrate levels is therefore a reduction in the rate of glycolysis. This reduced glycolysis, in turn, may cause accumulation of glucose-6-phosphate (G-6-P) in the muscle, which inhibits hexokinase activity and thus reduces muscle glucose uptake. Although this theory is attractive, it does not seem to explain the interaction between carbohydrate and fat metabolism during exercise of moderate to high intensities. It may be important though at rest and during very low intensity exercise.

A more recent theory about the regulation of carbohydrate and fat metabolism proposes that fat does not regulate carbohydrate metabolism, but rather that carbohydrate regulates fat metabolism. An increase in the rate of glycolysis decreases fat oxidation. Regulation of fat metabolism involves the transport of fatty acids into the mitochondria, which is controlled mainly by the activity of CPT I. CPT I is regulated by several factors, including the malonyl CoA (a precursor of FA synthesis) concentration. The high rate of glycogenolysis during high intensity exercise increases the amount of acetyl CoA in the muscle cell, and some of this acetyl CoA is converted to malonyl CoA by the enzyme acetyl CoA carboxylase (ACC). Malonyl CoA inhibits CPT I and could thus reduce the transport of fatty acids into the mitochondria. Reductions in intramuscular pH that may occur during high intensity exercise may also inhibit CPT I and, hence, FA transport into the mitochondria.

Another explanation is that a reduced free carnitine concentration limits the entry of fatty acids into the mitochondria. When glycogenolysis is accelerated, acetyl CoA accumulates during intense exercise and some of this acetyl CoA is bound to carnitine. As a result, the free carnitine concentration drops, and less carnitine is available to transport fatty acids into the mitochondria. Finally, it has been proposed that pyruvate derived acetyl CoA competes with the FA-derived acetyl CoA for entrance into the TCA cycle.

The rate of carbohydrate utilization during prolonged strenuous exercise is closely related to the energy needs of the working muscle. In contrast, fat utilization during exercise is not tightly regulated. No mechanisms closely match the metabolism of fatty acids to energy expenditure. Fat oxidation is, therefore, mainly influenced by fat availability and the rate of carbohydrate utilization. The importance of each of these factors may depend on the situation. For example, carbohydrate utilization may be a more important factor during exercise, whereas the availability of fatty acids may be more important at rest. A more detailed discussion of the regulation of fat and carbohydrate metabolism can be found in several recent review articles.

THE EFFECT OF EXERCISE DURATION ON FAT OXIDATION

Fat oxidation increases as the exercise duration increases. After several hours of strenuous exercise without eating, fat oxidation rates can increase from normal values around 0.4 g/minute up to 1 g/minute. The mechanism of this increased fat oxidation as exercise duration increases is not entirely clear but seems to be linked to the decrease in muscle glycogen stores. When glycogen stores become depleted later in exercise, plasma fatty acid concentrations are usually very high and can provide a source of fat for oxidation. Also, when carbohydrate availability is low this may relieve some of the inhibition on fatty acid transport into the mitochondria. Above, it was discussed how a high glycolytic flux can reduce the transport of fatty acids into the mitochondria. If glycolytic flux is reduced because the muscle is running out of glycogen, and pyruvate dehydrogenase (PDH) activity is reduced, this will reduce the formation of malonyl CoA, resulting in less inhibition of the CPT system. Ultimately this will allow more fatty acids to enter the mitochondria for oxidation.

FAT OXIDATION AND EXERCISE INTENSITY

Fat oxidation is usually the predominant fuel at low exercise intensities, whereas during high exercise intensities, carbohydrate is the main fuel source. In absolute terms, fat oxidation increases as the exercise intensity increases from low to moderate intensities, even though the percentage contribution of fat may actually decrease. For the transition from light-intensity to moderate-intensity exercise, the increased fat oxidation is a direct result of the increased energy expenditure. At higher intensities of exercise (>75% $\dot{V}O_2$max) fat oxidation is inhibited and both the relative and absolute rates of fat oxidation decrease to negligible values. Achten et al studied this relationship over a wide range of exercise intensities in a group of trained subjects and found that, on average, the maximal rates of fat oxidation were observed at 63% $\dot{V}O_2$max (Fig. 4.2A).

During exercise at 25% $\dot{V}O_2$max, most of the fat oxidized is derived from plasma fatty acids, and only small amounts are coming from intramuscular triglycerides. However, during moderate exercise intensity (65% $\dot{V}O_2$max), the contribution of plasma fatty acids declines, whereas the contribution of intramuscular triacylglycerols increases and provides about half of the fatty acids used for total fat oxidation. When the exercise intensity is further increased, fat oxidation decreases, even though the rate of lipolysis is still high. The blood flow to the adipose tissue may be decreased (because of sympathetic vasoconstriction), which may result in a decreased removal of fatty acids from adipose tissue. During high-intensity exercise, lactate accumulation may also increase the rate of re-esterification of fatty acids (and/or inhibit the transport of fatty acids into the mitochondria). As a result, plasma fatty acid concentrations are usually low during intense exercise.

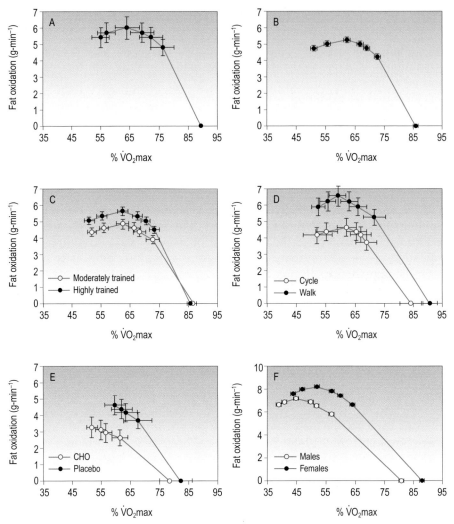

Figure 4.2 Fat oxidation rates versus exercise intensity expressed as percentage of maximal oxygen uptake. (A) Determined in moderately trained men, n = 11 (Achten et al 2002). (B) Determined in a large group of trained male cyclists with wide range of $\dot{V}O_2$max, n = 53 (Achten et al 2003a). (C) Determined in moderately (n = 26) and highly (n = 27) trained male cyclists ($\dot{V}O_2$max: 59 vs 72 mL/kg/minute) (Achten et al 2003a). (D) Determined during cycle-ergometer-based and treadmill-based test in moderately trained triathletes, n = 12 (Achten et al 2003b). (E) Determined in moderately trained cyclists after overnight fast and 45 minutes after ingestion of 75 g glucose, n = 11 (Achten & Jeukendrup 2003). (F) Determined in large group of individuals, treadmill-based test. Men, n = 157; women, n = 143 (Venables et al 2005).

However, this decreased availability of fatty acids can only partially explain the reduced fat oxidation observed in these conditions and an additional mechanism in the muscle is responsible for the decreased fat oxidation observed during high-intensity exercise. There is evidence that the decreased fat oxidation at higher intensities is not only related to fatty acid availability but also to the transport of fatty acids into the mitochondria. During high-intensity exercise, the oxidation of long-chain fatty acids is impaired, whereas the oxidation of medium-chain fatty acids is unaffected. Because the medium-chain fatty acids are less dependent on transport mechanisms into the mitochondria by CPT, these data provide evidence that carnitine-dependent FA transport is a limiting factor.

FAT OXIDATION AND TRAINING STATUS

Endurance training affects both substrate utilization and exercise capacity (Fig. 4.2C). Studies involving both animals and humans have established a marked adaptive increase in oxidative potential in response to increased regular physical activity. A consequence and probably contributing factor to the enhanced exercise capacity after endurance training is the metabolic shift to a greater use of fat and a concomitant sparing of glycogen. The contribution of fat to total energy expenditure increases after training at both the relative and the absolute exercise intensities. The adaptations that contribute to a stimulation of fat oxidation in trained subjects include increased mitochondrial density and an increase in the number of oxidative enzymes in trained muscle, which increases the capacity to oxidize fat. Some of the adaptations to endurance training include:

- increased mitochondrial density
- increased oxidative enzymes (citrate synthase, 3-hydroxyacyl CoA dehydrogenase (HAD)
- increased capillary density, which enhances FA delivery to the muscle
- increased FABP concentrations, which may facilitate uptake of fatty acids across the sarcolemma
- increased CPT activity, which facilitates the transport of fatty acids into the mitochondria.

Lipolysis in adipose tissue seems to be unaffected by training. After training, the rate of lipolysis at the same absolute exercise intensity does not seem to be affected. At the same relative exercise intensity, the rate of lipolysis is increased after training. An increased lipolysis of intramuscular triacylglycerol likely contributes to this increased whole-body lipolysis.

RESPONSE TO CARBOHYDRATE FEEDING

The fastest way to alter fat metabolism during exercise is probably by carbohydrate feeding (Fig. 4.2E). Carbohydrate increases the plasma insulin concentration, which reduces lipolysis and causes a marked reduction in fatty acid availability. In a study by Horowitz et al (1997) carbohydrate was ingested 1 hour before exercise. Both lipolysis and fat oxidation were reduced. Plasma fatty acid concentrations decreased to very low levels during exercise. However, when Intralipid was infused and heparin was injected to increase the plasma fatty acid concentrations, fat oxidation was only partially restored. These findings indicate that a reduced availability of fatty acids is indeed a factor that limits fat oxidation. However, because increasing the plasma fatty acid concentrations does not completely restore fat oxidation, other factors must play a role as well. These factors must be located inside the muscle itself.

When a large amount of glucose is ingested 1 hour before exercise, plasma insulin levels are very high at the start of exercise, whereas plasma fatty acid and glycerol concentrations are very low. This results in a 30% reduction in fat oxidation compared with no carbohydrate intake. In a study by Coyle et al (1997) trace amounts of labelled medium-chain or long-chain fatty acids were infused, and the oxidation rates of these fatty acids were determined. The oxidation of long-chain fatty acids appeared to be reduced, whereas the oxidation of medium-chain fatty acids appeared to be unaffected. Because medium-chain fatty acids are not as dependent on transport mechanisms into the mitochondria, but the long-chain fatty acids are highly dependent on this mechanism, these results provide evidence that this transport is an important regulatory step. Although the exact mechanisms are still unclear, carbohydrate feeding before exercise reduces fat oxidation by reducing lipolysis and plasma fatty acid availability and exerts an inhibiting effect on carnitine-dependent FA transport into the mitochondria.

FAT SUPPLEMENTATION DURING EXERCISE

The effects of eating fat before or during exercise have been studied as a method to increase FA availability and increase fat oxidation in order to reduce muscle glycogen breakdown. Initial studies looked at fatty meals mainly consisting of long-chain triacylglycerols (LCTs); later studies have also looked at alternative lipid fuels such as medium-chain triacylglycerols (MCTs).

INGESTION OF LONG-CHAIN TRIACYLGLYCEROLS

Nutritional fats include triacylglycerols (containing mostly C16 and C18 fatty acids), phospholipids and cholesterol, of which only triacylglycerols can contribute to any extent to energy provision during exercise. In contrast to carbohydrates, nutritional fats reach the circulation only slowly because they are potent inhibitors of gastric emptying. Furthermore, the digestion in the gut and absorption of fat are also rather slow processes compared with the digestion and absorption of carbohydrates.

Bile salts, produced by the liver, and lipase, secreted by the pancreas, are needed for lipolysis of the long-chain triacylglycerols (LCTs) into glycerol and

3 LC fatty acids or monoacylglycerol and 2 fatty acids. The fatty acids diffuse into the intestinal mucosa cells and are re-esterified in the cytoplasm to form LCTs. These LCTs are encapsulated by a coat of proteins – forming chylomicrons – to make them water soluble. These chylomicrons are then released in the lymphatic system, which ultimately drains in the systemic circulation. Exogenous LCTs enter the systemic circulation much slower than carbohydrates, which are absorbed as glucose (or to minor extents, as fructose or galactose) and directly enter the main circulation through the portal vein. Long-chain dietary fatty acids typically enter the blood 3 to 4 hours after ingestion.

The fact that these LC fatty acids enter the circulation in chylomicrons is also important, and the rate of breakdown of chylomicron-bound triacylglycerols by muscle is generally believed to be relatively low. The primary role of these triacylglycerols in chylomicrons may be the replenishment of intramuscular triacylglycerol stores after exercise. The intake of fat during exercise should, therefore, be avoided. Many so-called 'sports bars' or 'energy bars', however, contain relatively large amounts of fat. Food labels of these products should be checked when choosing an energy bar.

INGESTION OF MEDIUM–CHAIN TRIACYLGLYCEROLS

Medium-chain triacylglycerols (MCTs) contain fatty acids with a chain length of C8 or C10. MCTs are normally present in our diet in very small quantities and they have few natural sources. Intake via these sources is small and, therefore, MCTs are often consumed as a supplement. MCTs are sold as a supplement to replace normal fat as it is claimed that MCTs are not stored in the body and, therefore, could help athletes lose body fat. MCT supplements are fairly popular among body builders, they have been used as an alternative fuel source during exercise.

MCT is usually synthesized from coconut oil. Unlike most long-chain triacylglycerols (LCTs), MCTs are liquid at room temperature, partly because of the small molecular size of MCTs. MCTs are more polar and, therefore, more soluble in water. This greater water solubility and smaller molecular size has consequences at all levels of metabolism. MCTs are more rapidly digested and absorbed in the intestine than LCTs, MC fatty acids follow the portal venous system and enter the liver directly, whereas long-chain fatty acids pass into the lacteals and follow the slow lymphatic system.

MCT may, therefore, be a valuable exogenous energy source during exercise in addition to carbohydrates. Also, MCT ingestion may improve exercise performance by elevating plasma FA levels and sparing muscle glycogen because it increases the availability of plasma fatty acids, reduces the rate of muscle glycogen breakdown, and delays the onset of exhaustion. MCT added to carbohydrate drinks did not inhibit gastric emptying and the oxidation rates of orally ingested MCT are high. However, the maximal amount of oral MCT that is tolerated in the gastrointestinal tract is about 30 g, and this small amount limited the contribution of oral MCT to total energy expenditure to between 3% and 7%. When a large amount of MCT was ingested (86 g in 2 hours), subjects experienced gastrointestinal problems and their performance did not improve. In fact, MCT ingestion caused deterioration in performance compared with the placebo (water) treatment. MCT therefore does not appear to have the positive effects on performance that are often claimed.

FASTING

Fasting has been proposed as a way to increase fat utilization, spare muscle glycogen, and improve exercise performance. In rats, short-term fasting increases plasma adrenaline and noradrenaline concentrations, stimulates lipolysis, and increases the concentration of circulating plasma fatty acids. These effects, in turn, increase fat oxidation and 'spare' muscle glycogen, leading to a similar or even increased running time to exhaustion in rats. In humans, fasting also results in an increased concentration of circulating catecholamines, increased lipolysis, increased concentration of plasma fatty acids, and a decreased glucose turnover. Muscle glycogen concentrations, however, are unaffected by fasting for 24 hours when no strenuous exercise is performed. The effects on performance, however, are different in humans than in rats. Although fasting has been reported to have no effect on endurance capacity at low exercise intensities (45% $\dot{V}O_2max$), decreases in performance have been observed for exercise intensities between 50% and 100% $\dot{V}O_2max$. The observed decreased performance was not reversible by carbohydrate ingestion during exercise.

Some investigators argued that the effects observed in most of these studies were seen because, in the control situation, the last meal was provided 3 hours before the exercise to exhaustion. The effects, therefore, are of the feeding before exercise improving endurance capacity rather than of decreased performance after fasting. However, the studies that compared a prolonged fast (>24 hours) to a 12-hour fast also reported decreased performance and, thus, the conclusion that fasting decreases endurance capacity seems justified. The mechanism remains unclear, although certainly liver glycogen stores are substantially depleted after a 24-hour fast. Thus, euglycemia may not be as well maintained during exercise. Some degree of metabolic acidosis may also be observed after prolonged fasting. When hepatic glycogen stores are exhausted (e.g. after 12–24 hours of total fasting), the liver produces ketone bodies (acetoacetate, β-hydroxybutyrate and acetone) to provide an energy substrate for peripheral tissues. These keto-acids lower pH, although the acidosis is usually only mild.

EFFECTS OF A SHORT–TERM HIGH–FAT DIET

Diet also has marked effects on fat oxidation. Generally a high-carbohydrate, low-fat diet reduces fat oxidation, whereas a high-fat, low-carbohydrate diet increases fat oxidation. Some may argue that the results seen in most of these studies are the effects of the last meal, which is known to influence substrate utilization. However, it has been demonstrated that a high-fat, low-carbohydrate diet has a similar effect on substrate utilization, even after a day on a high-carbohydrate diet.

Christensen & Hansen (1939) showed that short-term exposure to a high-fat diet resulted in premature fatigue during exercise. After muscle biopsy techniques were redeveloped, a high-fat, low-carbohydrate diet was shown to result in decreased muscle glycogen levels, and this was the main factor causing lack of fatigue resistance during prolonged exercise. Plasma fatty acid concentrations are increased at rest and increase more rapidly when a low-carbohydrate diet is consumed. These changes in plasma fatty acid concentrations are attributed to changes in the rate of lipolysis. Not only plasma fatty acids but also plasma glycerol concentrations are increased after a low-carbohydrate diet. The decrease in muscle glycogen concentrations in combination with lower liver glycogen concentrations are likely responsible for the negative effects on performance that are usually observed compared with a high carbohydrate diet.

EFFECTS OF A LONG-TERM HIGH-FAT DIET

A 3-day to 4-day alteration in the dietary composition has been suggested to be an insufficient time to induce an adaptive response to the changed diet. A high-fat diet over a prolonged period, however, may result in a decreased utilization of carbohydrates and an increased contribution of fat to energy metabolism. In rats, adaptation to a high-fat diet leads to considerable improvements in endurance capacity. These adaptations can be attributed to the increased number of oxidative enzymes and a decreased degradation of liver glycogen during exercise. The results suggest that after adaptation to a high-fat diet, the capacity to oxidize fatty acids instead of carbohydrates is increased because of an adaptation of the oxidative enzymes in the muscle cell. These adaptations are much like the adaptations seen after endurance training.

One of the first studies that investigated the effects of prolonged high-fat diets on humans was conducted by Phinney et al (1980). They investigated exercise performance in obese subjects who followed a high-fat diet (90% of energy intake from fat) for 6 weeks. Before and after the diet, subjects exercised at 75% $\dot{V}O_2$max until exhaustion. Subjects were able to exercise as long on the high-fat diet as they did on their normal diet, but after the high-fat diet, fat became the main substrate. Results of this study, however, may have been influenced by the fact that these subjects were not in energy balance and lost 11 kg of body weight. So, although no differences were seen in the absolute $\dot{V}O_2$max before and after the dietary period, considerable differences were apparent in the relative exercise intensity.

The observed improvement in performance may have been an artefact rather than a positive effect of the adaptation period. Follow-up studies showed that adaptations to a high-fat diet occur (increased HAD activity, increased CPT I activity), but the diet had no ergogenic effect.

From a health perspective, eating large amounts of fat has been associated with the development of obesity and cardiovascular disease. Whether this association is also true for athletes has yet to be determined. Very few studies have described the effects of high-fat diets on cardiovascular risk factors in athletes who train regularly. Pendergast et al (1996) reported no changes in plasma LDL, HDL or total cholesterol levels in male and female runners with diets in the range of 17–40% fat. Although the risk of obesity and cardio-vascular diseases increases with the consumption of high-fat diets in sedentary people, regular exercise or endurance training seems to attenuate these risks. Exposure to high-fat diets has also been associated with insulin resistance, which has recently been linked to an effect of the intramuscular triacylglycerol pools on glucose uptake. However, these observations were made in obese subjects, and whether these results can be extrapolated to athletes is not clear, especially because athletes seem to have larger intra-muscular triacylglycerol stores and increased insulin sensitivity. Because little information is available about the negative effects of high-fat diets on athletes, and the effects of these diets on performance are unclear, we suggest caution when recommending high-fat diets to athletes.

In humans, Helge et al (1998) studied trained subjects who, after 7 weeks of adaptation to a high-fat diet (62% fat, 21% carbohydrate), changed to a high-carbohydrate diet (65% carbohydrate, 20% fat) for 1 week. A control group followed a high-carbohydrate diet for 8 weeks. Although exercise time to exhaustion increased from week 7 to week 8 in the group that received a high-fat diet followed by the high-carbohydrate diet, performance was less compared with the group that received the high-carbohydrate diet for 8 weeks. Because switching to a high-carbohydrate diet after 7 weeks of a high-fat diet did not reverse the negative effects, these authors concluded that the negative effects of 7 weeks of a high-fat diet on performance are not simply caused by a lack of carbohydrate as a fuel, but rather by suboptimal adap-tations to the training (i.e. improvements in endurance capacity were smaller compared with the high-carbohydrate diet).

Chronic effects of diet cannot be directly explained by substrate avail-ability. In the study by Burke et al (1999), for example, subjects consumed a high-fat diet or a high-carbohydrate diet for 5 days followed by 1 day on a high-carbohydrate diet. The one-day high-carbohydrate intake replenished glycogen stores in both conditions, and muscle glycogen concentrations were identical. Yet large differences existed in substrate utilization between the two diets. The respiratory exchange ratio (RER) changed from 0.90 to 0.82 after 5 days on a high-fat diet. After consuming a high-carbohydrate diet for one day, RER was still lower compared with baseline values (0.87). Because these changes were not caused by alterations in substrate availability, they are likely to be related to metabolic adaptations in the muscle.

Although the hypothesis that chronic high-fat diets may increase the capacity to oxidize fat and improve exercise performance during competition is attractive, little evidence indicates that it is true. The available studies that indicate a positive effect on performance were conducted at exercise intensities lower than the normal intensities during competition. Therefore, more well-controlled studies are needed to clarify the importance of the effect of dietary carbohydrate and fat content on athletic performance and, at this time, because little information is available about the negative effects of high-fat diets for athletes, caution should be exercised when recommending a high-fat diet to athletes.

SUPPLEMENTS THAT INCREASE FAT OXIDATION

There are many nutrition supplements on the market that claim to increase fat oxidation. These supplements include caffeine, carnitine, hydroxycitric acid (HCA), chromium, conjugated linoleic acid (CLA), ginseng, glucomannan, green tea, psyllium and pyruvate. There is limited to no evidence that these supplements actually increase fat oxidation during exercise. Caffeine is thought to stimulate lipolysis and the mobilization of fatty acids. Carnitine is believed to help transport fatty acids into the mitochondria. Pyruvate and dihydroxyacetone are often sold as supplements to increase fat oxidation. Similarly, the trace elements chromium and vanadium are claimed to promote fat oxidation and help weight loss.

GENDER DIFFERENCES

The majority of studies show that women rely more on fat oxidation and less on carbohydrate oxidation when exercising at the same relative exercise intensity as men. Most studies have compared respiratory exchange ratios of men and women at a certain relative intensity. For example, Tarnopolsky et al (1990) compared a group of men and women, matched for age, training status and performance. It was shown that women had significantly lower RER values during 90-minute running at 65% $\dot{V}O_2max$, indicating a greater relative contribution of fat to energy expenditure. It was also demonstrated that women had less muscle glycogen depletion than men during the exercise. Comparing fat oxidation in men and women at one exercise intensity has not always revealed the same results and several studies did not find gender differences in fat metabolism. This is likely due to the fact that a large inter-individual variation in fat oxidation exists and it is difficult to detect the gender differences from this large noise of the measurement. Another way of studying gender differences therefore is to measure fat oxidation over a wide range of intensities rather than a single exercise intensity. This approach was used in a recent study by Venables et al (2005). Fat oxidation (measured by gas exchange measurements) was measured in 300 volunteers (157 men and 143 women) and it was convincingly shown that women had higher rates of fat oxidation than men. Women had higher peak fat oxidation rates than men

(8.2 versus 7.1 mg/kg.minute) and this occurred at a slightly higher exercise intensity of 52 versus 45% $\dot{V}O_2$max, respectively (Fig. 4.2F). The exact mechanisms behind these gender differences in fat metabolism during exercise are not known but the effects observed have been attributed to the influence of the female sex hormone oestrogen on increasing the availability of lipids for substrate oxidation in the muscle. In addition it has also been suggested that the higher fat oxidation rates in women are related to differences in percent body fat, distribution of body fat, hormonal responses to exercise, hormone receptor type and sensitivity, an increased storage of intramuscular triacylglycerol in women and an increased expression of fatty acid transport proteins.

TYPE OF EXERCISE

Very few studies have compared the effect of different exercise modalities on fat oxidation. Recently Achten et al (2002) compared fat oxidation over a wide range of intensities during cycling versus running. Maximal fat oxidation rates were 28% higher during running compared with cycling (0.65 vs 0.47 g/minute) (Fig. 4.2D). However, the intensity which elicited maximal fat oxidation was not different between the cycle ergometer and treadmill test. Fat oxidation rates were significantly higher during the treadmill test compared to the cycle ergometer test between 55 and 80% $\dot{V}O_2$max.

Others have observed similar differences in substrate utilization between running and cycling. It is not clear why this difference in metabolism exists between these two exercise modes but it may be related to the muscle mass recruited during exercise. During cycling, the work rate will be shared by a smaller number of muscle fibres than during running. The metabolic stress per muscle fibre may be greater as a greater amount of energy per fibre is required and this would increase glycolytic flux and inhibit fat metabolism. There is little or no information available about fat oxidation rates during other exercise modalities.

LARGE VARIATION IN FAT OXIDATION BETWEEN INDIVIDUALS

Although factors like exercise intensity and duration, training status and nutrition can influence fat oxidation, they cannot predict fat oxidation rates in an individual. This is because there is a large inter-individual variation which is likely to be genetically determined. A recent large-scale study compared fat oxidation rates over a wide range of intensities in 300 men and women. A large variation was observed in maximal fat oxidation with oxidation rates ranging from 0.18 g/minute to 1.01 g/minute. One of the most important findings of this study was that gender and indices of an individual's level of fitness and activity such as $\dot{V}O_2$max and physical activity levels but not body fatness explained some of this inter-individual variation.

However, self-reported physical activity, $\dot{V}O_2$max and gender explained only 12% of the inter-individual variation in maximal fat oxidation during exercise. Another interesting finding is that each individual seems to have his or her own 'fat oxidation footprint'. The shape of the fat oxidation curves is characteristic for each individual. The fat oxidation curve may shift as a result of food intake or training but the shape of the curve seems to remain the same. Research is therefore needed into the causes of the inter-individual variation, especially because a low fat oxidation capacity might be a risk factor for the development of cardiovascular and metabolic diseases.

KEY POINTS

1. Fat oxidation during exercise is regulated by carbohydrate metabolism, which in turn is tightly regulated by exercise intensity and carbohydrate availability and is dependent on the metabolic machinery to oxidize fatty acids (mitochondria, oxidative enzymes, blood flow).
2. Fat oxidation during exercise is therefore influenced by exercise intensity and duration, diet, and training status.
3. Higher fat oxidation rates during exercise are generally reflective of good training status whereas low fat oxidation rates can reflect poor training status and might be a risk factor for obesity and insulin resistance.
4. Fat oxidation peaks at moderate intensities (around 63% $\dot{V}O_2$max in trained men and around 50% $\dot{V}O_2$max in the average population) and increases as exercise progresses but is suppressed by carbohydrate intake.
5. Fat oxidation is higher in women than in men.
6. The only effective way to increase fat oxidation is through exercise training; various supplements or dietary interventions do not have the desired effects.
7. There is a very large inter-individual variation in fat oxidation that is only partly explained by the factors mentioned above. There appears to be a large genetic component which needs further study since the rate of fat oxidation might be related to risk factors for cardiovascular and metabolic diseases.

References

Achten J, Jeukendrup AE 2003a The effect of pre-exercise carbohydrate feedings on the intensity that elicits maximal fat oxidation. Journal of Sports Science 21:1017–1024

Achten J, Jeukendrup AE 2003b Maximal fat oxidation during exercise in trained men. International Journal of Sports Medicine 24:603–608

Achten J, Gleeson M, Jeukendrup AE 2002 Determination of the exercise intensity that elicits maximal fat oxidation. Medicine and Science in Sports and Exercise 34:92–97

Achten J, Venables MC, Jeukendrup AE 2003 Fat oxidation rates are higher during running compared with cycling over a wide range of intensities. Metabolism 52:747–752

Burke LM, Angus DJ, Cox GR et al 1999 Fat adaptation with carbohydrate recovery promotes metabolic adaptation during prolonged cycling. Medicine and Science in Sports and Exercise 31:297

Christensen EH, Hansen O 1939 Arbeitsfähigkeit und Ernährung. Scandinavian Archives of Physiology 81:160–171

Costill DL, Coyle E, Dalsky G et al 1977 Effects of elevated plasma FFA and insulin on muscle glycogen usage during exercise. Journal of Applied Physiology 43:695–699

Coyle EF, Jeukendrup AE, Wagenmakers AJM, Saris WHM 1997 Fatty acid oxidation is directly regulated by carbohydrate metabolism during exercise. American Journal of Physiology 273:E268–E275

Greenhaff PL, Timmons JA 1998 Pyruvate dehydrogenase complex activation status and acetyl group availability as a site of interchange between anaerobic and oxidative metabolism during intense exercise. Advances in Experimental Biology and Medicine 441:287–298

Helge JW, Wulff B, Kiens B 1998 Impact of a fat-rich diet on endurance in man: role of the dietary period. Medicine and Science in Sports and Exercise 30:456–461

Horowitz JF, Mora-Rodriguez R, Byerley LO, Coyle EF 1997 Lipolytic suppression following carbohydrate ingestion limits fat oxidation during exercise. American Journal of Physiology 273:E768–E775

Jeukendrup AE 2002 Regulation of fat metabolism in skeletal muscle. Annals of the New York Academy of Science 967:217–235

Jeukendrup AE, Wallis GA 2005 Measurement of substrate oxidation during exercise by means of gas exchange measurements. International Journal of Sports Medicine 26 (suppl 1):S28–37

Jeukendrup AE, Saris WHM, Schrauwen P et al 1995 Metabolic availability of medium chain triglycerides co-ingested with carbohydrates during prolonged exercise. Journal of Applied Physiology 79:756–762

Jeukendrup AE, Thielen JJHC, Wagenmakers AJM et al 1998 Effect of MCT and carbohydrate ingestion on substrate utilization and cycling performance. American Journal of Clinical Nutrition 67:397–404

Pendergast DR, Horvath PJ, Leddy JJ, Venkatraman JT 1996 The role of dietary fat on performance, metabolism and health. American Journal of Sports Medicine 24:S53–S58

Phinney SD, Horton ES, Sims EAH et al 1980 Capacity for moderate exercise in obese subjects after adaptation to a hypocaloric, ketogenic diet. Journal of Clinical Investigation 66:1152–1161

Romijn JA, Coyle EF, Sidossis LS et al 1993 Regulation of endogenous fat and carbohydrate metabolism in relation to exercise intensity. American Journal of Physiology 265:E380–E391

Spriet LL 2002 Regulation of skeletal muscle fat oxidation during exercise in humans. Medicine and Science in Sports and Exercise 34:1477–1484

Tarnopolsky LJ, MacDougall JD, Atkinson SA 1990 Gender differences in substrate for endurance exercise. Journal of Applied Physiology 68(1):302–308

Venables MC, Achten J, Jeukendrup AE 2005 Determinants of fat oxidation during exercise in healthy men and women: a cross-sectional study. Journal of Applied Physiology 98:160–167

Chapter 5

Protein and amino acid requirements for athletes

Joanna L Bowtell

LEARNING OBJECTIVES

After studying this chapter, you should be able to:

1. Describe the concept of protein turnover and the process of protein synthesis, protein breakdown and amino acid oxidation.
2. Describe the methodologies used to measure protein turnover and to determine protein requirements.
3. Discuss the changes in protein turnover induced by endurance and resistance exercise.

4. Discuss the protein requirements for endurance and resistance trained athletes.
5. Critically evaluate the anabolic effects of consuming protein, amino acid, and carbohydrate supplements after exercise.

INTRODUCTION

Proteins are vital molecules, which have a number of important functions such as structural (collagen), contractile (myosin and actin), immune (antibodies) and regulatory (enzymes and hormones). This broad and diverse range of roles is possible due to the enormous variability in protein structure. Proteins are polymers of constituent amino acids. There are 20 different amino acids in total, with each amino acid comprised of an amino group (NH_2), carboxyl group (COOH) and a carbon chain. This carbon chain is different for each amino acid with, for instance, only a 2C chain for alanine whereas a larger amino acid such as leucine has a 5C chain. Nine of the 20 amino acids are classed as essential, i.e. must be obtained from the diet, as these amino acids cannot be synthesized by the tissues of the body in sufficient quantity to meet requirements. These are: histidine, isoleucine, leucine, valine, methionine, phenylalanine, threonine and tryptophan.

The structures of proteins vary at a number of levels: such as the size of the molecule, i.e. how many amino acids bonded together; the sequence in which the 20 different amino acids are joined together; as well as the three-dimensional structure.

Body proteins are in a constant state of turnover, with proteins continuously being broken down to release their constituent amino acids, and new proteins constantly synthesized from free amino acids (Fig. 5.1). Muscle

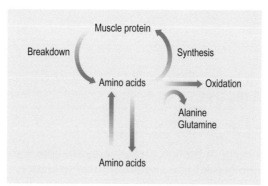

Figure 5.1 Schematic for the dynamic process of muscle protein turnover. Body proteins are constantly broken down, releasing their constituent amino acids into the free amino acid pool. Amino acids derived from the digestion and absorption of dietary protein and amino acids also feed into this pool. Free amino acids are either oxidized or used to synthesize new proteins.

contains approximately 50% of total body protein, with actin and myosin being the most plentiful muscle proteins (~65% total muscle protein), and muscle protein accounts for approximately 25% whole body protein synthesis at rest.

This constant degradation and synthesis of new proteins presumably allows removal of damaged proteins and synthesis of new proteins in response to cellular demands, thus allowing more rapid adaptation of the organism to environmental conditions.

PROTEIN SYNTHESIS

Proteins are synthesized in a two stage process: first transcription of the DNA into RNA and then translation of the RNA into the protein. DNA provides the comprehensive recipe book for all body proteins. A signal, nutritional, hormonal or mechanical, induces gene expression (transcription). The resultant RNA is processed within the cell nucleus and exported as messenger RNA (mRNA) into the cytosol. The mRNA is then translated into protein through the action of the ribosomes, in a triphasic process: initiation, elongation and termination. The mRNA encodes the sequence and number of amino acids required to form the protein, and amino acids are delivered to the ribosome through the action of an amino acid specific transfer RNA (tRNA), catalysed by tRNA synthases. The newly formed proteins can then be modified through processes such as glycosylation and phosphorylation (post-translational modification), which have important effects on the proteins' functions.

It is well accepted that repeated exercise, particularly resistance exercise, increases skeletal muscle mass through a greater elevation in protein synthesis than in protein breakdown. However, the mechanisms for these modifications are as yet relatively poorly understood. There are a number of candidates including increased calcium, increased levels of growth factors and mechanotransduction (conversion of mechanical energy into biological events). In the latter case, modification of the lipid bilayer (sarcolemma), and the cytoskeleton of the cell have all been suggested to be implicated in altering protein turnover as a result of force/tension development in the muscle (Hornberger & Esser 2004).

AMINO ACID OXIDATION

Oxidation of amino acids is not generally an important source of energy, usually supplying only 1–10% of energy requirements, although this contribution increases during starvation and prolonged glycogen-depleting exercise (Lemon & Mullin 1980, Vazquez et al 1988). Human skeletal muscle has the enzyme capacity to oxidize at least eight of the 20 amino acids (alanine, asparagine, aspartate, glutamate, isoleucine, leucine, lysine and valine), but during exercise branched chain amino acids (BCAA: isoleucine, leucine and valine) are predominantly oxidized. Oxidation of amino acids results in the loss of amino acids from the free amino acid pool, which in the case of essential amino acids such as the BCAA can only be replaced by consumption of dietary protein/amino acids.

Amino acids are first deaminated or transaminated to remove the amino group prior to decarboxylation or complete oxidation. BCAA are usually transaminated with 2-oxoglutarate (intermediate of the tricarboxylic acid cycle, TCA cycle) to form glutamate and the reciprocal oxo-acid. The oxo-acids are then oxidized via the action of branched-chain oxo-acid dehydrogenase (BCOADH). The mitochondral enzyme complex BCOADH catalyses the rate-limiting step in BCAA oxidation and it exists in active (dephosphorylated) and inactive (phosphorylated) forms. At rest, approximately 5–8% is in the active form and this increases to 20–25% during exercise (Bowtell et al 1998) due to decreases in the ATP:ADP ratio and in muscle pH (Kasperek 1989). Glycogen depletion also increases BCOADH activation hence BCAA oxidation is elevated during exercise especially in the glycogen-depleted state (Wagenmakers et al 1991); conversely glucose consumption during exercise suppresses BCAA oxidation (Bowtell et al 2000).

There is a close link between BCAA oxidation and gluconeogenesis and TCA cycle anaplerosis (increasing the concentration of TCA cycle intermediates). The glutamate derived from transamination of the BCAA is used to form either alanine via transamination with pyruvate (alanine aminotransferase) or glutamine via amination of glutamate (glutamine synthetase). The balance between synthesis of alanine or glutamine is dependent on the availability of pyruvate (high availability favouring alanine formation) and ammonia concentration (high availability favouring glutamine formation) (Akermark et al 1996). The formation of alanine recycles the 2-oxoglutarate used in the transamination of BCAA, which can then feed back into the TCA cycle (anaplerosis). Glutamine formation, however, results in a net drain of 2-oxoglutarate from the TCA cycle. It has been suggested that such drainage of TCA cycle intermediates in the glycogen-depleted state may contribute to the development of fatigue (Sahlin et al 1998). However, more recent evidence suggests that this is probably not the case (Gibala et al 2002).

Both alanine and glutamine are released from the muscle in significant quantities during endurance exercise (Akermark et al 1996), and are then taken up by the liver and kidneys and used for gluconeogenesis respectively (formation of new glucose) (Stumvoll et al 1998). Hence there is a strong logic that BCAA oxidation is elevated in conditions of low glycogen availability, since this increases the production and release of alanine and glutamine. In the liver alanine, in particular, is used to form new glucose, which is then released into the bloodstream to help to maintain blood glucose concentration. The amino group is removed from alanine and glutamine in this process and incorporated into urea (ureagenesis), which can then be harmlessly excreted from the body in the urine. This prevents the potentially harmful build-up of toxic ammonia, which could occur as a consequence of amino acid oxidation. The alanine-glucose and glutamine-glucose cycles thus fulfil two important functions: removal of amino groups derived from BCAA oxidation in the muscle, and provision of substrate to the liver and kidney for gluconeogenesis.

PROTEIN BREAKDOWN

There are three main pathways of protein degradation in skeletal muscle: lysosomal (cathepsin), and non-lysosomal (ubiquitin and calpain). The lysosomal pathway is involved in breakdown of proteins such as hormones and immune modulators (Dohm et al 1987). The ATP-dependent ubiquitin pathway is activated during starvation, muscle atrophy (wasting) and exercise (Finlay & Varshavsky 1985). The calcium activated neutral protease pathway (calpain) is involved in exercise-induced protein degradation (Belcastro 1993). The amino acids released from this breakdown of protein feed into the free amino acid pool, which can then be either oxidized or used to synthesize new proteins.

FREE AMINO ACID POOL

Protein synthesis and amino acid oxidation both drain amino acids from the free amino acid pool, whereas the breakdown of body protein and the digestion and absorption of dietary protein contribute amino acids to the free amino acid pool. Therefore the free amino acid pool size decreases when the rate of amino acid usage for protein synthesis and oxidation outstrips the rate of entry of amino acids into the pool via body protein breakdown and digestion and absorption of dietary protein/amino acids. It has been proposed that the maintenance of the free amino acid pool provides a strong link between protein synthesis and breakdown (Wolfe 2000); certainly amino acid availability is a potent driver for protein synthesis. After consumption of a protein meal when amino acid availability is high, protein synthesis rate is increased and protein breakdown rate reduced (McNurlan & Garlick 1989). Whereas in the fasted state when amino acid availability is low, protein breakdown rate is elevated and protein synthesis reduced (McNurlan & Garlick 1989). This creates a diurnal (cyclical 24-hour) protein turnover pattern associated with meal consumption, whereby in the fasted state there are net protein losses as protein breakdown rate exceeds that of protein synthesis (Fig. 5.2). However, in the fed state, protein synthesis rate is greater than protein breakdown, and hence there is a net protein gain. When dietary protein consumption is adequate, the fed state gains match or even exceed the fasted state losses and hence body protein mass is conserved or even increased (Pacy et al 1994). If protein intake is inadequate then the fasted state losses will exceed the fed state gains and hence a net body protein loss will occur (Price et al 1994). Since muscle is the most plentiful and labile body protein pool, it is likely that any such losses will be incurred by muscle protein.

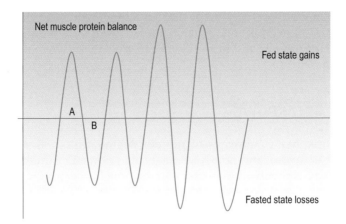

Figure 5.2   There is a diurnal cycle to protein turnover related to consumption of meals. In the fed state, muscle protein balance is positive (synthesis > breakdown), whereas in the fasted state muscle protein balance is negative (synthesis < breakdown). These gains and losses are in balance when dietary protein is adequate (area A = area B); increasing dietary protein increases the amplitude of the cycle (adapted from Price et al 1994).

FACTORS INFLUENCING PROTEIN TURNOVER

The impact of fuel availability on protein turnover has already been described to some degree, with increased protein breakdown and amino acid oxidation during exercise in conditions of low carbohydrate availability (glycogen depletion, no carbohydrate supplementation). In addition, suboptimal energy intake such as occurs during fasting and starvation is also associated with increased protein breakdown and amino acid oxidation (Todd et al 1984), presumably driven by the need to provide gluconeogenic precursors (alanine and glutamine) for the liver, to maintaining blood glucose concentration in the absence/deficit of dietary carbohydrate.

A number of hormones have key roles in the regulation of protein turnover. Insulin is the primary anabolic hormone (increases body protein), which suppresses protein breakdown and in the presence of abundant amino acids stimulates protein synthesis (Millward 1990). Thus the body protein gains that occur in the fed state, described earlier, relate in part to the increased availability of amino acids as well as the elevated concentration of insulin. Growth hormone (GH) and the growth factors (insulin-like growth factor-1, IGF-1; mechano growth factor, MGF) are also suggested to exert an anabolic effect (Goldspink & Harridge 2004). Recently, Healy et al (2003) demonstrated that 4-week GH supplementation exerted an anabolic effect on whole body protein turnover at rest, during and after exercise. Catecholamines (adrenaline/noradrenaline), glucagon and glucocorticoids are all catabolic hormones which enhance protein breakdown and suppress protein synthesis. It is evident if we examine the hormonal milieu during endurance exercise – reduced insulin and elevated catecholamines, glucagons and glucocorticoids – that a negative protein balance is likely to arise during endurance exercise. Indeed, endurance and resistance exercise are powerful modulators of protein turnover, both during and in recovery. These changes will be examined in more detail below.

One of the main questions that we will explore in this review is whether athletes have a greater requirement for dietary protein in order to optimize adaptations to their training regimen and hence performance. However, our capacity to answer this question is limited by the techniques currently available to measure protein metabolism and to determine protein requirements. We will first, therefore, examine these techniques and some of their limitations.

MEASUREMENT TECHNIQUES

There are three main categories of technique available: nitrogen balance, marker compounds, and stable isotope techniques. The first, nitrogen balance, provides gross information regarding nitrogen and hence protein balance over a 24-hour period. This technique is widely adopted as the means of estimating daily protein requirement. Secondly, a number of different compounds can be measured in blood and urine as proxy markers for protein breakdown. These techniques can indicate change in the rate of processes but a number of conceptual difficulties have been highlighted. Stable isotope techniques allow measurement of protein synthesis, protein breakdown and amino acid oxidation rates (collectively known as protein kinetics) in the whole body and specifically in skeletal muscle.

NITROGEN BALANCE

Proteins are the major nitrogen-containing molecules within our bodies, therefore with this classic technique, the amount of nitrogen consumed (1 g protein = 0.16 g nitrogen) is balanced against the amount of nitrogen excreted (urine, faeces, sweat and miscellaneous). When nitrogen balance is positive (nitrogen intake exceeds nitrogen excretion), whole body protein is increasing (anabolic state) and when negative, protein losses are occurring (catabolic state). In order to determine a safe protein intake, nitrogen balance is measured for a range of different protein intakes. A regression analysis is then performed on the data to ascertain at which protein intake a zero balance is achieved. The recommended daily intake for protein is then calculated as this zero balance protein intake plus a safety margin of 2 standard deviations, to account for any inter-individual variation.

There are a number of problems with this technique. First, it does not take into account the quality of the protein consumed, i.e. essential amino acid content. In addition, the technique is not reliable at the extremes of protein intake (low or high), which may potentially skew the regression analysis. For instance, the positive nitrogen balances that occur at high protein intakes have been suggested to be a technical artefact since the lean body mass gains that would be expected with a positive protein balance do not seem to occur (Millward et al 1994). In addition, at low protein intakes, the body enters an adapted or accommodated state in which amino acid recycling is more efficient and protein turnover rates are reduced (Millward et al 1994). Nitrogen balance may still be achieved; however, the ability to adapt to a change in environmental conditions or to maximize exercise training adaptations may be compromised.

MARKER COMPOUNDS

Urea
Urea is the body's waste product for nitrogen disposal, and is therefore generally believed to be representative of protein breakdown and amino acid oxidation. Certainly when consuming a high protein diet, protein turnover amino acid oxidation and plasma urea concentration and urinary urea excretion are all elevated in parallel. However, nitrogen derived from protein breakdown and amino acid oxidation is also incorporated into newly synthesized amino acids, e.g. alanine and glutamine, as well as into acute phase proteins such as plasma proteins. Therefore in some circumstances such as in response to exercise, urea production does not provide a good proxy marker for protein breakdown.

3–Methylhistidine
3-Methylhistidine (3-MH) is a breakdown product of myofibrillar (contractile) protein, and can be measured in both blood and urine to provide an index of myofibrillar protein breakdown. However, to employ this technique subjects must be on a meat free diet (otherwise 3-MH will be derived from digestion of dietary meat). In addition 3-MH is derived from the breakdown of smooth muscle present within the gut and vascular system and this may confound the quantitative accuracy of this technique (Rennie & Millward 1983).

Stable isotope techniques
Amino acids containing stable isotopes (13C, 15N or 2H) are infused intravenously in very small quantities and enable us to measure protein kinetics. Using mass spectrometry the level of isotope enrichment is measured within plasma (whole body measurements), skeletal muscle tissue (fractional muscle protein synthesis and breakdown); and for the arteriovenous model (a-v balance), samples from femoral artery and femoral vein as well as intramuscular fluid are analysed (muscle protein synthesis, breakdown and transmembrane amino acid transport). With recent advances it is now also possible to make synthesis and breakdown measurements within the different muscle

fractions, i.e. mitochondrial and myofibrillar proteins as well as mixed muscle protein. Although some further technological advances are necessary, it should shortly be possible to make measurements of the synthesis and breakdown rates of individual proteins (proteomics) such as actin or myosin.

EXERCISE–INDUCED CHANGES IN PROTEIN METABOLISM

Most of the evidence regarding changes in protein metabolism during exercise comes from stable isotope studies examining changes in whole body metabolism or changes in urea excretion. There are difficulties in applying stable isotope techniques over short time periods, such as during exercise. This is because isotopic enrichment of the plasma must reach steady state, and for measurements of protein synthesis, sufficient tracer amino acid must be incorporated into muscle protein to be accurately detected, all of which takes time, usually 1–2 hours. Therefore only a relatively small number of studies have examined changes in protein metabolism during exercise. It is evident from merely observing the phenotype of endurance and strength based athletes that training adaptations are vastly different for these different types of activity. Muscle hypertrophy predominates for strength athletes, with increases in mitochondrial volume and muscle capillarization being vital adaptations for endurance athletes. All such adaptations are, however, the result of synthesis/breakdown of proteins in response to the training stimulus. It should therefore be no surprise that profound changes in protein metabolism are induced by endurance and resistance exercise.

DURING ENDURANCE EXERCISE

There is good agreement between endurance exercise studies that amino acid oxidation rates are elevated, particularly leucine oxidation (Bowtell et al 1998, Hagg et al 1982, Lamont et al 2001, McKenzie et al 2000), which is most commonly used as the amino acid tracer. Lysine oxidation and urea excretion have also been shown to increase (Lamont et al 2001, Wolfe et al 1984), so that cumulatively, the evidence indicates that amino acid oxidation rates are increased during endurance exercise. However, energy requirements may increase by tenfold or more, compared to the only ~twofold increase in leucine oxidation. The rates of carbohydrate and fat oxidation increase to a greater degree than amino acid oxidation, so that the contribution to energy requirements from leucine oxidation is reduced during exercise (Lamont et al 2001). However, for the endurance athlete training intensively for several hours or more per day, the implications for dietary requirements of the oxidized amino acids may be significant, although McKenzie et al (2000) demonstrated that both leucine oxidation and BCOAD activation were lower during 90-minute exercise at 65% $\dot{V}O_2$max after 28 days' endurance training. This suggests that training may reduce the contribution of BCAA to energy requirements during exercise relative to the untrained individual. However, when exercising under conditions of low glycogen availability, low energy status and high metabolic stress ($>65\%$ $\dot{V}O_2max$), daily oxidation of amino acids for the athlete will likely exceed that of the sedentary individual.

Reduction in both whole body (Carraro et al 1990a, Knapik et al 1991, Rennie et al 1981, Wolfe et al 1982) and skeletal muscle (Carraro et al 1990b) protein synthesis have been reported during endurance exercise, although some studies suggest that whole body protein synthesis is unchanged (Carraro et al 1990a, Phillips et al 1993). Any decrease appears to be dependent upon intensity, duration and mode of exercise (Bylund-Fellenius et al 1984), and is probably related to magnitude of muscle force/tension, energy status of the muscle (ATP:ADP ratio), as well as total work done.

There is some controversy regarding the effect of endurance exercise upon whole body protein breakdown, with some studies indicating increased protein breakdown (Phillips et al 1993, Rennie et al 1981, Wolfe et al 1982) and others indicating no change (Carraro et al 1990a, Knapik et al 1991, Stein et al 1989). This may in part be related to feeding status since whole body protein breakdown tends to be unchanged in those studies performed in the fasted state but increased when subjects were in the fed state. In either case, unchanged or elevated protein breakdown during endurance exercise with reduced protein synthesis and increased amino acid oxidation a net loss of body protein occurs. This is confirmed by nitrogen balance studies, where a negative nitrogen balance is induced despite maintenance of constant protein intake and energy balance when unaccustomed exercise is performed (Gontzea et al 1975).

DURING RESISTANCE EXERCISE

There is far less evidence available in the literature regarding changes in protein metabolism during resistance exercise. This is presumably due to the brief nature of exercise, which creates methodological difficulties when applying stable isotope techniques. Tarnopolsky et al (1991) found that 1 hour of intense resistance exercise did not alter leucine oxidation rates or whole body protein breakdown or synthesis. More recently, Durham et al (2005) utilized the a-v balance stable isotope technique to examine changes in protein metabolism specifically in the exercising muscle during ~45 minutes of intense lower limb exercise. These authors demonstrated that there was no change in muscle protein turnover during resistance exercise.

RECOVERY FROM ENDURANCE EXERCISE

Amino acid oxidation rates return to pre-exercise levels rapidly after exercise, except in the case of eccentric exercise where leucine oxidation rates were reported to be elevated for up to 10 days (Fielding et al 1991). Whole body protein breakdown appears to be either decreased (Rennie et al 1981) or unchanged (Devlin et al 1990, Tipton et al 1996) during recovery from endurance exercise. 3-MH excretion data suggest that muscle protein breakdown is increased during recovery (see earlier discussion for methodological concerns) (Carraro et al 1990b).

Whole body protein synthesis appears to be increased after endurance exercise (Devlin et al 1990, Rennie et al 1981). Human muscle protein synthesis has been reported to be increased (Carraro et al 1990b) or unchanged (Tipton et al 1996) after endurance exercise. Training status provides one possible explanation for the discrepancy, since in the latter study the protein synthesis rate was measured in the deltoid muscle of trained swimmers before and after a 1.5-hour intensive swimming session, whereas in the former study vastus lateralis protein synthesis rate was measured before and after 4 hours walking at 40% $\dot{V}O_2$max in untrained subjects. Although deltoid muscle protein synthesis did increase by 41% in the trained swimmers after intense aerobic swimming, this did not attain statistical significance. Possibly a lesser overload was imposed upon the muscle of the trained subjects so that the increase in muscle protein synthesis post-exercise was not statistically significant. However, Short et al (2004) recently found that 4 months' cycle training (45 minutes at 80%HRpeak $\times$ 3/4 per week) increased mixed muscle protein synthesis by 22% in both young and elderly subjects. Also, a statistically significant 45% increase in muscle protein synthesis rate was observed 10 minutes after 45 minutes' walking at 40% $\dot{V}O_2$peak in both young and elderly subjects (Sheffield-Moore et al 2004). Studies in rats suggest that the muscle protein synthesis response in the early recovery phase is dependent upon exercise intensity and duration (Anthony et al 1999). More intense and prolonged exercise bouts exert a suppressive effect on muscle protein synthesis. However, synthetic rates recover within several hours post-exercise, although this rate of recovery also seems to be dependent upon intensity and duration of exercise.

RECOVERY FROM RESISTANCE EXERCISE

Many studies have demonstrated that mixed muscle protein synthesis is stimulated within 90 minutes of completing a bout of resistance exercise, and remains elevated for up to 48 hours in untrained subjects (Phillips et al 1997) (<36 hours trained subjects (MacDougall et al 1995)). The magnitude of the exercise-induced response also appears to be somewhat lessened by resistance training (~20%, (Phillips et al 2002)), although resting protein synthesis (~46%) and breakdown (~81%) rates were elevated by a period of resistance training (Phillips et al 2002). As suggested previously there appears to be a coupling between protein synthesis and breakdown rates (Wolfe 2000). It should therefore be no surprise that muscle protein breakdown rates are also elevated during recovery from resistance exercise (Phillips et al 1997). The increase in protein synthesis is, however, greater than the increase in protein breakdown, thus exerting a net anabolic effect (Biolo et al 1995, Phillips et al 1997).

Urinary 3-MH excretion rate has been shown to be increased or unchanged after resistance exercise (see earlier discussion for methodological concerns).

More recently a technique called microdialysis has been employed to directly measure the release of 3-MH from the muscle after resistance exercise (Trappe et al 2004). Microdialysis involves the placement of a small permeable sac (containing fluid isotonic with body fluids) directly over the muscle, under local anaesthetic. There was no increase in the release of 3-MH from the muscle into the interstitium after resistance exercise, which suggests that the elevation of muscle protein breakdown must largely be due to degradation of non-myofibrillar proteins.

Moore et al (2005) compared the effect of maximal shortening (concentric) or lengthening (eccentric) contractions on myofibrillar synthesis. Myofibrillar protein synthesis 4.5 hours after completion of lengthening contractions was significantly higher than after shortening contractions. However, after 8.5 hours' recovery myofibrillar protein synthesis was significantly higher after the shortening than lengthening contraction protocol. No data are available for muscle protein breakdown and it would also be interesting to observe a full 48 hours' recovery period to determine whether eccentric exercise might provoke a greater anabolic effect than concentric exercise.

In summary, endurance exercise exerts a catabolic effect during activity, but after a variable period of recovery post-exercise muscle protein synthesis is elevated so that an anabolic effect occurs, whereas for resistance exercise, no change in protein turnover occurs during exercise, but post-exercise a strong anabolic effect is exerted upon the exercised muscle. However, one must bear in mind that when exercise is completed in a fasted or post-absorptive state, protein balance will still be negative (Fig. 5.3). In order to convert the anabolic influence into positive protein balance or muscle protein gains, amino acids must be made available through protein/amino acid supplementation or consumption of a meal.

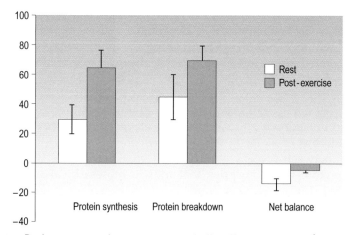

Figure 5.3 Resistance exercise exerts an anabolic effect on muscle (increasing protein synthesis); however, protein balance remains negative without consumption of protein or amino acids (adapted from Biolo et al 1995).

PROTEIN REQUIREMENTS FOR HABITUAL EXERCISERS

High-protein diets and protein and amino acid supplements are widely consumed by athletes in the belief that such practices will stimulate growth or maintenance of muscle mass and strength. If we consider the exercise-induced alterations of protein metabolism, it is possible to construct a rationale for some additional protein requirement in athletes. Endurance athletes may require additional protein to replace the amino acids oxidized during exercise, and to support the moderate elevation in muscle protein synthesis during recovery. Strength athletes may require additional protein to support muscle protein gains during recovery. However, there is still no consensus within the peer-reviewed scientific literature as to whether habitual exercise increases protein requirements. In the following sections, data from nitrogen balance and stable isotope studies will be evaluated to determine whether additional protein is necessary to achieve nitrogen/protein balance or may be beneficial for exercise performance.

PROTEIN REQUIREMENTS FOR ENDURANCE EXERCISE

Gontzea et al (1975) completed a 5-week nitrogen balance study in subjects consuming 1 g protein/kg body weight/day and 10% excess energy intake. For the first 2 weeks subjects were sedentary, and achieved a positive nitrogen balance as would be expected since protein intake was in excess of the recommended daily intake (RDI) for sedentary individuals (0.8 g/kg/day). Subjects then participated in exercise (6 × 20 minutes/day intense cycling) for 3 weeks, overload principles were not applied, i.e. duration/intensity of exercise remained constant for the 3-week period. For the first 2 weeks of the exercise programme subjects were in negative nitrogen balance, but by the third week nitrogen balance was again achieved (Fig. 5.4).

There are several possible interpretations of these data: protein requirement is certainly increased at least at the early stage of an endurance exercise programme, or by implication when training intensity/duration is increased. However, when the duration/intensity of exercise training remains constant it appears that the body's requirement for protein is not elevated. Alternatively, it may be that the body enters an accommodated/adapted state in order to conserve body protein in the face of a dietary deficit, and achieve protein balance. If this was the case then one might expect that the ability of the individual to adapt to the exercise training stimulus would be impaired. In order to answer this question, a longitudinal training study is required with several groups of sedentary subjects, completing a progressive endurance training programme whilst consuming different dietary protein intakes. Adequacy of protein intake would be assessed by improvement in exercise performance outcome measures, as well nitrogen balance/protein kinetics. No such study has yet been conducted, since the required duration and cost are prohibitive.

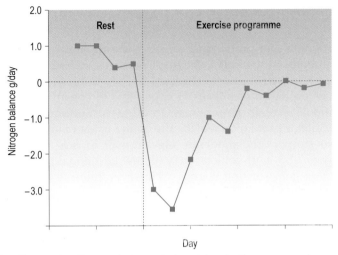

Figure 5.4 Change in nitrogen balance induced by starting an exercise programme, while maintained diet providing 1 g/kg/day protein and 10% excess energy intake (adapted from Gontzea et al 1975).

A number of nitrogen balance studies have been conducted to assess the protein requirement for endurance athletes. Meredith et al (1989) performed a nitrogen balance study in which six male endurance athletes (young and middle-aged) completed three trials during which subjects consumed 0.6 g/kg/day (below RDI for sedentary individuals), 0.9 g/kg/day or 1.2 g/kg/day for 10 days before nitrogen balance was measured. Regression analysis identified that on average zero balance was achieved at 0.94 g/kg/day (Fig. 5.5). When a 2 standard deviation safety margin was added in, the RDI for endurance athletes was 1.26 g/kg/day. Two further nitrogen balance studies confirmed that endurance trained male and female athletes were in negative nitrogen balance at protein intakes of both 0.86 g/kg/day (Phillips et al 1993) and 1 g/kg/day (Lamont et al 1990). Several nitrogen balance studies have been conducted on elite endurance trained athletes (Friedman & Lemon 1989, Tarnopolsky et al 1988), with identified RDI values ranging from 1.5 to 1.8 g/kg/day. Phillips et al (2004) conducted a regression analysis on the data from four such studies with moderate–elite endurance athletes and calculated RDI to be 1.11 g/kg/day. During such nitrogen balance studies it is vital that energy balance is maintained to avoid any confounding influence, and in addition sufficient time (minimum 10 days) must be allowed for subjects to adapt to the new level of dietary protein. Fed state gains are rapidly altered by change in dietary protein since they are dependent upon the level of amino acids provided. However, the losses incurred during fasting periods are slower to increase (increased protein intake) or decrease (decreased protein intake).

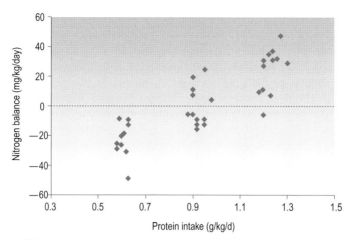

Figure 5.5 Nitrogen balance values for endurance trained athletes consuming three different levels of protein. Zero balance, calculated for each individual using linear regression, was 0.94 g/kg/day (adapted from Meredith et al 1989).

In summary, therefore, it seems that endurance athletes have a slightly greater protein requirement to achieve protein or nitrogen balance than sedentary individuals. In addition the magnitude of this elevation seems to be proportional to the training status of the athlete, and hence the stress to which the body is exposed as a consequence of the training load.

RESISTANCE TRAINED ATHLETES

As for endurance athletes a number of nitrogen balance studies have been completed to examine protein requirements for strength athletes. Tarnopolsky et al (1992) recruited two groups of male subjects: sedentary and strength trained (American football and rugby players) (each n = 7), with each subject completing three trials consuming 0.86, 1.4 or 2.4 g protein/kg/day. Protein requirement, identified via linear regression, was 0.89 g/kg/day for sedentary individuals and 1.76 g/kg/day for strength trained subjects. Stable isotope techniques were employed in tandem in this study and revealed that, at the low protein intake, strength trained athletes were in an accommodated state, i.e. whole body protein synthesis was reduced relative to the higher protein intakes. However, in an earlier study using a similar design, highly trained body builders (1.05 g/kg/day) were found to require only ~12% more protein than their sedentary counterparts (0.84 g/kg/day) (Tarnopolsky et al 1988), whereas Lemon et al (1992) found that the RDI for protein for novice body builders was 1.7 g/kg/day. In the face of this rather confusing picture, Phillips (2004) pooled and analysed the data from these three studies and calculated the RDI for strength trained athletes to be 1.33 g/kg/day or 66% higher than the RDI for sedentary individuals.

The discrepancy in RDIs between the studies may in part be accounted for by the diversity in training workloads of the different subject groups, quality of dietary protein, as well as variation in the period allowed for adaptation to the new protein intake levels. An additional problem alluded to earlier is the nitrogen balance technique itself. When consuming high protein intakes (~2.8 g/kg/day), highly positive nitrogen balances were achieved (~12–20 g nitrogen per day) equivalent to a body protein gain of ~75–125 g/day (Tarnopolsky et al 1988). This would equate to a gain in lean body mass of 0.3–0.5 kg per day when assuming a tissue water content of 75%. However, examination of lean body mass data clearly shows that such gains did not occur. Indeed, at the maximum steroid-induced rate of lean body mass accretion, the body protein gain can only account for 3% of the normal RDI (Millward et al 1994). It is therefore difficult to understand why protein requirement would be increased by 66–100%. Although, one study has demonstrated more rapid lean body mass gains in experienced weightlifters during a 6-week resistance training programme, when consuming 2.1 vs 1.2 g protein/kg/day (Burke et al 2001). Some studies have in fact indicated quite the opposite, that a strength training programme actually reduces protein requirement via improved protein metabolism efficiency (Butterfield & Calloway 1984, Campbell et al 1995).

Energy intake is a key determinant of protein requirement, with energy deficit increasing dietary protein need. This is an important issue to be considered by athletes required to make particular body weight categories, who often undergo a period of energy deficit to achieve the desired weight range. To conserve lean body mass during this period, athletes should increase their relative protein intake, and perform resistance training to preserve the exercised skeletal muscle.

In summary, nitrogen balance studies indicate that both endurance and strength athlete protein requirements are greater than those for the sedentary individual. However, this does not necessarily mean that we should recommend athletes to increase their protein intake. The training loads endured by both strength and endurance athletes require high energy intakes to achieve energy balance. In this situation, as long as 12–15% energy requirements are derived from protein, sufficient protein will be consumed to meet these targets without conscious consumption of a 'high protein diet'. Indeed, an analysis of data from studies with resistance trained athletes reveals that mean daily protein intake is 2.05 g/kg/day (Phillips 2004) (endurance athletes: 1.8 g/kg/day male; 1.2 g/kg/day female; both 14% energy intake (Tarnopolsky 2004)). These reported values are higher than any of the recommendations derived from the nitrogen balance studies.

Thus far we have considered only the amount of protein that athletes should consume; however, there is far more complexity to this topic! We must also consider the quality of protein consumed, the timing of ingestion, as well as the effect of combining protein and amino acids with other nutrients. There is good evidence from protein kinetics studies that such strategies exert a beneficial effect on the muscle protein synthesis response post-exercise.

PROTEIN QUALITY

The quality of protein is determined by the essential amino acid content. Complete protein foods such as eggs, meat and fish contain all of the essential amino acids in the correct balance to support protein synthesis. Grains, vegetables and fruits are incomplete protein foods, and must be consumed in an appropriate balance to obtain all of the essential amino acids in sufficient quantity. In addition, the speed of digestion and absorption should be considered for proteins just as for carbohydrates (glycaemic index), as well as the effect of consuming proteins with other macronutrients, which may also affect the digestibility and rate of absorption of amino acids. Amino acids from whey protein are absorbed into the bloodstream far more quickly than casein, so that casein provides a lower but more prolonged increase in blood amino acid concentration (Boirie et al 1997). At rest, casein protein ingestion resulted in more positive whole body protein balance than whey protein (Boirie et al 1997). However, studies comparing the effects of consumption of different proteins during recovery from exercise have not yet been conducted, and these are necessary to allow sports nutritionists to provide evidence-based recommendations to athletes. Indeed, the apparent importance of early consumption of amino acids after exercise (see below) may suggest that rapidly absorbed proteins such as whey may be more effective during recovery.

INGESTION OF AMINO ACIDS AFTER EXERCISE

In the earlier sections we examined the effect of exercise upon protein turnover, and concluded that due to a large elevation in muscle protein synthesis and a smaller increase in muscle protein breakdown, an anabolic effect is observed during recovery from exercise. However, when exercise is performed in the postabsorptive/fasted state, despite this anabolic influence, net muscle protein balance remains negative (Phillips et al 1997). The vital missing ingredients to push net muscle protein balance into the positive are amino acids.

Biolo et al (1997) observed that infusion of amino acids and prior resistance exercise exert additive effects on muscle protein synthesis. Subjects received 0.15 g mixed amino acids/kg/hour for 3 hours either at rest or after leg resistance exercise. The percentage change in protein breakdown rates from basal was not different between trials, which suggests that amino acids suppress the usual exercise-induced elevation in muscle protein breakdown. In addition, amino acid infusion increased muscle protein synthesis by ~150% at rest and by more than 250% after resistance exercise (Fig. 5.6). These

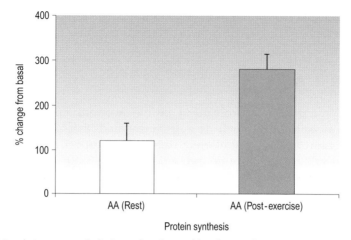

Figure 5.6   Intravenous infusion of amino acids after resistance exercise induces a positive protein balance (adapted from Biolo et al 1997).

findings led to an interest in determining whether consuming amino acids in the early post-exercise recovery period may enhance net muscle protein balance during recovery. Certainly, carbohydrate ingestion immediately post-exercise is known to stimulate glycogen synthesis and storage to a greater degree than when feeding was delayed by 2 hours (Ivy et al 1988).

Obviously to be a practical tool for athletes, amino acids must be ingested rather than infused but there were several concerns that this more practical amino acid delivery mode would not prove as effective. First, when ingested, amino acids must pass through the splanchnic bed before reaching the muscle, and splanchnic bed uptake of amino acids can account for between 20 and 90% of ingested amino acids (Matthews et al 1993). This means that a lower proportion of the amino acids consumed would reach the muscle. Secondly, there will be a longer delay before amino acids reach the muscle, while proteins are digested and absorbed or amino acids are absorbed.

However, Tipton et al (1999) subsequently established that the same effect was observed when amino acids were ingested rather than infused. Following leg resistance exercise on three different occasions, subjects consumed 40 g of either mixed amino acids (MAA) or essential amino acids (EAA) or a placebo solution ~225 minutes post-exercise. Net muscle protein balance was positive for both amino acid trials but as expected remained negative for the placebo trial. This was achieved through elevated protein synthesis and at least in the case of EAA consumption, suppression of muscle protein breakdown (did not attain statistical significance). More recently this group has confirmed that this acute effect of amino acid ingestion post-resistance exercise is reflective of the response over 24 hours (Tipton et al 2003). This supports the extrapolation of data from the acute effect of amino acid supplementation after resistance exercise to suggest that muscle protein (mass/strength) gains as a consequence of a chronic resistance training programme would be greater if combined with amino acid ingestion post-exercise.

Essential amino acids seem to be the key ingredient, since net protein balance during the second hour of recovery from leg resistance exercise after ingestion of 6 g EAA (Borsheim et al 2002) was double that observed after ingestion of 6 g MAA (containing 3 g EAA) (Miller et al 2003). However, there does seem to be an upper limit to the response to provision of amino acids. Tipton et al (1999) found no difference in muscle protein synthesis between trials when 40 g MAA (containing 20 g EAA) and 40 g EAA were consumed. This suggests that consuming more than 20 g EAA post-exercise will exert no additional effect; however, no studies have as yet precisely characterized the dose response and largest effective amino acid dose post-exercise.

Carbohydrate (cho) ingestion causes an elevation in blood glucose and insulin concentration: hyperglycaemia and hyperinsulinaemia. Insulin suppresses protein breakdown and at least in presence of abundant amino acids stimulates protein synthesis, thus exerting a protein anabolic effect. Ingestion of 1 g cho/kg immediately and 1 hour after resistance exercise reduced urinary nitrogen and 3-MH excretion, but neither muscle fractional synthetic rate nor whole body protein breakdown were affected (Roy et al 1997). More recently Borsheim et al (2004) confirmed that although cho ingestion (100 g) post-resistance exercise exerts an anabolic effect, primarily via a reduction in muscle protein breakdown, net protein balance remained negative.

One might expect that an optimal response would be achieved by combining EAA and carbohydrate supplements, reaping the benefit of both increased amino acid availability and hyperinsulinaemia. Ingestion of 6 g EAA + 35 g sucrose was found to create a positive protein balance when consumed after either 1 or 3 hours' recovery from resistance exercise (Rasmussen et al 2000). Perhaps surprisingly, in view of the hyperinsulinaemia, no suppression of muscle protein breakdown was observed but muscle protein synthesis was increased by ~400% above resting values. In this study it was not possible to answer the question of whether EAA + cho was more effective in promoting positive net protein balance, than EAA or cho alone since there were no EAA only or cho only conditions. Miller et al (2003) found that net protein balance during recovery from resistance exercise was 53 ± 6, 114 ± 38, and 71 ± 13 mg/leg/3 hours after ingestion of cho (~35 g sucrose), mix (both) and AA (~6 g MAA) respectively. This appears to suggest that the effects of amino acids and carbohydrate on protein turnover are broadly additive. However, Borsheim et al calculated that during the first hour of recovery from resistance exercise net protein balance after ingestion of 6 g EAA + 35 g cho (Rasmussen et al 2000) was not different from that achieved after consuming 6 g EAA alone (Borsheim et al 2002). It is clear that EAA are the vital ingredient; however, it would appear sensible to include cho in recovery supplements since cho certainly does not impair the protein synthetic response and will have the added value of facilitating glycogen re-synthesis, alongside improved protein kinetics.

Thus far all studies reported in this section have related to the beneficial effects of amino acid consumption after resistance exercise; however, similar benefits are observed after endurance exercise (during 3 hours' recovery from 60 minutes' cycling exercise at 60% $\dot{V}O_2$max) (Levenhagen et al 2002). Net protein balance was positive during recovery when supplement + protein (10 g casein protein + 8 g sucrose + 3 g milk fat) was consumed immediately post-exercise, but remained negative during the placebo (0 g casein protein + 0 g sucrose + 0 g milk fat), and supplement − protein (0 g casein protein + 8 g sucrose + 3 g milk fat) conditions. This positive balance was achieved via a ~fourfold elevation in muscle protein synthesis in protein condition versus supplement only condition.

In summary, consumption of essential amino acids with or without carbohydrate after exercise increases the exercise-induced elevation in muscle protein synthesis, so that muscle protein gains occur. The upper effective dose is somewhere between 6–20 g EAA, but it has not yet been precisely identified. Combining amino acids with carbohydrate does not seem to improve the net positive protein balance, but will have the added advantage of supporting muscle glycogen resynthesis during recovery.

TIMING OF INGESTION

The elevation in protein synthesis after resistance exercise has been observed within 90 minutes of the end of resistance exercise and lasts for up to 48 hours (Phillips et al 1997). Rasmussen (2000) demonstrated that muscle protein balance was equivalently positive whether consuming EAA + cho at 1 or 3 hours post-resistance exercise, suggesting that the beneficial effects are relatively independent of timing. However, Tipton et al (2001) found that consuming EAA + cho before exercise was more effective at promoting net muscle protein synthesis than consumption of the same supplement immediately post-exercise. This was primarily due to an earlier and more prolonged stimulation of muscle protein synthesis, most likely because amino acid delivery to the leg muscle will be maximized while blood flow is elevated during exercise.

During recovery from endurance exercise it appears that early feeding is critical to maximize net protein balance. Levenhagen (2001) found that when feeding was delayed to 3 hours after 60 minutes' cycling exercise at 60% $\dot{V}O_2$max, leg protein balance remained negative during the following 3 hours. When the supplement was consumed immediately post-exercise leg protein balance was positive over the following 3 hours and whole body protein synthesis was increased threefold. It appears therefore that in order to achieve net protein synthesis during recovery from exercise, EAA and cho should be consumed pre resistance exercise (if tolerable by the individual) and immediately post-endurance exercise.

To date there is only one study which has examined the chronic effect of timing of protein supplement consumption post-exercise (Esmarck et al 2001). Thirteen elderly men habitually consuming 1 g protein/kg/day completed a 12-week resistance exercise programme and received a protein supplement (10 g protein, 7 g cho, 3 g fat) either immediately after or 2 hours after each training session. There was a significant increase in the cross-sectional area of quadriceps femoris muscle (measurement via MRI) and also in the mean fibre area for the immediate feeding group but no significant change for the delayed feeding group. Dynamic strength increased for both groups but isokinetic strength increased by 15% only for the immediate feeding group. It appears therefore, at least in elderly men consuming an adequate protein diet, that chronic consumption of a protein supplement immediately post-exercise will promote muscle mass and strength gains. There is some evidence that muscle protein synthesis is less responsive to increased amino acid availability in elderly and young subjects (Volpi et al 2000), and it would therefore be helpful to confirm this finding in young sedentary subjects. However, in the interim, there are no contraindications for consumption of such moderate amounts of protein and it is likely that the protein anabolic effect will be significant.

PRACTICAL CONSIDERATIONS

Athletes should ensure that sufficient calories are consumed to maintain energy balance, and ~15% of these calories should be obtained from protein sources.

If athletes are in energy deficit to achieve weight loss, then the protein intake should be increased to 25–30% energy intake to prevent loss of muscle protein.

Any reduction in protein intake should be undertaken gradually. The fed state body protein gains will decrease immediately, but the losses incurred during the fasted state will take up to 10 days to decrease so that protein balance is re-established. During this time body protein, most likely muscle protein, will be lost.

Carbohydrate and essential amino acid supplements should be consumed either before or immediately after exercise to enhance the anabolic effects of exercise.

Consuming more than 20 g EAA does not induce any further benefit, and the optimal dose is somewhere between 6 and 20 g.

KEY POINTS

1. During endurance exercise there is a net loss of body protein, but during recovery, protein synthesis is increased to a greater degree than protein breakdown (anabolic effect).
2. Protein turnover is not altered during resistance exercise, but during recovery protein synthesis rates are increased for up to 48 hours, with a smaller increase in protein breakdown (anabolic effect).
3. Despite this anabolic effect during recovery from exercise, protein balance will remain negative until amino acids are provided.
4. Endurance and resistance trained athletes both have moderately higher protein requirements than sedentary individuals. However, as long as athletes are in energy balance protein requirements should be met when ~15% energy is derived from protein.
5. Consumption of essential amino acids, either before or immediately after exercise, enhances the increases in muscle protein synthesis which occur during recovery.

References

Akermark C, Jacobs I, Rasmusson M, Karlsson J 1996 Diet and muscle glycogen concentration in relation to physical performance in Swedish elite ice hockey players. International Journal of Sport Nutrition 6:272–284

Anthony JC, Anthony TG, Layman DK 1999 Leucine supplementation enhances skeletal muscle recovery in rats following exercise. Journal of Nutrition 129:1102–1106

Belcastro AN 1993 Skeletal muscle calcium activated neutral protease (calpain) with exercise. Journal of Applied Physiology 74:1381–1386

Biolo G, Maggi SP, Williams BD et al 1995 Increased rates of muscle protein turnover and amino acid transport after resistance exercise in humans. American Journal of Physiology 268:E514–E520

Biolo G, Tipton KD, Klein S, Wolfe RR 1997 An abundant supply of amino acids enhances the metabolic effect of exercise on muscle protein. American Journal of Physiology-Endocrinology and Metabolism 36:E122–E129

Boirie Y, Dangin M, Gachon P et al 1997 Slow and fast dietary proteins differently modulate postprandial protein accretion. Proceedings of the National Academy of Sciences of the USA 94:14930–14935

Borsheim E, Tipton KD, Wolf SE, Wolfe RR 2002 Essential amino acids and muscle protein recovery from resistance exercise. American Journal of Physiology 283:E648–E657

Borsheim E, Cree MG, Tipton KD et al 2004 Effect of carbohydrate intake on net muscle protein synthesis during recovery from resistance exercise. Journal of Applied Physiology 96:674–678

Bowtell JL, Leese GP, Smith K et al 1998 Modulation of whole body protein metabolism, during and after exercise, by variation of dietary protein. Journal of Applied Physiology 85:1744–1752

Bowtell JL, Leese GP, Smith K et al 2000 Effect of oral glucose on leucine turnover in human subjects at rest and during exercise at two levels of dietary protein. Journal of Physiology (London) 525(1):271–281

Burke DG, Chilibeck PD, Davison KS et al 2001 The effect of whey protein supplementation with and without creatine monohydrate combined with resistance training on lean tissue mass and muscle strength. International Journal of Sport Nutrition and Exercise Metabolism 11:349–364

Butterfield GE, Calloway DH 1984 Physical activity improves protein utilisation in young men. British Journal of Nutrition 51:171–184

Bylund-Fellenius A, Ojamaa KM, Flaim KE, Li JB 1984 Protein synthesis versus energy state in contracting muscles of perfused rat hind-limb. American Journal of Physiology 246:E297–E305

Campbell WW, Crim MC, Young VR et al 1995 Effects of resistance training and dietary protein intake on protein metabolism in older adults. American Journal of Physiology 268:E1143–E1153

Carraro F, Hartl WH, Stuart CA et al 1990a Whole body and plasma protein synthesis in exercise and recovery in human subjects. American Journal of Physiology 258:E821–E831

Carraro F, Stuart CA, Hartl WH et al 1990b Effect of exercise and recovery on muscle protein synthesis in human subjects. American Journal of Physiology 259:E470–E476

Devlin JT, Brodsky I, Scrimgeour A et al 1990 Amino acid metabolism after intense exercise. American Journal of Physiology 261:E249–E255

Dohm GL, Tapscott EB, Kasperek GJ 1987 Protein degradation during endurance exercise and recovery. Medicine and Science in Sports and Exercise 19:S166–S171

Durham WJ, Miller SL, Yeckel CW et al 2005 Leg glucose and protein metabolism during an acute bout of resistance exercise in humans. Journal of Applied Physiology 97:1379–1386

Esmarck B, Andersen JL, Olsen S et al 2001 Timing of postexercise protein intake is important for muscle hypertrophy with resistance training in elderly humans. Journal of Physiology (London) 535:301–311

Fielding RA, Meredith CN, O'Reilly KP et al 1991 Enhanced protein breakdown after eccentric exercise in young and older men. Journal of Applied Physiology 71:674–679

Finlay D, Varshavsky A 1985 The ubiquitin system: functions and mechanisms. TIBS 10:343–347

Friedman JE, Lemon PWR 1989 Effect of chronic endurance exercise on retention of dietary protein. International Journal of Sports Medicine 10:118–123

Gibala MJ, Peirce N, Constantin-Teodosiu D, Greenhaff PL 2002 Exercise with low muscle glycogen augments TCA cycle anaplerosis but impairs oxidative energy provision in humans. Journal Of Physiology (London) 540:1079–1086

Goldspink G, Harridge SDR 2004 Growth factors and muscle ageing. Experimental Gerontology 39:1433–1438

Gontzea I, Sutzescu R, Dumitrache S 1975 The influence of adaptation to physical effort on nitrogen balance in man. Nutrition Reports International 11:231–236

Hagg SA, Morse EL, Adibi SA 1982 Effect of exercise on rates of oxidation, turnover and plasma clearance of leucine in human subjects. American Journal of Physiology 242:E407–E410

Healy ML, Gibney J, Russell-Jones DL et al 2003 High dose growth hormone exerts an anabolic effect at rest and during exercise in endurance-trained athletes. Journal of Clinical Endocrinology and Metabolism 88:5221–5226

Hornberger TA, Esser KA 2004 Mechanotransduction and the regulation of protein synthesis in skeletal muscle. Proceedings of the Nutrition Society 63:331–335

Ivy JL, Katz AL, Cutler CL et al 1988 Muscle glycogen synthesis after exercise: effect of time of carbohydrate ingestion. Journal of Applied Physiology 64:1480–1485

Kasperek GJ 1989 Regulation of branched chain 2-oxo-acid dehydrogenase activity during exercise. American Journal of Physiology 256:E186–E190

Knapik J, Meredith C, Jones B et al 1991 Leucine metabolism during fasting and exercise. Journal of Applied Physiology 70:43–47

Lamont LS, Patel DG, Kalhan SC 1990 Leucine kinetics in endurance trained humans. Journal of Applied Physiology 69:1–6

Lamont LS, McCullough AJ, Kalhan SC 2001 Relationship between leucine oxidation and oxygen consumption during steady-state exercise. Medicine and Science in Sports and Exercise 33:237–241

Lemon PWR, Mullin JP 1980 Effect of initial muscle glycogen levels on protein catabolism during exercise. Journal of Applied Physiology 48:624–629

Lemon PWR, Tarnopolsky MA, MacDougall JD, Atkinson SA 1992 Protein requirements and muscle mass/strength changes during intensive training in novice bodybuilders. Journal of Applied Physiology 73:767–775

Levenhagen DK, Gresham JD, Carlson MG et al 2001 Postexercise nutrient intake timing in humans is critical to recovery of leg glucose and protein homeostasis. American Journal of Physiology 280:E982–E993

Levenhagen DK, Carr C, Carlson MG et al 2002 Postexercise protein intake enhances whole-body and leg protein accretion in humans. Medicine and Science in Sports and Exercise 34:828–837

MacDougall JD, Gibala MJ, Tarnopolsky MA et al 1995 The time course of elevated muscle protein synthesis following heavy resistance exercise. Canadian Journal of Applied Physiology 20:480–486

McKenzie S, Phillips SM, Carter SL et al 2000 Endurance exercise training attenuates leucine oxidation and branched-chain 2-oxo acid dehydrogenase activation during exercise in humans. American Journal of Physiology 278:E580–E587

McNurlan MA, Garlick PJ 1989 Influence of nutrient intake in protein turnover. Diabetes 5:165–189

Matthews DE, Marano MA, Campbell RG 1993 Splanchnic bed utilization of glutamine and glutamic acid in humans. American Journal of Physiology 264:E848–E854

Meredith CN, Zackin MJ, Frontera WR, Evans WJ 1989 Dietary protein requirements and body protein metabolism in endurance-trained men. Journal of Applied Physiology 66:2850–2856

Miller SL, Tipton KD, Chinkes DL et al 2003 Independent and combined effects of amino acids and glucose after resistance exercise. Medicine and Science in Sports and Exercise 35:449–455

Millward DJ 1990 The hormonal control of protein turnover. Clinical Nutrition 9:115–126

Millward DJ, Bowtell JL, Pacy P, Rennie MJ 1994 Physical activity, protein metabolism and protein requirements. Proceedings of the Nutrition Society 53:223–240

Moore DR, Phillips SM, Babraj JA, Smith KM, Rennie MJ 2005 Myofibrillar and collagen protein synthesis in human skeletal muscle in young men after maximal shortening and lengthening contractions. American Journal of Physiology-Cell Physiology 288:E1153–E1159

Pacy PJ, Price GM, Halliday D et al 1994 Nitrogen homeostasis in man: the diurnal responses of protein synthesis and degradation and amino acid oxidation to diets with increasing protein intakes. Clinical Science 86:103–118

Phillips SM 2004 Protein requirements and supplementation in strength sports. Nutrition 20:689–695

Phillips SM, Atkinson SA, Tarnopolsky MA, MacDougall JD 1993 Gender differences in leucine kinetics and nitrogen balance in endurance athletes. Journal of Applied Physiology 75:2134–2141

Phillips SM, Tipton KD, Aarsland A et al 1997 Mixed muscle protein synthesis and breakdown after resistance exercise in humans. American Journal of Physiology 273:E99–E107

Phillips SM, Parise G, Roy BD et al 2002 Resistance-training-induced adaptations in skeletal muscle protein turnover in the fed state. Canadian Journal of Physiology and Pharmacology 80:1045–1053

Price GM, Halliday D, Pacy PJ et al 1994 Nitrogen homeostasis in man: influence of protein intake on the amplitude of diurnal cycling of body nitrogen. Clinical Science 86:91–102

Rasmussen BB, Tipton KD, Miller SL et al 2000 An oral essential amino acid-carbohydrate supplement enhances muscle protein anabolism after resistance exercise. Journal of Applied Physiology 88:386–392

Rennie MJ, Millward DJ 1983 3-methylhistidine excretion and urinary 3-methylhistidine/creatinine ratio are poor indicators of muscle protein breakdown. Clinical Science 61:217–225

Rennie MJ, Edwards RHT, Krywawych S, Davies CTM 1981 Effect of exercise on protein turnover in man. Clinical Science 61:627–639

Roy BD, Tarnopolsky MA, MacDougall JD et al 1997 Effect of glucose supplement timing on protein metabolism after resistance training. Journal of Applied Physiology 82:1882–1888

Sahlin K, Tonkonogi M, Soderlund K 1998 Energy supply and muscle fatigue in humans. Acta Physiologica Scandinavica 162:261–266

Sheffield-Moore M, Yeckel CW, Volpi E et al 2004 Post exercise protein metabolism in older and younger men following moderate-intensity aerobic exercise. Amercian Journal of Physiology 287:E513–E522

Short KR, Vittone JL, Bigelow ML et al 2004 Age and aerobic exercise training effects on whole body and muscle protein metabolism. American Journal of Physiology 286:E92–E101

Stein TP, Hoyr RW, O'Toole M et al 1989 Protein and energy metabolism during prolonged exercise in trained athletes. International Journal of Sports Medicine 10:311–316

Stumvoll M, Meyer C, Perriello G et al 1998 Human kidney and liver gluconeogenesis: evidence for organ substrate selectivity. American Journal of Physiology 274:E817–E826

Tarnopolsky M 2004 Protein requirements for endurance athletes. Nutrition 20:662–668

Tarnopolsky MA, MacDougall JD, Atkinson SA 1988 Influence of protein intake and training status on nitrogen balance and lean body mass. Journal of Applied Physiology 64:187–193

Tarnopolsky MA, Atkinson SA, MacDougall JD et al 1991 Whole body leucine metabolism during and after resistance exercise in fed humans. Medicine and Science in Sports and Exercise 23:326–333

Tarnopolsky MA, Atkinson SA, MacDougall JD et al 1992 Evaluation of protein requirements of trained strength athletes. Journal of Applied Physiology 73:1986–1995

Tipton KD, Ferrando AA, Williams BD, Wolfe RR 1996 Muscle protein metabolism in female swimmers after a combination of resistance and endurance exercise. Journal of Applied Physiology 81:2034–2038

Tipton KD, Ferrando AA, Phillips SM et al 1999 Postexercise net protein synthesis in human muscle from orally administered amino acids. American Journal of Physiology 276:E628–E634

Tipton KD, Rasmussen BB, Miller SL et al 2001 Timing of amino acid-carbohydrate ingestion alters anabolic response of muscle to resistance exercise. American Journal of Physiology 281:E197–E206

Tipton KD, Borsheim E, Wolf SE et al 2003 Acute response of net muscle protein balance reflects 24-h balance after exercise and amino acid ingestion. American Journal of Physiology 284:E76–E89

Todd KS, Butterfield GE, Calloway DH 1984 Nitrogen balance in men with adequate and deficient energy intake at three levels of work. Journal of Nutrition 114:2107–2118

Trappe TA, Williams RS, Carrithers JA 2004 Influence of age and resistance exercise on human skeletal muscle proteolysis: a microdialysis approach. Journal of Physiology 554:803–807

Vazquez JA, Paul HS, Adibi SA 1988 Regulation of leucine catabolism by caloric sources. Journal of Clinical Investigation 82:1606–1613

Volpi E, Mittendorfer B, Rasmussen BB, Wolfe RR 2000 The response of muscle protein anabolism to combined hyperaminoacidemia and glucose-induced hyperinsulinemia is impaired in the elderly. Journal of Clinical Endocrinology and Metabolism 85:4481–4490

Wagenmakers AJM, Beckers EJ, Brouns F et al 1991 Carbohydrate supplementation, glycogen depletion and amino acid metabolism during exercise. American Journal of Physiology 260:E883–E890

Wolfe RR 2000 Protein supplements and exercise. American Journal of Clinical Nutrition 72:551S

Wolfe RR, Goodenough RD, Wolfe MH et al 1982 Isotopic analysis of leucine and urea metabolism in exercising humans. Journal of Applied Physiology 52:458–466

Wolfe RR, Wolfe MH, Nadel ER, Shaw JHF 1984 Isotopic determination of amino acid-urea interactions in exercise in humans. Journal of Applied Physiology 56:221–229

Chapter 6

Micronutrients important for exercise

Kathleen Woolf and Melinda M Manore

LEARNING OBJECTIVES

After studying this chapter, you should be able to:

1. Discuss how exercise may increase the need for micronutrients in active individuals.
2. Identify the micronutrients most likely to be low in the diets of active individuals and the dietary patterns that lead to low energy intakes.
3. Discuss the role that energy intake has on the intake of micronutrients.
4. Discuss the role zinc, iron, folate and vitamin B_{12} play in haemoglobin synthesis.
5. Describe the association between folate, vitamin B_{12} and vitamin B_6, and vascular disease.
6. Discuss the impact of poor iron status on exercise performance.
7. Describe the nutrients important for bone health and their function.

INTRODUCTION

Vitamins and minerals play important roles in maintaining the health of physically active individuals (Manore & Thompson 2000). For example, the

B vitamins are necessary in the energy-producing pathways of the body, while several micronutrients, including iron, zinc, copper, vitamin K, folate and vitamin B_{12}, are required for the production of healthy red blood cells. Other micronutrients are important for maintaining adequate immune function, protecting the tissues of the body from oxidative damage, maintaining bone health, and the building and repairing of muscle tissue.

Regular physical activity may alter the need or requirements for many of the vitamins and minerals in several ways (Manore & Thompson 2000). First, the metabolic pathways that produce energy are stressed during physical activity; thus, requirements for the nutrients used in these processes may be increased. Second, biochemical adaptations that occur with training in the tissues of the body may increase requirements of the micronutrients. Third, strenuous exercise may also increase the turnover or loss of a particular micronutrient in sweat, urine or faeces. Finally, additional micronutrients may be required to repair and maintain the higher lean tissue mass of the active individual.

When the current Dietary Reference Intakes (DRIs) for each of the micronutrients were established for the United States and Canada, there was inadequate information to calculate specific micronutrient recommendations for active individuals (IOM 1997, 1998, 2001) (see Table 6.1). If exercise increases the need for selected micronutrients, then athletes may have poorer micronutrient status while consuming the DRI for these nutrients or have poorer status compared to sedentary controls with similar dietary intakes. Athletes at greatest risk of poor micronutrient status are those who restrict energy intake for weight loss or are concerned about maintaining a low body weight (i.e. gymnasts, jockeys, wrestlers, figure skaters), or who eliminate selected food groups, such as dairy or meat. Individuals with these types of eating behaviour may need to use a multivitamin or mineral supplement or use fortified foods to improve overall micronutrient status.

This chapter will focus on those micronutrients for which the athlete or active individual is most at risk of deficiency. The B-complex vitamins involved in energy metabolism and blood health will be covered first followed by the minerals of special importance to active individuals. The DRIs for the micronutrients discussed in this chapter are provided in Table 6.1.

B-COMPLEX VITAMINS

B-complex vitamins have several important functions in the body including energy production, haemoglobin synthesis, adequate immune function and building and repair of muscle tissue. Manore (2000) reviewed the B-vitamin intakes in active individuals and athletes who recorded dietary intakes for at least 3 days. Results showed that mean intakes of B vitamins are typically normal for both male and female athletes, but examination of individual intakes showed that 10–60% of female athletes had intakes below recommended levels (Manore 2000, 2002). Low intakes of the B vitamins are closely associated with poor energy intakes, which is much more common in active

Table 6.1   Dietary Reference Intakes (DRIs) and Tolerable Upper Intake Levels (UL) for selected nutrients: recommended intakes for individuals 19–50 years[a,b]

Nutrient	Males RDA/AI	Females RDA/AI	UL	Adverse effects of high doses
Thiamin (mg/day)	1.2	1.1	ND[c]	Data are inadequate to assess risk
Riboflavin (mg/day)	1.3	1.1	ND[c]	Data are inadequate to assess risk
Vitamin B_6 (mg/day)	1.3	1.3	100	No adverse effect of ↑ food B_6; ↑ supplemental B_6 can cause sensory neuropathy (difficulty walking)
Folate (µg/day)	400	400	1000	No adverse effect of fortified food folic acid; ↑ supplemental folic acid can mask vitamin B_{12} deficiency
Vitamin B_{12} (µg /day)	2.4	2.4	ND[c]	Data are inadequate to assess risk; no adverse effect of ↑ food B_{12}
Calcium (mg/day)	1000*	1000*	2500	Kidney stones, blocks absorption of other nutrients (iron, zinc); high blood calcium and renal problems
Iron (mg/day)	8	18	45	Toxic levels negatively affect the cardiovascular, central nervous, kidney, liver and blood systems. High iron intake also reduces zinc absorption
Magnesium (mg/day)	400–420	310–320	350	Diarrhoea; adverse effects are only related to high doses from supplements, not food
Zinc (mg/day)	11	8	40	Suppression of immune response, decreased high-density lipoprotein (HDL) cholesterol and reduced copper status

[a]This table summarizes Recommended Dietary Allowances (RDAs) and Adequate Intakes (AIs). The AIs are followed by an asterisk (*).
[b]Source: Institute of Medicine, Food and Nutrition Board 1997, 1998, 2001. A complete table of RDAs and AIs for all life stages groups can be found at http://www.iom.edu.
[c]ND = none determinable due to lack of data.

women than men. In general, active males have better nutrient intakes, not because they select a more nutrient-dense diet, but because their energy intake can easily be 2–3 times that of an active female. See Table 6.2 for the specific functions of the B vitamins related to exercise.

THIAMIN

Thiamin is important for the metabolism of carbohydrates, fats and proteins, especially the branched chain amino acids (BCAAs) (leucine, isoleucine and

Table 6.2 Exercise-related functions of micronutrients that may be low in the diets of active individuals and athletes

Micronutrient	Function	Food sources
Thiamin	Serves as a coenzyme [TPP (thiamin pyrophosphate)] in reactions in the energy pathways	Whole grains and enriched grain products, pork, liver, dark green vegetables and nuts
Riboflavin	Participates in electron transfer in energy metabolism	Milk and dairy products, organ meats, whole grains and enriched grain products, eggs and nuts
Vitamin B_6	Involved in amino acid metabolism (such as transamination) and in glycogen breakdown	Animal foods, such as meats, fish and poultry
Folate	Required for cell division and cell regeneration in cells such as the red blood cells	Plant sources and organ meats
Vitamin B_{12}	Involved in the recycling of folate and in neural tissue	Found only in animal foods
Calcium	Component of bone; required for muscle contraction, nerve transmission and blood coagulation	Dairy products and some vegetables, fortified juices and cereals
Iron	Component of haemoglobin and myoglobin; also a constituent of cytochromes and enzyme complexes	Meat, fish, poultry, whole grains and fortified foods
Magnesium	Required for proper functioning of many reactions in the body	Whole grains, legumes and leafy vegetables
Zinc	Component of many enzyme systems in the body, especially the building and repair of muscle tissue	Organ meats, other red meats, seafood, poultry, pork, dairy products, whole grains and leafy vegetables

valine) (Manore & Thompson 2000). The active form of this micronutrient, thiamin pyrophosphate (TPP), serves as a coenzyme in many key reactions in the energy-producing pathways of the body, which are stressed during physical activity. For example, TPP is required by pyruvate dehydrogenase, the enzyme that converts pyruvate to acetyl CoA, and by α-ketoglutarate dehydrogenase in the tricarboxylic acid (TCA) cycle. Thus, thiamin is critical to aerobically metabolize carbohydrates and fats. In addition, thiamin is also needed for BCAA metabolism, which increases with physical activity, especially endurance exercise.

Requirements. Thiamin is found in a variety of foods, such as whole grains and enriched grain products, pork, liver, nuts, legumes and green leafy vegetables. Athletes at risk for poor thiamin status are those who restrict dietary intake or select highly refined diets. The Recommended Dietary Allowance (RDA) for thiamin is 1.1 and 1.2 mg/day for adult females and males, respectively (IOM 1998). No Tolerable Upper Intake Level (UL) has been established for thiamin (IOM 1998).

Assessment of status.   To assess nutritional status of a nutrient, dietary intake data and biochemical measures (blood and urine) are typically determined. For thiamin, biochemical status is typically determined by assessing activity of erythrocyte transketolase located in the red blood cell. The assessment marker, erythrocyte transketolase activity coefficient or ETKAC, is measured by determining the activity of erythrocyte transketolase before and after the coenzyme (thiamin) is added. The more enzyme activity that is generated when additional thiamin is added is an indication of poor or marginal thiamin status (Manore 2000). Thiamin is also needed at two steps of the pentose phosphate pathway, a pathway that generates ribose-5-phosphate needed in the production of ATP. One of these steps requires erythrocyte transketolase.

Researchers have examined the dietary intakes of thiamin in active individuals and found that intakes are adequate, except where energy intake is low. For example, Beshgetoor & Nichols (2003) and Ziegler et al (1999) reported normal mean intakes of thiamin in their athletes. Beshgetoor & Nichols (2003) measured the thiamin intakes in diets of supplementing and non-supplementing female athletes and found that mean intakes of thiamin exceeded the 1998 RDA for both groups of athletes. Ziegler et al (1999) measured the dietary intakes of thiamin in male and female adolescent figure skaters and found mean intakes to be normal, with only 7% of males and 13% of females to have thiamin intakes less than two-thirds the RDA for thiamin. Thus, athletes that participate in sports that emphasize leanness, such as figure skating, need to be examined for poor nutrient intakes.

Although dietary intakes for thiamin are typically above recommended guidelines, exercise or vigorous physical activity may alter nutrient requirements and result in marginal or poor status in some active individuals. Fogelholm and colleagues at the University of Helsinki have done a series of studies examining thiamin status in active males and females (see Manore 2000 review). Two studies using either Finnish male athletes or Nordic skiers did not document poorer status in athletes using ETKAC compared to control subjects. This research is supported by others (Raczynski & Szczepanska 1993) who examined thiamin status in 1918 elite Polish athletes (males and females combined) from 1987 to 1992 and found little risk of thiamin deficiency, with only 2% in all athletes having poor status, ranging from 0 to 3% over a 6-year period. Conversely, a third study by Fogelholm and colleagues documented 12% of the athletes they examined with marginal thiamin status (males and females combined). Thus, there is documentation, although limited, in the research literature that some athletes have poor thiamin status based on blood assessments.

Although we have limited data on the prevalence of poor thiamin status in active individuals, we do know that thiamin deficiency can impair athletic performance. Using a controlled metabolic feeding study, van der Beek et al (1994) depleted male athletes of thiamin, riboflavin and vitamin B_6 over a 3-week period by feeding commonly consumed processed foods. They found that exercise performance decreased significantly after vitamin depletion, with significant increases in lactic acid production. Thiamin functions in the conversion of pyruvate into acetyl CoA; thus, a deficiency of thiamin could impair metabolism of carbohydrates and result in the accumulation of lactic acid. In general, if thiamin status is good, supplementation with addition thiamine does not improve exercise performance. Although poor thiamin status can definitely impact exercise performance, the incidence of thiamin deficiency appears to be low in active individuals.

RIBOFLAVIN

Riboflavin is an essential component of two important coenzymes, flavin adenine dinucleotide (FAD) and flavin mononucleotide (FMN). These coenzymes participate in the transfer of electrons in energy metabolism, amino acid metabolism and steroid hormone production (Manore 2000, Manore & Thompson 2000). Thus, riboflavin is important for exercise because it assists with the transfer of electrons that come from the energy pathways to the electron transport chain for formation of ATP. Finally, riboflavin is involved in the conversion of vitamin B_6 to its active form (Manore 2000).

Requirements. Adequate riboflavin intakes can easily be achieved by regularly consuming milk and milk products, eggs, whole grains and cereals, lean meats and broccoli. As with thiamin, those athletes at risk of poor thiamin status are those that restrict dietary intake or select highly refined diets. The RDA for riboflavin is 1.1 and 1.3 mg for adult females and males, respectively, while a UL for riboflavin has not been established (IOM 1998).

Assessment of status. Riboflavin status is typically assessed by measuring the activity of erythrocyte glutathione reductase, similar to the assessment of ETKAC used for thiamin (Manore 2000). Activity of this enzyme is the most sensitive marker of riboflavin status and is the method typically utilized in exercise studies examining riboflavin status.

Most cross-sectional studies comparing riboflavin status in active and sedentary individuals have found that riboflavin intake by athletes is adequate to meet dietary guidelines. For example, Beshgetoor & Nichols (2003) found that mean intakes for riboflavin for female master athletes (cyclists and runners) exceeded the 1998 RDA of 1.1 mg/day. However, like thiamin, athletic performance can be impaired by riboflavin deficiency. When van der Beek et al (1994) fed a diet low in thiamin, riboflavin and vitamin B_6 until blood levels indicated deficiency, lactate threshold and exercise performance decreased. Thus, supplemental riboflavin is only beneficial for those individuals in poor riboflavin status. For example, in a study of children 12–14 years, supplementation with riboflavin improved riboflavin status and level of physical fitness as assessed by a bicycle ergometer (see Manore 2000 for a review).

Because riboflavin is so critical for energy metabolism during exercise, research suggests that athletes may need more riboflavin than the general population. Based on data from metabolic studies examining the effects of exercise, dieting or dieting plus exercise on riboflavin requirements, riboflavin needs are higher in females engaging in exercise for fitness compared to sedentary controls (see Manore 2000 for a review of this literature). In the 1980s, a series of metabolic studies that examined the riboflavin status of active young women were completed at Cornell University. In the first metabolic study, researchers found that moderate physical activity (20–50 minutes/day, 6 days/week) increased riboflavin requirements to 1.4 mg/1000 kcal (1998 Recommended Dietary Allowance [RDA] = 1.1 mg/day for adult women) (IOM 1998). Two subsequent metabolic studies also found that dieting (1200–1250 kcal/day) and dieting plus fitness exercise increased riboflavin requirements in active women. In these studies, 1.16 mg of riboflavin/1000 kcal (1.4 mg/day) was required to maintain good riboflavin status when subjects were dieting for weight loss and exercising (3 hours/week at 75–85% of maximal heart rate). Even active elderly women (2.5 hours' exercise/week) eating a weight-maintenance diet (1800–2000 kcal/day) required 1.8 mg/day of riboflavin to maintain good status. Based on these studies, it appears that exercise, dieting and dieting plus exercise increase the need for riboflavin above the 1998 RDA for active women (Manore 2000). However, it should be noted that these subjects performed moderate exercise (2.5–5 hours/week) for fitness. Unfortunately, no metabolic studies have examined riboflavin status in female athletes who participate in strenuous exercise and competitive sports. However, if moderately active females have an increased need for riboflavin, then female athletes who are even more active, would have just as great a need, if not higher. Exercise has also been shown to further decrease riboflavin status in individuals with marginal riboflavin status. Thus, based on the research to date, athletes may need more riboflavin than the general population and more than the current RDA.

VITAMIN B$_6$

Vitamin B$_6$ plays an important role in the metabolic pathways required for exercise, principally amino acid metabolism and glycogen breakdown (Manore 2000, Manore & Thompson 2000). The active form of vitamin B$_6$ is pyridoxal phosphate (PLP), which plays an important role in protein associated transamination and deamination reactions. The breakdown of glycogen is regulated through glycogen phosphorylase, which also requires PLP.

Requirements.   Good sources of vitamin B$_6$ include animal foods such as meat, fish and poultry, and plant foods, such as bananas, navy beans and walnuts. The RDA for vitamin B$_6$ for men and women 19–50 years is 1.3 mg, while the UL for vitamin B$_6$ is 100 mg (IOM 1998).

Assessment of status. Several blood and urine indicators are used in the assessment of vitamin B_6 status, including plasma PLP and urinary levels of a B_6 metabolite, 4-pyridoxic acid. Activity of the transaminase enzymes in the blood is also used to determine status (Manore 2000).

Manore (2000) reviewed the research examining vitamin B_6 intakes and status in active individuals, especially female athletes (Manore 2002). While few studies report poor mean dietary intakes of vitamin B_6 by athletes, numerous studies report a certain number of their individual athletes with poor vitamin B_6 status (range = 5–60%) (Hansen & Manore 2005, Manore 2000). For example, Telford et al (1992) studied 86 male and female athletes before and after an 8-month training period. Roughly half of the subjects (n = 42) consumed a multivitamin/mineral supplement and half took a placebo (n = 44). They found that 60% of the athletes had poor baseline vitamin B_6 status while consuming their typical diets. At the end of the 8-month study, 41% of the athletes on the placebo had poor vitamin B_6 status. Raczynski & Szczepanska (1993) also examined vitamin B_6 status in 1753 elite male and female Polish athletes from the year 1987 to 1992. The risk of vitamin deficiency averaged 9% in all athletes over the 6-year period, with a range of 4–15%. The highest prevalence of vitamin B_6 deficiency was in endurance athletes (13%), while athletes in team sports had the lowest prevalence rate (10%). They also observed that the risk of vitamin B_6 deficiency was highest in pre-Olympic years (16%) and lowest in Olympic years (3%), suggesting that some athletes had poor vitamin B_6 status while consuming their typical diets.

Recent metabolic research studies, done after the 1998 RDA for vitamin B_6 was established, have documented that ~1.5–2.3 mg/day of vitamin B_6 is required to maintain good vitamin B_6 status in sedentary individuals (Hansen & Manore 2005). This level of vitamin B_6 intake is higher than the current RDA of 1.3 mg/day for men and women (IOM 1998). It has also been well documented that exercise alters vitamin B_6 metabolism by increasing blood concentrations of PLP (Manore 2000). An increase in PLP in the blood increases the probability that PLP will be converted to 4-pyridoxic acid and lost in the urine. Thus, exercise may increase the turnover and loss of vitamin B_6 from the body. Research has documented higher 4-pyridoxic acid losses in active individuals compared to sedentary controls or periods of inactivity; higher 4-pyridoxic acid losses have also been documented after strenuous physical activity (Hansen & Manore 2005, Manore 2000). Using 4-pyridoxic acid excretion concentrations, researchers have calculated that marathon runners lost approximately 1 mg of vitamin B_6 during a race (26.2 miles). Thus, based on the current research literature, active individuals may require 1.5–2.5 times the current RDA (approximately 2.0–3.0 mg/day) for vitamin B_6 to maintain good B_6 status (Hansen & Manore 2005, Manore 2000).

FOLATE

Folate is required for a number of enzymes that are critical for DNA synthesis and amino acid metabolism (Manore & Thompson 2000). In addition, folate's role in assisting with cell division makes it a critical nutrient for growth, the synthesis of new cells, such as the red blood cells, and for the repair of damaged cells and tissues. Thus, it is easy to see that folate requirements might be higher with exercise, since damaged muscle tissue needs to be repaired. Finally, folate, vitamin B_{12} and vitamin B_6 are closely interrelated in the metabolism of methionine, an essential amino acid. If these key B vitamins are not available, homocysteine, an intermediate metabolite in methionine metabolism, increases. High blood levels of homocysteine have been associated with an increased risk of cardiovascular disease, and are discussed later in this chapter.

Requirements.   Rich sources of dietary folate include leafy green vegetables, fortified cereals and grains, nuts, legumes, liver and brewer's yeast. If these types of foods are not consumed in the diet, dietary supplementation may be required. The RDA for folate is 400 µg per day for adults, while the UL for folate is 1000 µg per day (IOM 1998).

Assessment of status.   Folate status is assessed by measuring serum folate and red blood cell folate concentrations. With a folate deficiency, the ability to make red blood cells becomes impaired and can eventually lead to megaloblastic anaemia, as the megaloblasts fail to replicate into functional red blood cells. This results in large red blood cells that cannot effectively transport oxygen. Another measure of folate status is mean corpuscular volume (MCV), which is an indication if the red blood cells have increased in size.

Active men typically have adequate intakes of folate due to high-energy intakes (Manore & Thompson 2000). Conversely, Manore (2002) reviewed the research examining dietary intakes of folate in active women and found intakes consistently low, ranging from 126 to 364 µg/day. For example, using 7-day weighed food records, Beals & Manore (1998) reported mean folate intakes for their female athletes (n = 48) to be less than 400 µg/day of folate. Ziegler et al (1999) also found poor mean dietary intakes of folate for male (234 µg/day) and female (275 µg/day) figure skaters, which can be attributed to lower energy intakes.

Research examining the folate status in athletes is limited. When Beals and Manore (1998) examined folate status in their female athletes (~50% reported supplementing), 8% of their athletes were in poor folate status (plasma folate ≤6.8 nmol/L). In this study, supplementation appeared to be a significant contributor to the adequate folate status of the athletes, since folate intakes from food were low. It is recommended that all athletes, both males and females, increase their daily intake of folate to the current RDA of 400 µg/day.

VITAMIN B_{12}

Vitamin B_{12} is part of coenzymes that assist with DNA synthesis, which is necessary for the formation of red blood cells. A deficiency in vitamin B_{12} can lead to pernicious anaemia, which is characterized by large red blood cells similar to that seen with folate deficiency (Manore & Thompson 2000).

Vitamin B_{12} is also essential for the nervous system because it helps maintain the sheath that coats nerve fibres. If these nerve fibres are damaged or altered the conduction of nervous signals is interrupted, causing numerous neurological problems. As mentioned earlier, adequate levels of vitamin B_{12}, folate and vitamin B_6 are also necessary for the metabolism of methionine and keeping blood levels of homocysteine low (Manore & Thompson 2000).

Requirements.   The best dietary sources include meats, fish, poultry, shellfish, eggs, milk and milk products. Because vitamin B_{12} is found almost exclusively in animal products, an athlete following a vegetarian diet needs to include food sources that will provide vitamin B_{12}. Fortunately, many vegetarian food products are fortified with vitamin B_{12}. The risk of poor vitamin B_{12} status is low in active individuals unless animal products are avoided and no supplementation is occurring. The RDA for vitamin B_{12} for adults is 2.4 µg per day, while a UL for vitamin B_{12} has not been determined (IOM 1998).

Assessment of status.   Assessment of vitamin B_{12} status includes measuring the vitamin B_{12} transport proteins, transcobalamin II and haptocorrins, and measuring the concentration of vitamin B_{12} bound to the transport protein (holotranscobalamin II and holohaptocorrins). Additionally, serum vitamin B_{12} and MCV can also be used.

Limited research has examined vitamin B_{12} dietary intakes and status in active individuals. Beals and Manore (1998) examined vitamin B_{12} status in their female athletes and found no athlete with poor vitamin B_{12} status; however, about half of the athletes reported taking a multivitamin supplement. In an earlier study, Telford et al (1992) reported that 3% of their athletes had poor vitamin B_{12} status, but they did not report vitamin B_{12} intakes. Finally, Ziegler et al (1999) found the vitamin B_{12} intakes in their male and female figure skaters were less than that reported by the Third National Health and Nutrition Examination Survey (NHANES III), a national survey measuring the dietary intakes of adults in the United States.

As mentioned earlier, elevated blood homocysteine concentrations are considered another risk factor for cardiovascular disease. Numerous research studies show a strong inverse relationship between blood homocysteine concentrations and dietary intake and/or blood measures of folate, vitamin B_{12} and vitamin B_6; however, little is known about the effects of exercise on blood homocysteine concentrations. Research examining the effect of chronic exercise on homocysteine found that highly active individuals (men and women) had significantly lower homocysteine concentrations than their sedentary counterparts; however, many of these studies have not reported B vitamin intake or status. Conversely, recent research has documented the effects of acute strenuous endurance exercise on blood homocysteine concentrations and found that running a marathon significantly increased homocysteine concentrations, while mountain biking (120 km) or running 100 km had no effect (Herrmann et al 2003). These same researchers also found that training volume impacts blood homocysteine. It has been hypothesized that the combined effects of chronic physical exercise and a high folate and vitamin B_{12}

intake could help reduce plasma homocysteine concentrations and possibly prevent many chronic diseases. Clearly, more research is needed to determine the impact of physical activity on homocysteine concentrations and B vitamin status for athletes.

MINERALS

Athletes, especially female athletes, may have poor intakes of many minerals including calcium, iron, magnesium and zinc (Manore 2002). These low intakes are typically attributed to reduced energy intakes or the restriction of animal products, such as meat, fish, poultry, and dairy products, in the diet. Because meat products are rich sources of iron, zinc and magnesium, and dairy products are good sources of calcium, it is not surprising that dietary intakes of these nutrients are low. Unfortunately, mineral bioavailability is typically low compared to vitamins; thus, improving mineral status requires more time than improving vitamin status. For the athlete, minerals are needed for heart and muscle contractions, enzyme activation, function of the energy pathways, protection against free radicals, and the synthesis of haemoglobin, myoglobin and cytochromes. This section will briefly discuss the research literature for minerals that may be problems for athletes. Table 6.2 lists the functions of minerals that may be low in the diets of active individuals and athletes.

CALCIUM

Calcium serves both a structural and functional role in the body. Calcium is the major mineral found in bone and teeth and participates in muscle contraction, blood clotting and neurotransmitter release. Although calcium is thought of as a primary mineral associated with bone, there are many nutrients associated with good bone health including adequate energy and protein intakes, other minerals (fluoride, magnesium, zinc, copper and manganese) and vitamins (vitamins D, K and C) (Manore & Thompson 2000). In addition, a variety of hormones such as oestrogen, cortisol and thyroid can impact calcium absorption and bone health. Finally, menstrual dysfunction can negatively impact bone growth and maintenance and is a major factor in the poor bone health seen in some active women.

Requirements.   Dairy products are rich sources of dietary calcium. Sardines, oysters, clams, tofu, calcium-fortified foods and dark green leafy vegetables are also good sources of this mineral. The 1997 Dietary Reference Intake (DRI) Adequate Intake (AI) for calcium is 1000 mg/day for adult males and females 19–50 years of age, while the UL for adult men and women is 2500 mg/day (IOM 1997).

Assessment of status.   There are no blood biochemical assessment measures for calcium; however, over 99% of the body's calcium is found in the bones. Therefore, the determination of bone mineral density (BMD) provides an assessment of bone calcium and is the standard currently used to measure total body bone health. In general, good nutrition and physical activity, especially weight bearing activities, improve BMD.

Most females in the United States consume less than the recommended amount of calcium, while intakes for men are adequate. For example, dietary intake data from the NHANES III indicate that young adult females (20– 29 years) in the United States consume approximately 778 mg/day (IOM 1997). As a woman gets older, calcium intakes appear to decrease, with women 30 years or older consuming approximately 760 mg/day. The dietary intakes of calcium for men, however, are typically better; mean intakes are over 1000 mg/day for men 20–39 years of age.

Female athletes, like their sedentary counterparts, also have poor calcium intakes, especially if they eliminate dairy foods from their diet. In general, research studies examining calcium intake in female athletes (both high school and collegiate) report mean intakes ranging from 500 to 1623 mg/day; most studies report mean intakes of calcium below 1000 mg/day (Beals & Manore 1998, Haymes & Clarkson 1998). As expected, female athletes in sports that emphasize thinness (e.g. figure skating, ballet, gymnastics, and track and field events) report the lowest intakes of dietary calcium. For example, it is not unusual for collegiate athletes to have low calcium intakes, yet make no attempt to compensate their diet with additional calcium, either from calcium supplements or non-dairy calcium sources. For example, Beshgetoor & Nichols (2003) also found that mean calcium intakes in non-supplementing female master athletes were only 79% of the 1997 DRI, while Ziegler et al (1999) found that United States female figure skaters consumed only 62% of recommended amounts.

Unfortunately, inadequate intake of calcium increases the risk for poor BMD and stress fractures, especially in female athletes with poor energy intake and/or menstrual dysfunction (Manore 2002, Manore & Thompson 2000). Thus, female athletes need to consume adequate calcium in either dairy foods, calcium fortified products, or supplements. If an athlete is lactose intolerant, adequate calcium should be consumed through the use of other calcium-rich foods and calcium supplements. Optimal calcium absorption and good bone health cannot occur without adequate intakes of vitamin D and normal blood oestrogen concentrations. For athletes that live in northern climates and who exercise primarily indoors, vitamin D status may be poor. For these athletes, a calcium supplement fortified with other bone building nutrients may be recommended. In addition, adequate protein and energy are also important for bone health.

IRON

Iron has many important functions for the athlete; the principal one is the transport of oxygen in the iron-containing proteins haemoglobin from the lungs to the tissues of the body and myoglobin in the muscle (Manore & Thompson 2000). Iron is also a cofactor for enzymes located in the electron transport chain and enzymes required for carbohydrate and protein metabolism.

Requirements.   Two forms of iron are found in the diet: haem iron and non-haem iron. Haem iron is typically found in meat, fish or poultry, while non-haem iron is found in foods such as breads, grains, legumes, vegetables and fruit. Haem iron has a much higher absorption rate than non-haem iron. The current RDA is 18 mg for adult women and 8 mg for adult men (IOM 2001). Because pre-menopausal women lose more iron than men with the monthly menstrual cycle, requirements for younger women are higher than men. The UL for iron is 45 mg per day (IOM 2001).

Assessment of status.   Iron status is typically determined by measuring blood iron parameters, which are used to define stages of iron deficiency (Manore & Thompson 2000). The three stages of iron deficiency are iron depletion, iron deficiency erythropoiesis, and iron deficiency anaemia. Ferritin is the most commonly used assessment of body iron stores and iron depletion is characterized by ferritin concentrations <20 µg/L. Iron deficiency erythropoiesis is characterized by a decrease in plasma iron, an increase in total iron binding capacity, and a decrease in transferrin saturation. Iron deficiency anaemia is characterized by low haemoglobin, haematocrit, and red blood cells that are decreased in number and size.

Normal or high ferritin levels do not always guarantee adequate iron stores. Ferritin is an acute-phase protein and may therefore vary in certain conditions without changes in iron storage. For example, infection, inflammation and other conditions can cause an increase in serum ferritin levels and then mask iron depletion. Because physical activity can be accompanied by an inflammation-like response, it can cause an increase in ferritin levels and make assessment of iron difficult. Soluble transferrin receptor is a marker of iron stores and increases when iron stores are depleted. However, it does not increase in response to inflammation and has recently been used to assess iron status in physically active individuals.

In late 1980s and early 1990s, studies documented that typical dietary iron intakes of female athletes were less than the 1989 RDA of 15 mg/day (Haymes & Clarkson 1998). More recent studies report higher iron intakes in female athletes from diet alone (Beals & Manore 1998); however, there is still a high prevalence of iron depletion (e.g. low serum ferritin concentrations) even when mean dietary intakes are between 17 and 22 mg/day, close to or above the 2001 RDA of 18 mg/day (IOM 2001). Thus, although iron intakes may be at recommended amounts, much of this iron is from non-haem fortified foods, such as highly fortified breakfast cereal, energy and breakfast bars, and fat-free or low-fat snacks, which are poorly absorbed; non-haem iron has a much lower bioavailability in the body. Thus, increasing intake from haem iron sources can improve iron status.

Iron deficiency is one of the most prevalent nutrient deficiencies observed in the female athlete (Haymes & Clarkson 1998). The research literature reports that approximately 15–60% of female athletes have poor iron stores (e.g. low serum ferritin concentrations) compared to 20–30% in the general female population (Haymes & Clarkson 1998). Poor iron status is less common among male athletes than female athletes, but may still be a problem for some male athletes, especially in those that participate in thin-build sports or limit intake of haem iron.

Female athletes have low body stores of iron for a number of reasons. First, female athletes may have poor dietary intakes of iron because they avoid foods high in haem iron, such as meat, fish and poultry. Also, if energy intake is restricted, total daily iron intakes will decrease unless the individual is supplementing. Second, many female athletes follow vegetarian diets, which provide no haem iron; therefore, the bioavailability of the dietary iron that is consumed is reduced. Thus, even though the diet may appear to have adequate iron, the availability of the iron in the diet is poor. Finally, physical activity may increase iron losses in sweat, faeces and urine; furthermore, female athletes have additional iron losses through menstrual blood losses.

To illustrate the prevalence of poor iron status in active individuals, both men and women, Dubnov & Constantini (2004) examined iron depletion, with and without anaemia, in 103 top-level male and female basketball players. They found that iron depletion, defined as a ferritin level $<20\,\mu g/L$, was found in 22% of their participants (15% males; 35% females), while iron deficiency anaemia (ferritin $<12\,\mu g/L$; transferrin saturation $<16\%$; haemoglobin $<12\,g/dl$) was present in 3% of males and 14% of females. Because of the high incidence of iron depletion in active individuals, assessment of iron status, including types of dietary iron sources, should be routinely completed in the athlete. Poor iron status will negatively impact exercise performance by potentially decreasing oxygen-carrying capacity of haemoglobin and decreasing activity of iron-dependent mitochondrial enzymes. Other research has documented that iron depletion will impair any adaptation to aerobic or endurance capacity after exercise training.

Research has demonstrated that supplementation of iron in iron-depleted athletes (e.g. those with low ferritin levels) will improve performance (Brutsaert et al 2003, Friedmann et al 2001). For example, Friedmann et al (2001) randomly assigned 40 young iron-depleted elite female athletes to either iron or a placebo for 12 weeks; the iron-supplemented women had an increase in maximal aerobic performance. In another study, iron supplementation for just 6 weeks improved performance in muscle fatigue in iron-depleted women (Brutsaert et al 2003). Thus, athletes, especially female athletes, are at risk for poor iron status, and may need an iron supplement, even though dietary iron intakes appear adequate. However, iron supplementation in athletes that are not iron depleted does carry the risk for inducing haemochromatosis, especially male athletes.

MAGNESIUM

Magnesium functions as a cofactor for multiple enzymes throughout the body and is required for enzymes of glycolysis, TCA cycle and beta-oxidation (Manore and Thompson 2000). Thus, magnesium plays an important role in the metabolism of carbohydrates, proteins and fats. Magnesium is also required for muscle contraction, protein synthesis and the immune system. Finally, magnesium is part of the structural component of bone. Like iron, athletes can have increased losses of magnesium through sweat and urine, especially with prolonged physical activity (Haymes & Clarkson 1998).

Requirements.   For optimal health and performance, athletes need to include good sources of magnesium in the diet, such as whole grains and cereals, beans and legumes, meat, fish, milk and yogurt, and some nuts (almonds and sunflowers), vegetables (broccoli, green beans, carrots and potatoes) and fruits (bananas). The magnesium density of the typical American diet is ~120 mg of magnesium per 1000 kcal; thus, it is easy to see that by reducing energy intake, magnesium intake will decrease unless special care is taken to consume magnesium dense foods. The RDA for magnesium is 400 mg/day for men 19–30 years; the RDA for older men (31–70 years) is 420 mg/day (IOM 2001). For women 19–30 years, the RDA is 310 mg/day; the RDA for older women (31–70 years) is 320 mg/day (IOM 2001). The UL for magnesium for adults is 350 mg/day from supplements only, and does not include intake from food or water (IOM 2001).

Assessment of status.   Currently, there is not a single biochemical marker to assess magnesium status; thus, status is typically determined by measuring serum or urinary magnesium concentrations. Research studies document magnesium intakes of athletes also to be at or above two-thirds of the RDA (310–320 mg/day) (IOM 1997, Manore & Thompson 2000). As mentioned above, if energy intake is restricted, magnesium intakes can be low. Beals & Manore (1998) reported that 54% of a group of female athletes with subclinical eating disorders (consuming only 1989 kcal/day; 8322 kJ) consumed less than 100% of the RDA for magnesium and 8% of the female athletes consumed less than 66% of RDA. Conversely, in athletes with a higher energy intake (consuming 2293 kcal/day; 9594 kJ), only 17% of the athletes consumed less than the RDA for magnesium and none consumed less than two-thirds the RDA. Other studies also document the importance of energy intakes on dietary magnesium intake in female athletes (see Manore 2002 for a review of this literature). Numerous studies have documented low magnesium intakes in active women with low energy intakes. Although limited in the research literature, some investigators have found low magnesium intakes in male athletes involved in thin-build sports, such as ski jumpers, runners and figure skaters, compared to controls. For example, Ziegler et al (1995) reported low intakes of magnesium in their male figure skaters.

Intense exercise, such as a marathon, has been associated with a shift in body stores of magnesium and an increased loss of magnesium in the urine. Thus, increased losses and poor dietary intakes of magnesium can reduce the body stores of magnesium and affect sports performance. However, no research indicates that magnesium supplementation will improve exercise performance in individuals with good magnesium status.

ZINC

Zinc is involved as a cofactor in many enzyme reactions, including those involved in energy pathways, protein digestion, haem production, anti-oxidant function, and protein and nucleic acid metabolism (Manore & Thompson 2000). Zinc is also important for the repair of tissue. Like the other minerals, physical activity can result in increased losses of zinc through sweat and urine, especially with prolonged physical activity. Exercise may also induce changes in blood zinc concentrations.

Requirements. Small amounts of zinc are found in many foods, including both animal and plant products; however, if energy intakes are restricted, it is difficult to consume adequate minerals unless good food choices are made. Animal foods are better sources of zinc than plant foods. Good sources of zinc include organ meats, other red meats, seafood, poultry, milk and milk products, whole grains, and leafy and root vegetables. The RDA for zinc for adult men and women is 11 and 8 mg/day, respectively, while the UL for zinc for adult men and women is 40 mg/day (IOM 2001).

Assessment of status. As with magnesium, there are no good assessment parameters for zinc; however, plasma and serum zinc are most commonly used for zinc assessment. The body can lose zinc in the urine and sweat.

Dietary intakes of male athletes typically indicate that they are at or above the RDA. However, research has documented that mean dietary zinc intakes of active women are below the RDA of 8 mg/day (Beals & Manore 1998, IOM 2001). These lower intakes of zinc are usually associated with lower energy intakes and lower intakes of animal products. As reviewed by Manore (2002), case studies on amenorrhoeic athletes found that only one of the four women consumed the RDA for zinc. For these women, meat intake was limited to less than two servings per week. Athletes who avoid animal products and limit intakes of whole or fortified cereals and grains may need zinc supplements. Beals & Manore (1998) documented that reduced energy intake can impact zinc intake; female athletes with low energy intakes did not consume the RDA for zinc.

SUMMARY

Micronutrients play important roles in maintaining the health of the active individual and assuring that energy can be produced for physical activity. Athletes who have poor or marginal nutrition status for a micronutrient may have decreased ability to perform exercise at high intensities. Long periods of poor nutrition status, such as poor calcium or iron intakes, can have serious consequences for the athlete and active individual. To obtain adequate status of these micronutrients, nutrient rich foods, such as whole grains, fruits and vegetables, and lean meats and dairy, should be selected and energy intake should be adequate to maintain weight. Athletes who have poor diets, especially those restricting energy intakes, may want to consider supplementing with a multivitamin or mineral.

KEY POINTS

1. Exercise may alter the need for micronutrients due to increased losses and turnover, muscle tissue repair and maintenance and adaptations to metabolic pathways stressed during exercise.
2. Micronutrients most likely to be low in the diets of active individuals include the B vitamins and selected minerals (calcium, iron, magnesium, zinc).
3. Low energy intake can result in low micronutrient intakes, especially if diets are less than 1800–1900 kcal/day.
4. Haemoglobin synthesis requires folate and vitamin B_{12} for cell division and growth and iron and zinc for haem formation.
5. Folate, vitamin B_6 and vitamin B_{12} are important for methionine metabolism. When adequate B vitamins are not available blood levels of homocysteine increase, with higher levels associated with increased risk of cardiovascular disease.
6. Iron depletion and iron deficiency anaemia can both decrease the ability to work due to decreased oxygen transport to the muscles and inadequate iron for electron transport enzymes.
7. Calcium, magnesium, vitamin D and protein are all important nutrients for bone growth and maintenance.

References

Beals KA, Manore MM 1998 Nutritional status of female athletes with subclinical eating disorders. Journal of the American Dietetic Association 98:419–425

Beshgetoor D, Nichols JF 2003 Dietary intake and supplement use in female master cyclists and runners. International Journal of Sport Nutrition and Exercise Metabolism 13:166–172

Brutsaert TD, Hernandez-Cordero S, Rivera J et al 2003 Iron supplementation improves progressive fatigue resistance during dynamic knee extensor exercise in iron-depleted, nonanemic women. American Journal of Clinical Nutrition 77:441–448

Dubnov G, Constantini NW 2004 Prevalence of iron depletion and anemia in top-level basketball players. International Journal of Sport Nutrition and Exercise Metabolism 14:30–37

Friedmann B, Weller E, Mairbaurl H, Bartsch P 2001 Effects of iron repletion on blood volume and performance capacity in young athletes. Medicine and Science in Sports and Exercise 33:741–746

Hansen CM, Manore MM 2005 Vitamin B_6. In: Wolinsky I et al (eds) Sports nutrition. Vitamins and trace elements. 2nd edn. CRC Press, Boca Raton FL, p 81–91

Haymes EM, Clarkson PM 1998 Minerals and trace minerals. In: Berning JR, Steen SN (eds) Nutrition and Sport and Exercise. 2nd edn. Aspen Publishers, Gaithersburg MD, p 77–107

Herrmann M, Schorr H, Obeid R et al 2003 Homocysteine increases during endurance exercise. Clinical Chemistry and Laboratory Medicine 41:1518–1524

IOM (Institute of Medicine), Food and Nutrition Board 1997 Dietary reference intakes: Calcium, phosphorus, magnesium, vitamin D, and fluoride. National Academy Press, Washington DC

IOM (Institute of Medicine), Food and Nutrition Board 1998 Dietary reference intakes: Thiamin, riboflavin, niacin, vitamin B_6, folate, vitamin B_{12}, pantothenic acid, biotin, and choline. National Academy Press, Washington DC

IOM (Institute of Medicine), Food and Nutrition Board 2001 Dietary reference intakes: Vitamin A, vitamin K, arsenic, boron, chromium, copper, iodine, iron, manganese, molybdenum, nickel, silicon, vanadium, and zinc. National Academy Press, Washington DC

Manore MM 2000 Effect of physical activity on thiamine, riboflavin, and vitamin B_6 requirements. American Journal of Clinical Nutrition 72:598S–606S

Manore MM 2002 Dietary recommendations and athletic menstrual dysfunction. Sports Medicine 32:877–901

Manore MM, Thompson JA 2000 Sport nutrition for health and performance. Human Kinetics, Champaign IL

Raczynski G, Szczepanska B 1993 Longitudinal studies on vitamin B_1 and vitamin B_6 status in Polish elite athletes. Biology of Sport 10:189–194

Telford RD, Catchpole EA, Deakin V et al 1992 The effect of 7 to 8 months of vitamin/mineral supplementation on the vitamin and mineral status of athletes. International Journal of Sport Nutrition 2:123–134

van der Beek EJ, van Dokkum W, Wedel M et al 1994 Thiamin, riboflavin and vitamin B_6: Impact of restricted intake on physical performance in man. Journal of the American College of Nutrition 13:629–640

Ziegler, PF, Nelson, JA, Jonnalagadda SS (1999) Nutritional and physiological status of US national figure skaters. International Journal of Sport Nutrition 9:345–360

Chapter **7**

Maintenance of fluid balance in sport and exercise

Susan Shirreffs

LEARNING OBJECTIVES

After studying this chapter, you should be able to:

1. Have an understanding of the science behind the recommendations for drinking before, during and after exercise.
2. Understand the role of electrolytes in fluid balance
3. Understand the role of carbohydrate consumption in fluid balance.
4. Appreciate the differences in optimizing and maintaining fluid balance during and after exercise.

INTRODUCTION

BODY WATER

In healthy individuals, water is the largest single component of the body and the total body water content varies from approximately 45–70% of the total body mass, corresponding to about 31–49 litres for a 70-kg man. Although body water content varies greatly between individuals, the water content of the various tissues is maintained relatively constant. The body water can be divided into two components – the intracellular fluid (ICF) and the extracellular fluid (ECF); the intracellular fluid is the major component and comprises approximately two-thirds of total body water. The extracellular fluid can be further divided into the interstitial fluid (that between the cells) and the plasma, with the plasma volume representing approximately one quarter of the extracellular fluid volume. Although water balance is regulated around a range of volumes rather than a finite set point, its homeostasis is critical for virtually all physiological functions.

To further assure proper regulation of physiological and metabolic functions, the composition of the individual body water compartments must also be regulated. A wide range of electrolytes and solutes are dissolved in varying concentrations within the body fluids. The major cations (positively charged electrolytes) in the body water are sodium, potassium, calcium and magnesium; the major anion (negatively charged electrolytes) is chloride. Sodium is the major electrolyte present in the extracellular fluid, while potassium is present in a much lower concentration: in the intracellular fluid, the situation is reversed, and the major electrolyte present is potassium, with sodium found in much lower concentrations. It is critical for the body to maintain this distribution of electrolytes because maintenance of the transmembrane electrical and chemical gradients is of paramount importance for assuring the integrity of cell function and allowing electrical communication throughout the body.

THERMOREGULATION AND BODY WATER LOSSES

Exercise elevates the metabolic rate and only about 20–25% of the energy made available by the metabolic pathways is used to perform external work, with the remainder being dissipated as heat. When the energy demand is high, as occurs during periods of physical activity, high rates of heat production result. To limit the potentially harmful rise in core temperature, the rate of heat loss must be increased accordingly. The evaporation of 1 litre of water from the skin will remove 2.4 MJ (580 kcal) of heat from the body. As an example, for a 2-hour 30-minute marathon runner with a body mass of 70 kg, to balance the rate of metabolic heat production by evaporative heat loss alone would require sweat to be evaporated from the skin at a rate of about 1.6 litres per hour. At such high sweat rates, an appreciable amount of sweat drips from the skin without evaporating, and a sweat secretion rate of about 2 litres per hour is likely to be necessary to achieve this rate of evaporative heat loss. This is possible, but would result in the loss of 5 litres of body water, corresponding to a loss of more than 7% of body mass for the 70-kg runner. Water is also lost by evaporation from the respiratory tract. During hard exercise in a hot dry environment, this can amount to a significant water loss, although it is not generally considered to be a major heat loss mechanism in man.

In most activities, the energy demand varies continuously; average sweat losses for various sporting activities are well categorized. Even at low ambient temperatures, high sweat rates are sometimes observed when the energy demand is high, so it cannot be concluded that dehydration is a problem only when the ambient temperature and humidity are high. Sweat loss is, however, closely related to the environmental conditions, and substantial fluid deficits are much more common in the summer months and in tropical climates. Body mass losses of 6 litres or more are reported for marathon runners in warm-weather competition. This corresponds to a water deficit of about 8% of body mass, or about 12–15% of total body water. In spite of the large variation among individuals, sweating rate has been found to be related to running speed in a heterogeneous group of marathon runners.

SWEAT ELECTROLYTES

Electrolyte losses in sweat are a function of sweating rate and sweat composition, and both of these vary over time as well as being substantially influenced by the exercise intensity, environmental conditions, and the physiology of the individual. Added to this variability is the difficulty in obtaining a reliable estimate of sweat composition, and these methodological problems have contributed at least in part to the diversity of the results reported in the literature. In spite of the variability in the composition of sweat, however, it is invariably hypotonic with respect to plasma, and the major electrolytes are sodium and chloride, as in the extracellular space. It is usual to present the electrolyte composition of sweat in mmol per litre, and the extent of the sodium losses in relation to daily dietary intake in grams. Loss of 1 litre of sweat with a sodium content of 50 mmol per litre represents a loss of 2.9 grams of sodium chloride. The athlete who sweats 5 litres in a daily training session will therefore lose almost 15 grams of salt. Even allowing for a reduced sweat sodium concentration and a decreased urinary output when sodium losses in sweat are large, this salt loss is large in comparison to normal intake, and it is clear that the salt balance of individuals exercising regularly in the heat is likely to be precarious.

When exercise is undertaken or when an individual is exposed to a warm environment, the additional heat load is lost largely due to sweating and this can increase greatly the individual's daily water loss and therefore the amount that must be consumed. Sweat rates in the order of 2 to 3 litres per hour can be reached and maintained by some individuals for a number of hours and it is not impossible for total losses to be as much as 10 litres in a day. These losses must of course be replaced and when they are so extreme, the majority must be met from fluid consumption rather than food ingestion. A variety of drink types and flavours are likely to be favoured by individuals who have extreme losses to replace.

OPTIMIZING FLUID BALANCE BEFORE EXERCISE

For a person undertaking regular exercise, any fluid deficit that is incurred during one exercise session can potentially compromise the next exercise session if adequate fluid replacement does not occur. In a healthy individual, the kidneys excrete any excess body water; therefore, ingesting excess fluid before exercise is generally ineffective at inducing pre-exercise hyper-hydration. To overcome this, ingestion of either salt or glycerol solutions has been investigated as possible means of minimizing the usual diuresis when a euhydrated individual ingests excess water. A limited amount of temporary hyperhydration occurs when drinks with high concentrations (more than 100 mmol/L) of sodium are ingested, but there are problems of palatability with high sodium drinks and nausea and vomiting with salt tablets. Glycerol has been shown to be an effective hyperhydrating agent. Several studies have suggested that ingesting 1.0–1.5 g glycerol/kg body mass, together with a large volume of water, can significantly increase water retention and improve cycling time to fatigue. Others have observed no differences in thermoregu-latory or performance parameters. In addition, there have been a number of reports of side-effects with glycerol ingestion that preclude this technique as a method of pre-exercise hyperhydration. A review of hyperhydration and glycerol by Latzka & Sawka (2000) came to the conclusion that 'if euhy-dration is maintained during exercise-heat stress then [pre-exercise] hyper-hydration appears to have no meaningful advantage'. However, the practice of drinking in the hours before exercise is effective at ensuring euhydration before exercise if there is any possibility that slight hypohydration is present.

The 1996 American College of Sports Medicine practical recommendation of ingesting 400–600 mL of water 2 hours before exercise to allow the kidneys time to regulate total body water volume has been used to help ensure euhy-dration before laboratory studies. The resulting data of urine osmolality or specific gravity and serum osmolality or hormone measures indicate that the practice is generally effective at achieving euhydration in such circumstances.

OPTIMIZING FLUID BALANCE DURING EXERCISE

In exercise lasting longer than about 30–40 minutes, carbohydrate depletion, elevation of body temperature and reductions in the circulating fluid volume are all potentially important factors in causing fatigue. Clearly all of these can be manipulated by the ingestion of fluids, but this section will not consider either carbohydrate depletion or carbohydrate ingestion during exercise as this is covered elsewhere in this volume in considerable depth (Chapter 3). The exceptions to this, which will be discussed here, relate to the effects carbohydrate ingestion can have on both the rates of water availability in the body from drinks and on water movement across the walls of the intestine.

WHOLE BODY HYDRATION STATUS, ENVIRONMENTAL TEMPERATURE AND ENDURANCE EXERCISE PERFORMANCE

It is frequently recommended (ACSM 1996) that athletes be encouraged to drink fluids at a rate that matches their sweat rate. However, these are general guidelines and they must be viewed with some caution in some circumstances. For example, an athlete with a sweat rate in the order of 3 litres per hour is likely to find it impractical to drink at such high rates.

As humans we are designed to cope with a small amount of both hypo-hydration and hyperhydration: we regulate our body water content over a range of about 0.2% of our body weight on a daily basis (Greenleaf 1992). Therefore, it could feasibly be suggested that a 70-kg athlete is euhydrated if he gains or loses up to 140 mL of water. However, it is also clear that if the extent of hypohydration becomes too great, exercise performance and capacity are reduced. Additionally, it is important to consider the extent to which hypohydration can be tolerated without heat illness. Sam Cheuvront and his colleagues (2003) have surveyed the literature with these questions in mind and the available evidence led the authors to conclude that in situations of exercise in a warm environment (defined as an ambient temperature greater than 30°C), dehydration to the extent of 2–7% of body mass consistently decreased endurance exercise performance. However, the extent of the performance decrements was highly variable, ranging from a reduction of only 7% to a 60% decline. However, a less consistent picture was gleaned when the endurance exercise was undertaken in temperature conditions. It was concluded that in these situations dehydration by 1–2% of body mass had no effect on endurance exercise performance when the exercise duration was less than 90 minutes, but when the level of dehydration was greater than 2% of body mass and the exercise duration was greater than 90 minutes endurance exercise performance was impaired.

So to summarize, dehydration by 2% of body mass during exercise in a hot environment (31–32°C) clearly impairs endurance performance, but when exercise is performed in a temperate environment (20–21°C), dehydration by 2% of body mass appears to have a lesser and insignificant effect on endurance performance. Taken together, these findings suggest that athletes are advised to try to offset dehydration as much as possible when exercising intensely in a hot environment (e.g. 31–32°C) for durations approaching 60 minutes and longer. However, when the environment is temperate (20–21°C), athletes may be better able to tolerate 2% dehydration without significant performance decrement or risk of significantly added hyperthermia compared with exercise with full fluid replacement. In cold environments, dehydration by more than 2% may be tolerable.

DRINK CARBOHYDRATE CONTENT AND FLUID BALANCE

Clearly the most effective drink composition and the optimum amount of fluid ingested during exercise will depend on individual circumstances. However, water is not the optimum fluid for ingestion during endurance exercise, and there is compelling evidence that drinks containing added substrate and electrolytes are more effective. However, while increasing the carbohydrate content of drinks will increase the amount of fuel which can be supplied, it will tend to decrease the rate at which water can be made available (Vist & Maughan 1995). This must be a consideration for fluid balance during exercise. Where provision of water is the priority, the carbohydrate content of drinks and their total osmolality should be low, thus restricting the rate at which substrate is provided. The composition of drinks to be taken will thus be influenced by the relative importance of the need to supply fuel and water, which in turn depends on the intensity and duration of the exercise task, on the ambient temperature and humidity, and on the physiological and biochemical characteristics of the individual athlete. Carbohydrate depletion will result in fatigue and a reduction in the exercise intensity which can be sustained, but is not normally a life-threatening condition. However, disturbances in fluid balance and temperature regulation have potentially more serious consequences, and it may be, therefore, that the emphasis for the majority of participants in endurance events should be on proper maintenance of fluid and electrolyte balance.

DRINK SODIUM CONTENT

The available evidence indicates that the only electrolyte that should be added to drinks consumed during exercise is sodium, which is usually added in the form of sodium chloride, but which may also be added as sodium citrate or other salts. The use of citrate rather than chloride helps stabilize pH and affects taste. Sodium will stimulate sugar and water uptake in the small intestine and will help to maintain extracellular fluid volume as well as maintaining the drive to drink by keeping plasma osmolality high. Most soft drinks of the cola or lemonade variety contain virtually no sodium (1–2 mmol/L), and drinking water (even mineral water) is also essentially sodium-free; sports drinks commonly contain 10–25 mmol/L sodium, and oral rehydration solutions intended for use in the treatment of diarrhoea-induced dehydration have higher sodium concentrations, in the range 30–90 mmol/L. A high sodium content may be important in stimulating jejunal absorption of glucose and water, but it tends to make drinks unpalatable. Drinks intended for ingestion during or after exercise, when thirst may be suppressed and large volumes must be consumed, should have a pleasant taste in order to stimulate consumption.

Hyperthermia and hypernatraemia can be relatively common in endurance events held in the heat, and often affect the less well prepared participants. It has, however, become clear that a small number of individuals at the end of very prolonged events may be suffering from hyponatraemia: this may be associated with either hyperhydration or hypohydration. The total number of reported cases is rather small, and the great majority of these have been associated with ultramarathon or prolonged triathlon events; there are few reports of cases of exercise-associated hyponatraemia where the exercise duration is less than 4 hours. The dangers of ingestion of excessive volumes of fluid without adding salt have long been recognized in various industrial settings, including foundry workers and ships' stokers. It is also well recognized that the inclusion of sodium salts in drinks ingested in these situations is a simple and effective preventive measure. Many of the drinks consumed in endurance events, whether plain water, soft drinks, or sports beverages, have little or no electrolyte content. Even among the drinks intended for consumption by sports men and women during prolonged exercise, most have a low electrolyte content, with sodium concentrations typically in the range of 10–25 mmol/L. This is adequate in most situations, but may not be so when sweat losses and fluid intakes are high. Some supplementation with sodium chloride in amounts beyond those normally found in sports drinks may be required in extremely prolonged events where large sweat losses can be expected and where it is possible to consume large volumes of fluid. This can be achieved by eating solid food. It remains true, however, that electrolyte replacement during exercise is not a priority for most participants in most sporting events. Extra salting of food is an effective strategy for athletes living and training hard in hot weather conditions.

CARDIOVASCULAR, METABOLIC AND PERFORMANCE EFFECTS

Many of the published studies investigating the effects of fluid ingestion on exercise performance have failed to include appropriate control trials that allow the separate effects of water replacement and substrate provision to be assessed. Generally, the studies in the literature have reported either no effect of fluid ingestion on exercise performance or a beneficial effect. In many cases, the absence of a statistically significant effect simply reflects the variability in the assessment methods used and inadequate subject numbers. There seems to be a lessened hyperthermia and cardiovascular drift during prolonged moderate intensity exercise which is attributed to fluid replacement during the exercise. The studies that have reported adverse effects of fluid ingestion on exercise performance have generally been studies in which the fluid ingestion has resulted in gastrointestinal disturbances.

Drinking plain water can improve performance in endurance exercise, but there are further performance improvements when carbohydrate and electrolytes are added. A study that attempted to distinguish between the effects of carbohydrate provision from the water replacement properties of a drink was that conducted in Austin, Texas by Below and colleagues (Below et al 1995). In it, eight men undertook the same cycle ergometer exercise on four separate occasions. After 50 minutes' exercise at 80% of $\dot{V}O_2max$, a performance test at a higher exercise intensity (completion of set amount of work as quickly as possible) was completed; this test lasted approximately 10 minutes. On each of the four trials, a different beverage consumption protocol was followed during the 50 minutes' exercise; nothing was consumed during the performance tests. The beverages were electrolyte-containing water in a large (1330 mL) and small (200 mL) volume and carbohydrate-electrolyte (79 g) solutions in the same large and small volumes; the electrolyte content of each beverage was the same and amounted to 619 mg (27 mmol) and 141 mg (3.6 mmol) of sodium and potassium respectively. The results of the study indicated that performance was 6.5% better after consuming the large volume of fluid in comparison to the smaller volume and was 6.3% better after consuming carbohydrate-containing rather than carbohydrate-free beverages; the fluid and carbohydrate each independently improved performance and the two improvements were additive. The mechanism for the improvements in performance with the large fluid replacement versus the small fluid replacement was attributed to a lower heart rate and oesophageal temperature when the large volume was consumed.

OPTIMIZING FLUID BALANCE AFTER EXERCISE

The main factors influencing the post-exercise rehydration process are the volume and composition of the fluid consumed. The volume consumed will be influenced by many factors, including the palatability of the drink and its effects on the thirst mechanism, although with a conscious effort some people can still drink large quantities of an unpalatable drink when they are not thirsty. The ingestion of solid food, and the composition of that food, may also be important, but there are many circumstances in which solid food is avoided between exercise sessions or immediately after exercise.

DRINK COMPOSITION

Sodium
Plain water is not the ideal post-exercise rehydration beverage when rapid and complete restoration of fluid balance is necessary and where all intake is in liquid form. Early studies in the area established that the high urine flow that followed ingestion of large volumes of electrolyte-free drinks did not allow individuals to remain in positive fluid balance for more than a very short time. They also established that the plasma volume was better maintained when electrolytes were present in the fluid ingested, an effect attributed to the presence of sodium in the drinks. In none of these studies, however, could the mechanism of the action be identified, as the drinks used differed from each other in several respects, including flavouring, carbohydrate and electrolyte content. The first studies to investigate the mechanisms of post-exercise rehydration showed that the ingestion of large volumes of plain water after exercise-induced dehydration resulted in a rapid fall in plasma osmolality and sodium concentration, leading to a prompt and marked

diuresis caused by a rapid return to control levels of plasma renin activity and aldosterone. Therefore, the replacement of sweat losses with plain water will, if the volume ingested is sufficiently large, lead to haemodilution. The fall in plasma osmolality and sodium concentration that occurs reduces the drive to drink and stimulates urine output and has potentially more serious consequences such as hyponatraemia. Sodium is the major ion in the extracellular fluid, thus it is intuitive that sweat sodium losses should be replaced if plasma volume is to be restored or maintained. In a systematic investigation of the relationship between whole-body sweat sodium losses and the effectiveness of beverages with different sodium concentrations in restoring fluid balance, Shirreffs & Maughan (1998) showed that, provided that an adequate volume is consumed, euhydration is achieved when the sodium intake is greater than the sweat sodium loss.

The addition of sodium to a rehydration beverage is therefore justified on the basis that sodium is lost in sweat and must be replaced to achieve full fluid balance restoration. It has also been demonstrated that a drink's sodium concentration is more important than its osmotic content for increasing plasma volume after dehydration. Sodium also stimulates glucose absorption in the small intestine via the active co-transport of glucose and sodium, which creates an osmotic gradient that acts to promote net water absorption. This sodium can either be consumed with the drink or be secreted by the intestine. Furthermore, sodium has been recognized as an important ingredient in rehydration beverages by an inter-association task force on exertional heat illnesses because sodium plays a role in the aetiology of exertional heat cramps, exertional heat exhaustion and exertional hyponatraemia.

Potassium

Potassium is the major ion in the intracellular fluid. Potassium may therefore be important in achieving rehydration by aiding the retention of water in the intracellular space. An initial study investigating this, thermally dehydrated rats by approximately 9% of their body mass and then gave them free access to rehydration solutions consisting of isotonic sodium chloride (NaCl), isotonic potassium chloride (KCl) or tap water. While the rats drank substantially more NaCl than KCl, they urinated only slightly more after consuming the NaCl. The best rehydration was achieved with the NaCl treatment. In this study, whole-body net fluid balance was influenced by the rats' taste preferences for the beverages, in addition to the effects of the drinks on urine production. With the NaCl drink, 178% of the extracellular volume losses were restored, compared with only 50% with the KCl drink. The intracellular volume recovery did not differ significantly between groups but did tend to be higher in the KCl group. The author suggested that, in the extracellular space, restoring sodium concentration is more important than volume restoration but volume restoration has priority in the intracellular fluid. Also, the role of potassium in restoring intracellular volume is more modest than sodium's role in restoring extracellular volume. This topic was subsequently investigated in men dehydrated by approximately 2% of body mass by exercise who then ingested a glucose beverage (90 mmol/L), a sodium-containing beverage (NaCl 60 mmol/L), a potassium-containing beverage (KCl 25 mmol/L) or a beverage containing all three components. All drinks were consumed in a volume equivalent to the mass loss, but a smaller volume of urine was excreted following rehydration when each of the electrolyte-containing beverages was ingested compared with the electrolyte-free beverage. Therefore, there was no difference in the fraction of ingested fluid retained 6 hours after finishing drinking the drinks that contained electrolytes. This may be because the beverage volume consumed was equivalent to the volume of sweat lost and, because of the ongoing urine losses, the participants were dehydrated throughout the entire study, even immediately after the drinking period. The volumes of urine excreted were close to basal values and significant further reductions in output may not have been possible when both sodium and potassium were ingested. An estimated plasma volume decrease of 4.4% was observed with dehydration over all trials, but the rate of recovery was slowest when the KCl beverage was consumed. Potassium, therefore, may be important in enhancing rehydration by aiding intracellular rehydration, but further investigation is required to provide conclusive evidence.

Other electrolytes

The importance of including magnesium in sports drinks has been the subject of much discussion. Magnesium is lost in sweat and many believe that this causes a reduction in plasma magnesium concentrations which has been implicated in muscle cramp. Even though there can be a decline in plasma magnesium concentration during exercise, it is most likely to be due to compartmental fluid redistribution rather than to sweat loss. There does not, therefore, appear to be any good reason for including magnesium in post-exercise rehydration and recovery sports drinks. Sodium is the most important electrolyte in terms of recovery after exercise. Without its replacement, water retention is hampered. Potassium is also included in sports drinks in concentrations similar to those in sweat. Although there is strong evidence for the inclusion of sodium, this is not the case with potassium. There is no evidence for the inclusion of any other electrolytes.

VOLUME TO BE CONSUMED

Obligatory urine losses persist after exercise, even in the dehydrated state, because of the need for elimination of metabolic waste products. Respiratory and transcutaneous losses also contribute to an ongoing loss of water from the body. The volume of fluid consumed after exercise-induced or thermal sweating must therefore be greater than the volume of sweat lost if effective rehydration is to be achieved. This contradicts earlier recommendations that after exercise athletes should match fluid intake exactly to the measured body mass loss. Shirreffs et al (1996) examined the effect of drink volumes equivalent to 50, 100, 150 and 200% of the sweat loss consumed after exercise-induced dehydration equivalent to approximately 2% of body mass. To investigate the possible interaction between beverage volume and its sodium content, a relatively low sodium drink (23 mmol/L) and a moderately high sodium drink (61 mmol/L) were compared. Participants were unable to return to euhydration when they consumed a volume equivalent to, or less than, their sweat loss, irrespective of the drink composition. When a drink volume equal to 150% of the sweat loss was consumed, participants were slightly hypohydrated 6 hours after drinking when the test drink had a low sodium concentration, and they were in a similar condition when they drank the same beverage in a volume of twice their sweat loss. With the high sodium drink, enough fluid was retained to keep the participants in a state of hyperhydration 6 hours after ingesting the drink when they consumed either 150% or 200% of their sweat loss. The excess would eventually be lost by urine production or by further sweat loss if the individual resumed exercise or moved to a warm environment. Calculated plasma volume changes indicated a decrease of approximately 5.3% with dehydration. At the end of the study period, the general pattern was for the increases in plasma volume to be a direct function of the volume of fluid consumed, with the increase tending to be greater for those individuals who ingested the high sodium drink. Additionally, evidence has recently emerged suggesting that the rate of drinking a large rehydration bolus can have important implications for the physiological handling of the drink. Drinking a large single bolus of fluid has the potential to induce a greater decline in plasma sodium concentration and osmolality, which, in turn, have the potential to induce a greater diuresis.

BEVERAGE PALATABILITY AND VOLUNTARY FLUID INTAKE

In most scientific studies in this area, a fixed volume of fluid is consumed; in everyday circumstances, however, intake is determined by the interaction of physiological and psychological factors. When the effect of palatability and solute content of beverages in promoting rehydration after sweat loss was studied, participants drank 123% of the sweat volume losses with flavoured water and 163% and 133% when the solution had 25 and 50 mmol/L sodium. Three hours after starting the rehydration process, the participants had a better whole-body hydration status after drinking the sodium-containing beverages than the flavoured water. In a similar study, participants drank a greater volume of sports drink and orange juice/lemonade mixture than of either water or an oral rehydration solution, reflecting their taste preferences. As expected, urine output was greatest with the low electrolyte drinks that were consumed in the largest volumes (the sports drink and the orange juice/lemonade mixture), and was smallest after drinking the oral rehydration solution.

These studies demonstrate the importance of palatability for promoting consumption, but also confirm earlier results showing that a moderately high electrolyte content is essential if the ingested fluid is to be retained in the body. The benefits of the higher intake with the more palatable drinks were lost because of the higher urine output. Other drink characteristics, including carbonation, influence drink palatability and therefore need to be considered when a beverage is being considered for effective post-exercise rehydration.

FOOD AND FLUID CONSUMPTION

In many cases, there may be opportunities to consume solid food between exercise bouts; this should be encouraged unless it is likely to result in gastrointestinal disturbances. Maughan et al (1996) examined the role of solid food intake in promoting rehydration from a 2.1% body mass sweat loss with consumption of either a solid meal plus flavoured water or a commercially available sports drink. The volume of fluid in the meal plus water was the same as the volume of sports drink consumed. The amount of urine produced after food and water ingestion was almost 300 mL less than that when the sports drink was consumed. Plasma volume decreased by approximately 5.4% with dehydration and was restored to the same extent with both rehydration processes. Although the quantity of water consumed with both rehydration methods was the same, the meal had a greater electrolyte content (63 mmol Na^+ and 21 mmol K^+ vs 43 mmol Na^+ and 7 mmol K^+) and it is most probable that the greater efficacy of the meal plus water treatment in restoring whole-body water balance was a consequence of the greater total cation content causing a smaller volume of urine to be produced. Subsequent studies have also highlighted a role for food products in post-exercise fluid balance restoration.

INTRAVENOUS REHYDRATION

Intravenous fluid therapy has, in the last few years, been used as a rehydration method for dehydrated athletes in cases where it has not been necessary for medical treatment. The argument for its use is based upon perceived health, performance or other benefits over and above those that can be achieved with oral rehydration. In the scientific literature, comparisons have been made between oral and intravenous rehydration from very moderate dehydration on subsequent exercise performance and found no difference in exercise capacity. Similarly, a series of papers reporting a study investigating partial rehydration (from approximately 4% to 2% dehydration) concluded that subsequent exercise performance was better when rehydration occurred irrespective of whether it was by mouth or intravenously. These papers showed that during the subsequent exercise, rectal temperature was lower and heart rate tended to be lower when rehydration had been achieved orally. There is, however, evidence that the sensation of thirst remains higher after partial intravenous rehydration than after partial oral rehydration (flavoured drink with 77 mmol/L Na^+), which is more likely to promote subsequent drinking as required. In combination, these studies provide data both to support and refute intravenous rehydration, particularly when a subsequent exercise bout is to be performed. One potentially practical use of selecting intravenous rehydration over drinking is the case in which significant dehydration is incurred over a short time frame and with a brief rest period before subsequent exercise. For example, a trained and heat-acclimated athlete can sweat at a rate in excess of 2 litres/hour. Assuming that one of two or more daily training sessions lasts 2 hours and 50% of sweat losses are replaced during exercise, a 2-litre deficit occurs and 3–4 litres of fluid must be consumed (150–200% of deficit) to fully restore fluid balance before the next workout. The challenge to rehydrate orally and then perform again could, when limited time is available, be better achieved with intravenous rehydration.

CONCLUSIONS

Substantial whole-body alterations in both fluid and electrolyte balance can occur during or as a result of exercise. These are primarily a result of sweat losses during the exercise but can clearly be modified or prevented by water consumption, either with or without accompanying electrolytes.

For a person undertaking regular exercise, any fluid deficit that is incurred during one exercise session can potentially compromise the next exercise session if adequate fluid replacement does not occur. As such, fluid replacement after exercise can frequently be thought of as hydration before the next exercise bout. However, additional specific issues in this area include ensuring euhydration before exercise and inducing a temporary hyperhydration with sodium salts or glycerol solutions.

During exercise, if it is possible, fluid should be ingested at a rate that is similar to sweat rate, unless sweat losses are very small or they are moderate and the environment is cool. Additionally, during exercise, fluid should never be ingested at rates in excess of sweat rate. As such, body weight (and water content) should not increase during exercise. Consideration should also be given to including sodium in drinks to be consumed during exercise if it lasts more than 2 hours or if the athlete knows they will have high sodium losses.

Complete restoration of fluid balance after exercise is an important part of the recovery process, and becomes even more important in hot, humid conditions. If a second bout of exercise has to be performed after a relatively short interval, the rate of rehydration is of crucial importance. Rehydration after exercise requires not only replacement of volume losses, but also replacement of the electrolytes, primarily sodium, lost in the sweat. Drinks intended specifically for rehydration should probably have a higher electrolyte content than drinks formulated for consumption during exercise. The addition of an energy source does not appear necessary for rehydration, although a small amount of carbohydrate may improve the rate of intestinal uptake of sodium and water, and will improve palatability. The volume of beverage consumed should be greater than the volume of sweat lost to allow for the ongoing obligatory urine losses, and palatability of the beverage is a major issue when large volumes of fluid have to be consumed.

Intravenous rehydration after exercise has been investigated to a lesser extent and its role for fluid replacement in the dehydrated but otherwise well athlete remains open to discussion.

DEFINITIONS

- Euhydration: in water balance.
- Dehydration: the process of losing water.
- Rehydration: the process of regaining water.
- Hypohydration: the steady state of reduced water.
- Hyperhydration: the steady state of increased water.
- Hyponatraemia: low plasma sodium concentration
- Hypernatraemia: high plasma sodium concentration.

KEY POINTS

1. The primary factors influencing the post-exercise rehydration process are the volume and composition of the fluid consumed.
2. The volume consumed will be influenced by many factors, including the palatability of the drink and its effects on the thirst mechanism. Despite this, however, with a conscious effort some people can still drink large quantities of an unpalatable drink when they are not thirsty.
3. Post-exercise rehydration can only be achieved if a fluid volume greater than the sweat volume lost is consumed.
4. Replacement of the sodium lost in sweat is a pre-requisite for retention of drinks consumed after exercise. There is no strong conclusive evidence for the necessary inclusion of any other electrolytes.
5. Plain water is not an effective post-exercise rehydration drink UNLESS sodium is ingested at the same time via solid food.

References

ACSM (American College of Sports Medicine) 1996 Position stand on exercise and fluid replacement. Medicine and Science in Sports and Exercise 28:i–vii

Below RP, Mora-Rodriguez R, Gonzalez-Alonso J, Coyle EF 1995 Fluid and carbohydrate ingestion independently improve performance during 1 h of intense exercise. Medicine and Science in Sports and Exercise 27:200–210

Broad EM, Burke LM, Cox GR et al 1996 Body weight changes and voluntary fluid intakes during training and competition sessions in team sports. International Journal of Sport Nutrition 6:307–320

Burke LM, Hawley JA 1997 Fluid balance in team sports: guidelines for optimal practices. Sports Medicine 24:38–54

Cheuvront SN, Carter III R, Sawka N 2003 Fluid balance and endurance performance. Current Sports Medicine Reports 2:202–208

Coyle EF 2004 Fluid and fuel intake during exercise. Journal of Sports Sciences 22:39–55

Latzka WA, Sawka MN 2000 Hyperhydration and glycerol: thermoregulatory effects during exercise in hot climates. Canadian Journal of Applied Physiology 25:536–545

Maughan RJ, Leiper JB, Shirreffs SM 1996 Restoration of fluid balance after exercise-induced dehydration: effects of food and fluid intake. European Journal of Applied Physiology and Occupational Physiology 73(3-4):317–325

Shirreffs SM, Maughan RJ 1997 Whole body sweat collection in man: an improved method with preliminary data on electrolyte content. Journal of Applied Physiology 82:336–341

Shirreffs SM, Maughan RJ 1998 Volume repletion following exercise-induced volume depletion in man: replacement of water and sodium losses. American Journal of Physiology 274:F868–F875

Shirreffs SM, Taylor AJ, Leiper JB, Maughan RJ 1996 Post-exercise rehydration in man: effects of volume consumed and sodium content of ingested fluids. Medicine and Science in Sports and Exercise 28:1260–1271

Shirreffs SM, Armstrong LE, Cheuvront SN 2004 Fluid and electrolyte needs for preparation and recovery from training and competition. Journal of Sports Sciences 22:57–63

Vist GE, Maughan RJ 1995 The effect of osmolality and carbohydrate content on the rate of gastric-emptying of liquids in man. Journal of Physiology (London) 486(2):523–531

Chapter **8**

Antioxidants and free radicals

Graeme L Close and Frank McArdle

LEARNING OBJECTIVES

After studying this chapter, you should be able to:

1. Define what free radicals are and how are they formed in vivo.
2. Understand the difference between free radicals and reactive oxygen species (ROS).
3. Discuss the sites of ROS formation and their effects on target cells.

4. List some of the key free radicals produced during exercise and how they are formed.
5. Discuss the role of ROS as signalling molecules.
6. Describe what an antioxidant is, and how they are classified.
7. Discuss the effects of antioxidant supplementation on redox regulated transcription factors.
8. Critically evaluate the effects of antioxidants on athletic performance.
9. Critically assess the role of exercise-induced free radical production.
10. Critically address the question 'is oxidative stress a problem for athletes?'.

INTRODUCTION

Mammalian skeletal muscle is capable of producing a large number of free radicals and it is well recognized that a major source of this free radical production occurs during oxygen flux through the mitochondria. Throughout exercise this oxygen flux through the mitochondria can increase 100-fold, potentially resulting in an increased risk of 'oxidative stress', muscle injury and fatigue. However, skeletal muscle is well equipped to deal with this oxidative stress by possessing a number of antioxidant species including both endogenous and exogenous antioxidants. It is only when there are an increased number of free radicals, or a depletion of antioxidant levels that 'redox balance' is disturbed and the cell becomes vulnerable to free radical attack (Fig. 8.1). The purpose of this chapter is to investigate the production of free radicals during exercise and critically evaluate what their role is within the muscle cell. Furthermore, the role of antioxidant supplementation to prevent exercise-induced free radical production will also be examined.

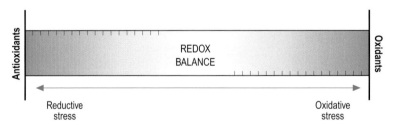

Figure 8.1 Effects of oxidant/antioxidant balance on oxidative/reductive stress. When there is a balance of oxidants and antioxidants homeostasis is achieved, this being known as 'redox balance'. However, when the number of oxidants is greater than antioxidant defences the cell is under 'oxidative stress' and conversely when the number of antioxidants is greater than the oxidants the cell is under 'reductive stress'.

STRUCTURE AND FUNCTION OF FREE RADICALS

The mere fact that oxygen is essential for human survival somewhat eclipses the reality that oxygen is a toxic mutagenic gas. It has long been established that energy production in animals involves the 'oxidizing of fuels', such as carbohydrates and fats. This production of energy is not a direct reaction of oxygen with the 'fuel' but rather a transfer of electrons where molecular oxygen is the final electron acceptor. In air, oxygen exists as a diatomic molecule and should really be called dioxygen. In its ground state, dioxygen has two unpaired electrons with identical spins in its outer shell. This results in the reduction of oxygen being more complicated than most other elements. In this state, oxygen cannot be reduced in one step and therefore the univalent reduction of oxygen is preferred (reduction of oxygen one electron at a time). This univalent reduction of oxygen results in the production of reactive intermediates commonly referred to as 'free radicals'.

A free radical is any species capable of independent existence that contains at least one unpaired electron in its outer shell, and is conventionally depicted as a heavy superscript dot ($R^{\bullet}$) indicating where the unpaired electron is located. For example, the hydroxyl radical is written as $^{\bullet}OH$ showing that the unpaired electron is on the oxygen. Free radicals are formed in one of three ways:

1. The addition of a single electron to a non-radical molecule ($A + e \rightarrow A^{\bullet}$).
2. The loss of a single electron from a non-radical ($A - e \rightarrow A^{\bullet}$).
3. Homolytic fission, i.e. the cleavage of a covalent bond resulting in one electron from the pair shared remaining with each atom ($A : B \rightarrow A^{\bullet} + B^{\bullet}$). (Halliwell & Gutteridge 1999)

Electron transfer (addition or loss of a single electron) is more common than homolytic fission due to the high energy input that is required for homolytic fission to occur (usually through extreme heat, UV light or ionizing radiation) (Cheeseman & Slater 1993). Free radicals are chemically extremely reactive since the unpaired electron attempts to stabilize itself by pairing with another electron. The extent of the reactivity depends upon what the radical is presented with. If the radical meets another radical, a termination reaction occurs and the two radicals become a non-radical:

$$A^{\bullet} + B^{\bullet} \rightarrow AB$$

However, if a radical meets a non-radical, a new radical is formed, thus producing a radical chain:

$$A^{\bullet} + B \rightarrow A + B^{\bullet}$$

This is the most likely scenario since most biological molecules in vivo are non-radicals. The radical chain continues until a termination reaction takes place. The termination reaction can be either when the radical meets another radical, or when it meets an antioxidant (any product that prevents damage by molecular oxygen). Antioxidants will be discussed in more detail later in this chapter.

Free radical reactions result in electrons being removed from the chemical bonds that hold structures together. Radicals are capable of attacking all major structures including proteins, lipids, carbohydrates and nucleic acids, causing irreparable damage to the cell and its genetic material. Importantly, in an exercise setting, lipids are particularly susceptible. Since cell membranes are rich sources of polyunsaturated fatty acids, cell membranes are readily attacked by free radicals, potentially resulting in exercise-induced muscle damage. The destruction of lipid membranes (lipid peroxidation) is said to be especially damaging as it proceeds as a self-perpetuating chain reaction. Lipid peroxidation always results in the formation of reactive aldehydes and these aldehydes can diffuse from the original site of damage to other parts of the cell. Consequently ROS have the ability to cause skeletal muscle damage at either the site of origin or elsewhere. A schematic representation of the bioactivity of free radicals can be seen in Figure 8.2.

TERMINOLOGY IN THE STUDY OF FREE RADICALS

The terms Reactive Oxygen Species (ROS) and free radicals are often used interchangeably in the literature although there is a subtle yet distinct

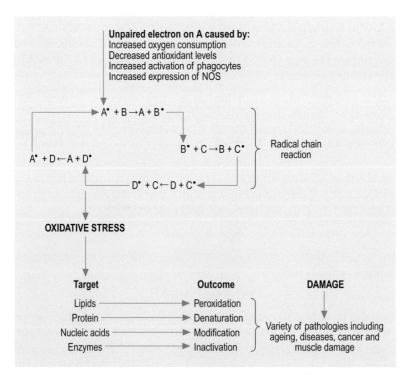

Figure 8.2 Schematic representation of the consequences of free radical chain reactions.

difference between the two. A free radical must contain at least one or more unpaired electrons whereas ROS is a term used to describe both free radicals such as the superoxide anion radical ($O_2^{\bullet-}$), nitric oxide (NO), peroxyl ($RO_2^{\bullet}$) and hydroxyl radical ($^{\bullet}OH$) as well as some non-radical derivatives of $O_2^{\bullet-}$ such as hypochlorous acid (HOCl), singlet oxygen ($^1O_2$), hydrogen peroxide (H_2O_2) and ozone (O_3).

Table 8.1 shows examples of ROS and their major sources.

The generation of ROS causes 'oxidative stress', which is defined as the harmful influence of in vivo oxidation due to an alteration in the body's antioxidant:oxidant ratio.

FREE RADICAL PRODUCTION AND EXERCISE

BRIEF HISTORY OF FREE RADICAL PRODUCTION FOLLOWING EXERCISE

The first evidence of exercise-induced oxidative stress came from Al Tappel's laboratory in the late 1970s. This work demonstrated that there was increased release of pentane (a marker of oxidative stress) in the breath of exercising rats. Interestingly, in these early days of exercise-induced free radical research there were attempts to prevent this production of free radicals through antioxidant intervention due to the assumption that the production of free radicals was deleterious to health. Tappel's group demonstrated that treatment of the rats with the antioxidant vitamin E reduced the observed increase in pentane production and this was presumed to be advantageous.

The next major breakthrough came in 1982 when Kelvin Davies produced the first direct evidence of free radical production by exercising muscle using electron paramagnetic (EPR) spectroscopy. This study demonstrated an increased EPR signal in contracting muscle and liver in rats post-exercise. For the next decade there were many studies reporting equivocal findings on

Table 8.1   Examples of major reactive oxygen species in skeletal muscle and their primary source of origin (modified from Lawler & Powers 1998)

ROS	Primary source
Hydroxyl radical ($^{\bullet}OH$)	$O_2^{\bullet-}$ H_2O_2
Superoxide anion ($O_2^{\bullet-}$)	Electron transport chain Xanthine oxidase Phagocytes
Nitric oxide (NO)	Nitric oxide synthase (NOS)
Peroxynitrite ($ONOO^-$)	$O_2^{\bullet-}$ NO
Hydrogen peroxide (H_2O_2)	$O_2^{\bullet-}$

free radical production by skeletal muscle following exercise. Most of these studies reported changes in indirect markers of oxidation in tissues and blood of exercising subjects, such as malonaldehyde (MDA), oxidation of protein thiols, F2-Isoprostanes, glutathione status etc. However, in 1992 Mike Reid's group in Kentucky (USA) published a landmark study, providing clear evidence of superoxide release from contracting diaphragm muscle. This was the first study to show a specific free radical produced from contracting muscle.

Today, the field of free radical production by skeletal muscle is considerable, highlighted by the fact that entering the keywords 'free radical' and 'muscle' into the scientific search engine 'pubmed' produces over 10 500 hits. Work from our laboratory has spent several years attempting to identify specific ROS produced following skeletal muscle contraction, and using the novel technique of in vivo microdialysis we have now demonstrated that following a period of isomeric contractions in animal models, superoxide, hydrogen peroxide and hydroxyl are all released into the extracellular fluid (Close et al 2005a).

EXAMPLES OF SPECIFIC ROS PRODUCED DURING EXERCISE

Superoxide anion ($O_2^{\bullet-}$)

Superoxide is the one electron reduction product of oxygen and is formed in almost all aerobic cells.

$$O_2 + e^- \rightarrow O_2^{\bullet-}$$

Superoxide is produced deliberately by phagocytes, assisting in the inactivation of viruses and bacteria, although it can also be formed from 'accidents of chemistry'. A major cellular source of superoxide is electron leakage from the mitochondria and endoplasmic reticulum. In aqueous solutions superoxide is not particularly reactive although it is dangerous to biological systems as it can be easily converted to more potent ROS, including H_2O_2 by superoxide dismutase and spontaneous dismutation that can then result in the generation of the extremely potent hydroxyl radical.

Hydrogen peroxide (H_2O_2)

Hydrogen peroxide is not strictly a free radical although it can react to generate more reactive free radicals. In vivo, most of the hydrogen peroxide generated is produced enzymaticaly by the dismutation of superoxide (as seen below):

$$2O_2^{\bullet-} + 2H^+ \xrightarrow{\text{Superoxide dismutase}} H_2O_2 + O_2$$

Hydrogen peroxide can also be produced by oxidase enzymes in vivo including xanthine oxidase. In its molecular structure, hydrogen peroxide resembles water and is extremely diffusible within and between cells. Although hydrogen peroxide is a weak oxidizing agent (and has been described as less reactive than superoxide), it can readily be converted to more potent radicals, such as hydroxyl, and is therefore extremely cytotoxic. In biological systems, hydrogen peroxide can be long lived and is able to travel a considerable distance. Hydrogen peroxide, unlike superoxide which requires anion channels, is able to cross cell membranes, resulting in oxidative stress at sites distant to its origin. Although the major cytotoxicity of hydrogen peroxide is through its conversion to hydroxyl, hydrogen peroxide can itself cause the inactivation of several enzymes. An example of this is that glyceraldehyde-3-dehydrogenase, which is an important enzyme in glycolysis, is inactivated by hydrogen peroxide and therefore chronic exposure of cells to hydrogen peroxide can result in ATP depletion and therefore potentially premature fatigue.

Hydroxyl radical ($^{\bullet}$OH)

Hydroxyl is one of the most reactive of all known ROS. It was originally suspected that hydroxyl was formed directly by the reaction of superoxide with hydrogen peroxide in a reaction termed the 'iron catalysed Haber–Weiss reaction':

$$O_2^{\bullet-} + H_2O_2 \xrightarrow{\text{Fe–Catalysed}} {}^{\bullet}OH + OH^- + O_2$$

However, it has since been shown that the rate constant for this reaction in aqueous solutions is virtually zero. In vivo, hydroxyl is more likely to occur via Fenton chemistry as seen below:

$$O_2^{\bullet-} + Fe^{3+} \rightarrow Fe^{2+}$$
$$Fe^{2+} + H_2O_2 \rightarrow {}^{\bullet}OH + OH^- + Fe^{3+}$$

Hydroxyl radicals have an extremely short half-life (Table 8.2) and thus do not migrate any significant distance within the cell. Therefore, when hydroxyl is formed in vivo it reacts with and damages any molecule in its immediate vicinity including proteins, carbohydrates, DNA and lipids at a diffusion-limited rate.

Nitric oxide (NO)

Nitric oxide is synthesized from the amino-acid L-arginine by vascular endothelial cells, certain cells in the brain, and phagocytic cells. Despite the

Table 8.2   Some of the major ROS and their relative half-lives

ROS	Half-life
Superoxide ($O_2^{\bullet-}$)	10^{-6} seconds
Hydroxyl ($^{\bullet}$OH)	10^{-12} seconds
Nitric oxide (NO)	~30 seconds
Hydrogen peroxide (H_2O_2)	Minutes

fact that nitric oxide is a free radical, it is usually written as NO with the absence of the superscript dot. This is probably a result of the unpaired electron being delocalized between the nitrogen and the oxygen atom. Nitric oxide is continuously generated in quiescent skeletal muscle by nitric oxide synthase (NOS) and this production increases during exercise. Nitric oxide is often useful in skeletal muscle acting as a vasodilator and an important neurotransmitter as well as being involved in the killing of parasites by macrophages. However, over-production of nitric oxide can be cytotoxic, both directly and by its reaction with superoxide, to form peroxynitrite ($ONOO^-$), a ROS that is more potent than either of its parent species.

SITE OF ROS PRODUCTION IN SKELETAL MUSCLE

In order to allow a greater understanding into the role of free radicals following exercise, it is necessary to identify their site of production. However, identification of the site of ROS production is extremely difficult, largely due to the rapid half-lives of ROS and the fact that there are multiple pathways of ROS generation in skeletal muscle. These pathways include the mitochondrial electron transfer system, xanthine oxidase within endothelial cells, NAD(P)H oxidase, infiltrating phagocytes and nitric oxide from nitric oxide synthase.

Oxidative phosphorylation takes place in the mitochondria where molecular oxygen undergoes a four-electron reduction catalysed by cytochrome oxidase. It has been estimated that approximately 95–98% of the total oxygen consumption is reduced in this way (Halliwell 1994). The remaining 2–5% may undergo a one-electron reduction, resulting in the formation of superoxide. If superoxide then undergoes a further one-electron reduction, hydrogen peroxide is produced. McCord (1985) estimated that for every 25 oxygen molecules reduced by 'normal' respiration, one free radical is produced. Therefore, increased oxygen flux through the mitochondria electron transport chain could result in the increased production of ROS. It is therefore not surprising that the mitochondria have a well-developed system for protection against ROS, possessing a specific mitochondrial superoxide dismutase (MnSOD) to prevent against superoxide mediated degeneration of biomolecules.

During exercise there is increased oxygen demand. Oxygen consumption during intense exercise can rise up to 15-fold resting levels and more importantly, oxygen flux in an active muscle can increase up to 100-fold, placing greater demands on MnSOD and the other antioxidant defences; consequently this pathway is considered to be the major source of ROS both by quiescent and active skeletal muscle.

A further source of ROS production during exercise is xanthine oxidase. Xanthine oxidase is localized in the capillary endothelium of most human tissues including skeletal muscle, where it serves to catalyse the oxidation of hypoxanthine to xanthine as well as the oxidation of xanthine to uric acid. McCord (1985) proposed that during ischaemia there is an activation of a calcium-dependent protease that results in the formation of xanthine oxidase from xanthine dehydrogenase as well as the breakdown of ATP with the formation of AMP via the adenylate kinase reaction. AMP is then further metabolized to hypoxanthine, this being a substrate for xanthine dehydrogenase and xanthine oxidase. Xanthine oxidase may then use molecular oxygen as an electron acceptor, resulting in the formation of xanthine and superoxide.

Furthermore, several cells in the immune system can also produce large quantities of ROS, including monocytes/macrophages, eosonophils and neutrophils. Interestingly, all of these cells demonstrate significant activation during and following various forms of exercise. The ability of neutrophils to produce ROS and specifically target these against microorganisms is absolutely essential in host-defence. ROS are produced by neutrophils to attack bacteria, viruses and, in the case of exercise-induced muscle damage, to attack degenerated cells. Once inside the muscle tissue, and when the neutrophils are exposed to a phagocytic stimulus, there follows an 'oxidative' or 'respiratory' burst which is characterized by an increase in oxygen consumption. In this oxidative burst, molecular oxygen is initially reduced to superoxide by the activation of the NAD(P)H oxidase and then further reduced to hydrogen peroxide. Catalysed by myeloperoxidase, hypochlorous acid (HOCl) may then be subsequently formed from hydrogen peroxide. Further reactions can then result in the production of the highly reactive hydroxyl either through the Fenton reaction or from the reaction of superoxide with hypochlorous acid.

MEASUREMENT OF ROS

Many of the discrepancies in the literature regarding ROS production and exercise may be attributed to the difficulties and inaccuracies in the measurement of ROS. It is difficult to directly detect ROS in biological systems, largely because they exist in low concentrations, react almost immediately at their formation sites, and therefore have no capacity to accumulate (Table 8.2).

There are currently many methods available to assess ROS generation although the vast majority of these involve the measurement of end products of ROS reactions, such as products of lipid peroxidation (e.g. malonaldehyde), products of DNA oxidation (e.g. 8-hydroxydeoxyguanosine) or end products of protein oxidation (e.g. production of protein carbonyls or loss of thiols). These end products are often referred to as 'footprints' of ROS reactions.

Other commonly cited methods of detecting ROS activity involve the assessment of endogenous antioxidant levels such as glutathione peroxidase and catalase. Depletion of endogenous antioxidant levels would suggest an antioxidant response to an oxidative challenge. One of the only techniques available to directly detect free radicals involves electron paramagnetic resonance (EPR) spectroscopy. It is beyond the scope of this chapter to fully describe EPR spectroscopy and therefore the reader is referred to Symons (1978). Briefly, the basic feature of EPR is the ability to detect and characterize the presence of an unpaired electron. When an unpaired electron is exposed to an external magnetic field it aligns itself either parallel or antiparallel to that field, creating two possible energy levels. Transition between these different energy levels can be induced by absorption of a photon of appropriate frequency, creating an absorption spectra, and this can be detected by EPR and the specific species identified by their spectra.

Despite the known advantages of EPR, its use in exercising humans is still limited to a few studies (e.g. Ashton et al 1999, Bailey et al 2003, Close et al 2004). The reason for this is that EPR is expensive, time consuming and requires significant expertise. Jackson (1999) suggested that in view of a lack of any gold standard of free radical assessment, where possible a multi-assay approach should be used, measuring:

1. Endogenous antioxidant levels
2. 'Footprints' of free radical activity such as MDA, and
3. A direct measure of free radicals using EPR spectroscopy.

ROS AS SIGNALLING MOLECULES

It should now be clear that skeletal muscle generates a number of ROS during contraction, including superoxide, hydrogen peroxide, nitric oxide and hydroxyl. If this was unregulated then the effects of increased ROS production by repeated bouts of exercise on target cells would be disastrous. Therefore skeletal muscle has the unique ability to adapt to the oxidative stress of exercise and this adaptation is crucial to the survival of this tissue. An inability of these terminally differentiated muscle cells to adapt in this way would be catastrophic.

There is now compelling evidence to suggest that ROS themselves act as signalling molecules, both directly and indirectly, to control the activity of multiple transcription factors leading to modulation of the expression of genes controlled by these factors (for a review see Close et al 2005b). These transcription factors include HSF1, NFkB, AP-1 NRF-1, Tfam and PGC-1, which are all crucial in the adaptive responses to exercise.

The transcription factors NFkB and AP-1 result in the increased production of antioxidant enzymes such as catalase, superoxide dismutase and glutathione peroxidase. These antioxidant enzymes are the main cellular defence against ROS damage. The role of these antioxidant defence proteins will be discussed in detail later in this chapter.

HSF1 results in the increased production of a highly conserved family of proteins known as heat shock proteins (HSPs) which are also involved in protecting the muscle cell. In unstressed skeletal muscle, HSPs are present in low levels and in this situation are thought to act as molecular chaperones, binding to newly synthesized proteins and ensuring that these newly synthesized proteins are correctly folded and function correctly. Work in our labs has demonstrated that increased production of superoxide during exercise results in a transient and reversible oxidation of protein thiol groups within the muscle which is accompanied by an increased production of HSPs in skeletal muscle (for a review see Close et al 2005b). This transient and reversible oxidation of protein thiols may be the signal for the activation of adaptive responses, especially HSPs. This hypothesis is supported by further studies from our laboratory. We initially demonstrated that there is increased muscle HSP content following an acute period of non-damaging exercise in humans with an associated increase in ROS production. However, this increase in HSPs was attenuated following vitamin C supplementation which attenuated ROS production.

NRF-1, PGC-1 and Tfam are redox regulated transcription factors crucial in adaptation to physical exercise. Part of the adaptive response that occurs with training is mitochondrial biogenesis resulting in improved athletic performance. Studies from 'Pepe' Vina's laboratories in Valencia (Spain) have suggested that attenuation of ROS by antioxidant supplementation prevents mitochondrial biogenesis and diminishes the observed training effect. This will be discussed in more detail later in this chapter.

In summary, increased production of ROS appears to initiate a cascade of adaptive responses producing changes in the expression of a number of cytoprotective proteins, which provide additional protection to the muscle. Furthermore, there is also some evidence to suggest that mitochondrial biogenesis which is crucial to increased fitness associated with exercise training may also occur through ROS regulated transcription factors. Therefore, it is becoming increasingly evident that ROS play a crucial physiological role in skeletal muscle, acting as signals for the muscle cell to adapt, as well as the more often cited pathological role. Furthermore, prevention of ROS production following exercise may prevent ROS working as signalling molecules. This will be discussed in more detail later in this chapter.

STRUCTURE AND FUNCTION OF ANTIOXIDANTS

The first living organisms on earth survived under an atmosphere containing little oxygen and essentially were anaerobic. Rising atmospheric oxygen concentration, due to the evolution of photosynthetic organisms, resulted in many of these anaerobes becoming extinct. The few remaining anaerobes have adapted to the current oxygen concentration of 21% by restricting themselves to environments where oxygen could not penetrate. Not all animals did this and a second line of defence was developed, this being the evolution of an antioxidant system to protect them against the toxicity of atmospheric oxygen (Halliwell 1994).

By definition an antioxidant is any compound (usually organic) that prevents or retards oxidation by molecular oxygen, thus conferring some protection from the damaging effects caused by ROS. Cellular antioxidant defences may be categorized as either enzymatic or non-enzymatic. Primary enzymatic antioxidants include superoxide dismutase (SOD), glutathione peroxidase (GPX) and catalase. As well as the primary enzymatic antioxidants, there are also a number of enzymes that do not directly prevent or remove ROS, but play a significant role in the supply of substrates and reducing power for primary enzymatic antioxidants. Such enzymes include glutathione reductase (GR), glucose-6-phosphate dehydrogenase (G6PDH) and glutathione sulphur-transferase (GST). Non-enzymatic antioxidants include ascorbate, α-tocopherol and β-carotene, and have the ability to directly scavenge certain radicals including superoxide and the more potent hydroxyl radical.

Antioxidants can also be classified according to where they are synthesized. These include antioxidants that are synthesized endogenously under oxidative stress, for example glutathione, and those that cannot be synthesized endogenously and must therefore be taken in through diet, for example, ascorbic acid or α-tocopherol. This system of classification emphasizes the importance of nutrition on cellular antioxidant stores. Endogenous antioxidants work in concert with their exogenous counterparts, providing defences against ROS. Endogenous antioxidant supplies are not able to completely prevent oxidative stress and consequently dietary antioxidants are essential to maintain cellular redox balance.

EXAMPLE OF SPECIFIC ANTIOXIDANTS

Ever since data were produced that demonstrated exercise could induce an oxidative stress, and the assumption that this was damaging, many workers have used a variety of antioxidant compounds in order to reduce this stress. The compounds described below are just a few examples of the many used.

VITAMIN C

Vitamin C is the generic name for substances that provide the biological activity of L-ascorbic acid ($C_6H_6O_8$). Vitamin C is a water-soluble, dietary antioxidant present in the cytosolic compartment of the cell and the extra-cellular fluid, and is known to be a powerful inhibitor of lipid peroxidation in plasma. The putative effect of vitamin C occurs though both direct and indirect methods. Vitamin C can function directly as an antioxidant, interacting with superoxide and hydroxyl, although it is better known for its relationship with vitamin E. The spatial arrangement of vitamin C allows it to scavenge aqueous phase vitamin E radicals generated in the cell membrane during oxidative stress, through its ability to rapidly donate electrons to vitamin E radicals. After donating an electron, vitamin C can then be oxidized to a semihydroascorbate (SDA) radical, this being a much less reactive substance. SDA radicals are then either converted directly to ascorbate by the enzyme SDA reductase, using nicotinamide adenine dinucleotide (NADH) or indirectly converted to vitamin C in the presence of glutathione. Ascorbate also acts indirectly through its ability to regenerate oxidized vitamin E.

It should also be noted that in high concentrations vitamin C can also act as a pro-oxidant. The pro-oxidant effects of vitamin C occur through its ability to reduce ferric iron (Fe^{3+}) to its ferrous form (Fe^{2+}) (Powers et al 2004). As previously shown, the ferrous from of iron is an important catalyst in many redox reactions, for example the production of hydroxyl from hydrogen peroxide via Fenton chemistry ($Fe^{2+} + H_2O_2 \rightarrow {}^{\bullet}OH + OH^- + Fe^{3+}$).

VITAMIN E

Naturally occurring Vitamin E is in fact not one compound but a complex mixture of eight closely related molecules known at tocopherols and tocotrienols. Of all of these molecules, α-tocopherol has been shown to be the most effective antioxidant, and the terms vitamin E and α-tocopherol have now become freely transposable in both scientific and commercial forums. Due to the chemical structure of α-tocopherol, it is highly hydrophobic, and thus lipid soluble. As a result of this, it tends to associate with lipids in biological systems and has its primary function in lipid-rich environments such as various cellular and intracellular membranes.

When a lipid molecule is oxidized, this oxidation is propagated to adjacent lipid molecules, via radical formation, in a chain reaction, which results in the oxidation of many target molecules. α-Tocopherol has been demonstrated to be the major chain-breaking antioxidant in lipid membranes, thus stopping the oxidative chain reaction and limiting the propagation of oxidative damage to the lipid membrane involved.

The chemistry involved in 'chain breaking' relies on the fact that α-tocopherol reacts much more quickly with lipid radicals than do lipids, thus, rather than lipid radical to lipid molecule propagation of oxidation, lipid radical to α-tocopherol takes place. The resulting α-tocopheryl radical is reconverted to α-tocopherol mostly by the ascorbate system, but other compounds including glutathione and ubiquinol may be involved. This chemistry demonstrates complex interactions between the different arms of the antioxidant defences, and the heavy dependency that exists between them.

α-Tocopherol can also act as a free-radical scavenger of other reactive species, including singlet oxygen, superoxide and hydroxyl radicals, thus blocking the start of lipid oxidation, before the chain reaction occurs.

Analysis of the structure of α-tocopherol reveals the presence of two functional groups, a chromanol ring group and a phytol side chain (Fig. 8.3). Both of these groups are essential for the natural antioxidant activity of α-tocopherol, with the phytol side chain anchoring α-tocopherol into lipid membranes, thus bringing the 'antioxidant' chromanol head group into close association with these lipids where it can exert its major effects.

GLUTATHIONE

Glutathione is a naturally occurring tripeptide (glutamine-cysteine-glycine) and is the most abundant source of non-protein thiol groups in most organ systems. Glutathione can act as a direct antioxidant by reaction with free radicals, or indirectly in cooperation with antioxidant enzyme systems.

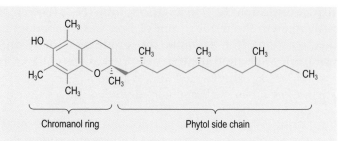

Figure 8.3 Structure of vitamin E.

It has been shown that glutathione can react directly with various free-radical species. These include both carbon centred and hydroxyl radicals. The mechanism of these reactions involves the donation of a hydrogen atom by glutathione to the reactive species.

The indirect antioxidant effects of glutathione centre around its role as a cofactor for the antioxidant glutathione peroxidase enzyme family (Fig. 8.4). These enzymes are able to metabolize both hydrogen peroxide and organic peroxides, again, by hydrogen atom donation supplied by reduced glutathione. During this process two molecules of glutathione are used and oxidized glutathione is formed. Oxidized glutathione is a dimmer of reduced glutathione that have been linked via a disulphide bridge between their cysteine residues. This oxidized glutathione is then recycled to the reduced form by glutathione reductase, which uses NADPH to donate hydrogen atoms back to the oxidized glutathione, resulting in the production of two molecules of the reduced

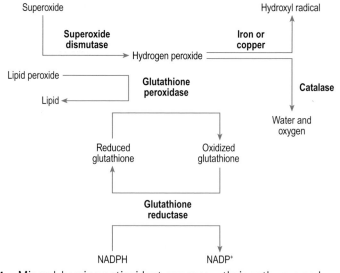

Figure 8.4 Mineral-bearing antioxidant enzymes – their pathways and interconnections.

form. Glutathione has also been implicated in the recycling of various other cellular antioxidants.

Supplementation with glutathione has no effect of cellular glutathione levels, as it is hydrolysed to its constituent amino acids at the gut level. However, studies have shown that supplementation with N-acetylcysteine (a cysteine, thus glutathione precursor) will maintain glutathione levels during periods of oxidative stress.

LIPOIC ACID (THIOCITIC ACID; 1,2-DITHIOLANE-3-PENTANOIC ACID)

Lipoic acid is a naturally occurring thiol-containing compound, normally found in association with a mitochondrial enzyme complex responsible for the decarboxylation of α-keto acids. The tight association to this enzyme complex, coupled with the very low levels of 'free' lipoic acid observed in body tissues and fluids, has prompted the argument that lipoic acid does not act as a natural antioxidant in vivo (Packer 1994).

However, many in vitro studies have shown that a 'free' lipoic acid/ dehydrolipoic acid couple is an extremely powerful and effective reducing agent, capable of directly reducing oxidized glutathione back to its active form, regenerating ascorbate (vitamin C) from oxidized dehydroascorbate, and reducing the α-tocopheryl radical back to active α-tocopherol (vitamin E). Theoretically, lipoic acid may also regenerate α-tocopherol indirectly due to its action on dehydroascorbate, with the reformed ascorbate then reducing the α-tocopheryl radical back to active α-tocopherol in a coupled reaction.

Lipoic acid may also act as an indirect antioxidant by reducing free-radical generation, rather than mopping up preformed oxidants. This effect is due to the fact that lipoic acid has some affinity for both iron and copper ions, producing complexes in which the metal ions are poorly available for free-radical generating reactions such as the Fenton reaction.

These in vitro studies, together with the fact that dietary administration has no obvious toxic effects, have prompted the use of supranutritional levels of lipoic acid in various animal and human trials, aimed at elevating the tissue and body fluid levels of 'free' lipoic acid, thus allowing this compound to exert its numerous antioxidant properties.

ANTIOXIDANT MINERALS

Mineral ions can be found in association with various antioxidant enzymes, including catalase (iron), the superoxide dismutase family of enzymes (manganese, copper, zinc) and the glutathione peroxidase family of enzymes (selenium). These enzymes tend to work in cooperation and are capable of detoxifying many reactive species including superoxide, hydrogen peroxide, and various other organic peroxides (Fig. 8.4).

Under normal circumstances, the metal ions present in these enzymes are at optimal concentration, and manipulation of intake will result in no great change in their enzyme activity. However, selenium is an exception to this rule. It is thought that selenium intake in various parts of the world is suboptimal (including the UK, various parts of mainland Europe and New Zealand), with a resultant decrease in the activity of the enzyme activities associated with it.

As stated previously, the main antioxidant enzymes associated with selenium are the glutathione peroxidase family. This family comprises of at least four discrete enzymes, each with their own genes. These are cytosolic glutathione peroxidase, circulating glutathione peroxidase, phospholipids hydroperoxide glutathione peroxidase, and gastrointestinal glutathione peroxidase. Although their site of synthesis and amino acid sequence differs, they have a common role in the detoxification of reactive oxidants.

One property of this enzyme family which sets it aside from the other mineral-containing antioxidant enzymes is the mode of incorporation of the selenium into their peptide structure. Other mineral-containing enzymes hold the mineral within their structure by chelation using molecular forces; however, the selenium-containing glutathione peroxidases have a quite different method. These enzymes (and all other selenoproteins) incorporate selenium within their peptide chain as the selenium analogue (selenocysteine) of the sulphur amino acid cysteine. This incorporation is directed at the level of the gene, which uses a specific nucleotide triplet to direct the insertion of a selenocysteine residue into the growing peptide chain. Without exception, this residue is always placed at the active site of the enzyme and plays a critical role in the detoxifying function of these enzymes.

As can be seen in Figure 8.4, the activity of all of the glutathione peroxidase family is dependent on the availability of both reduced glutathione (consequently glutathione reductase activity), the levels of total glutathione and the availability of NADPH. This again demonstrates the cooperation between various metabolic pathways, and how the manipulation of one may influence the activity of another.

However, it has been demonstrated that supplementation with selenium will significantly increase the activity of many of the antioxidant enzymes associated with it. The interpretation of this assay of activity (as with all others) should be made with care, as it is an in vitro test, and does not evaluate other in vivo factors which may limit in vivo enzyme activity.

EXERCISE-INDUCED OXIDATIVE STRESS – IS THIS A PROBLEM FOR ATHLETES?

As previously stated, during exercise the oxygen flux through mitochondria can increase by up to 100 times resting levels. It would therefore seem logical that this automatically places athletes at an increased risk of oxidative stress, especially those engaged in regular aerobic endurance training such as cyclists, rowers and distance runners. Since we have already stated that oxidative stress can destroy lipid membranes, cause DNA mutations, inactivate enzymes and denature proteins, it would appear that athletes are subjecting themselves to significant cytotoxic stress every time they train or compete.

However, anecdotal evidence suggests that this is clearly not the case. It is generally accepted that regular aerobic exercise is beneficial to health and can result in increased lifespan and, therefore, increased exercise is unlikely to be detrimental to health. The reason for this is due to the cellular adaptation that occurs following an oxidative stress. As previously stated, increased exposure to ROS causes the up-regulation of a number of redox regulated transcription factors resulting in increased cellular content of anti-oxidant defence systems. It would therefore appear that the body is able to up-regulate antioxidant defences to deal with increased oxidative stress, maintaining redox balance and homeostasis. However, the question regarding antioxidant supplementation and exercise performance is a little more confusing.

ANTIOXIDANTS AND ATHLETIC PERFORMANCE – DEFICIENCIES AND SUPPLEMENTATION IN ATHLETES

Many research groups have investigated the feasibility that deficiencies in antioxidant defences could be detrimental to performance. For example, Davies et al (1982) looked at ROS responses from vitamin E deficient rats following exercise to exhaustion. The authors reported that vitamin E deficient rats had a 40% reduction in endurance performance compared with that of non-deficient controls. Similar findings have also been reported by other groups, for example Packer et al (1986) in exercising guinea pigs, and Coombes et al (2002) in exercising rats. It should be noted though that all of these studies were performed in animal models, and interestingly, such results have not been replicated using human subjects. Recently, however, Watson et al (2005) reported increased ratings of perceived exertion in human subjects following 2 weeks of dietary antioxidant restriction; although it must be stressed that no significant effects on exercise performance were noted in terms of either time to exhaustion or changes in aerobic capacity. Therefore it should be concluded that despite the greater oxidative stress and ratings of perceived exertion observed by Watson et al (2005), antioxidant restriction had no significant effects on performance. Even Bunnell et al (1975), whose study involved humans being vitamin E deficient for 13 months, dropping blood levels of tocopherol from 1.42 to 0.81 mg/100 mL, reported no significant effects on muscle strength.

The differences observed between animals and humans could be due to differences in responses between rodents or humans, although it is more likely a result of the differing levels of depletion between human and animal studies. It would appear that antioxidant restriction only affects performance at extreme clinically deficient levels and such dietary restriction is both unethical and dangerous; consequently, extreme vitamin deficient diets do not occur in human trials. An example of this can be seen by comparing the dietary restriction protocols of Watson et al (2005) and Coombes et al

(2002). Watson et al (2005) restricted their humans subjects to no more than 1–2 portions of fruit or vegetables per day whereas the diets imposed by Coombes et al (2002) involved their rats being fed a diet containing no vitamin E at all for 12 weeks, this being a far more severe depletion of vitamin E.

Powers et al (1988) highlighted the extreme nature of the vitamin deficiency needed to affect exercise performance in humans. The authors investigated the running performance in Gambian children who had evidence of clinical vitamin deficiencies. Children were given a vitamin mixture including vitamin C, riboflavin and ferrous sulphate for 9 weeks prior to performing an exercise test. The results demonstrated that supplementing antioxidants to antioxidant deficient children had no significant effects on running performance, suggesting that performance was not restricted by the clinical vitamin deficiencies.

There is growing evidence to suggest that excessive vitamin C supplementation may actually prevent adaptation to training. Vina et al (2005) studied the effects of 12 weeks of daily vitamin C supplementation (500 mg/kg body weight) during a 12-week training period, on the running performance of rats. Data suggest that this excessive supplementation with vitamin C not only did not improve performance, but moreover supplementation prevented improvements in performance capacity compared with placebo-fed controls. The authors concluded that ROS production is necessary for mitochondrial biogenesis associated with exercise training and therefore supplementation with antioxidants may impair adaptation to the training due to inactivation of transcription factors. It should be stressed, however, that the doses given in this research were far in excess of doses given to human subjects and therefore until this is repeated using physiological doses some caution should be exerted when interpreting these data.

There is also evidence in animal studies that high levels of antioxidant supplementation may be detrimental to exercise performance. For example, Coombes et al (2001) demonstrated that vitamin E supplementation (10 000 U/kg) combined with alpha lipoic acid (1.6 g/kg) for 8 weeks depressed force production at low frequencies (<40 Hz) compared with placebo-fed controls. Similarly, Marshall et al (2002) fed racing greyhounds 1 g per day of vitamin C and reported that supplementation slowed the greyhounds by 0.2 seconds, which equated to 3 metres over a 500-metre race.

It would therefore appear that extremely low levels of dietary antioxidants could impair performance; however, such levels are never observed in athletes and moreover, levels so low would have a multitude of negative effects, not simply adverse athletic ability. Therefore there appears to be no need for athletes consuming a healthy diet to supplement antioxidants in an attempt to directly improve athletic performance, and furthermore, excessive supplementation could impair performance and/or inhibit mitochondrial biogenesis and production of HSPs associated with the training (Fig. 8.5).

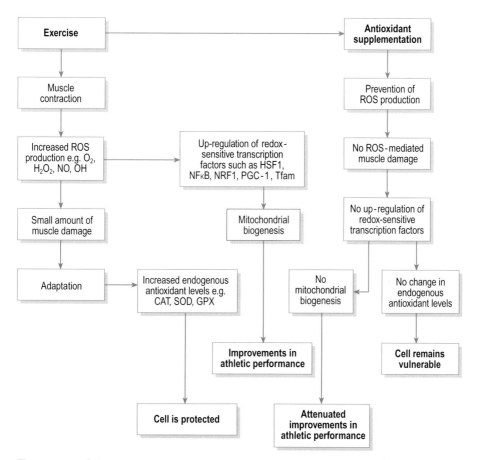

Figure 8.5   Schematic showing proposed interaction between exercise, ROS production and cellular adaptation.

ANTIOXIDANT SUPPLEMENTATION AND EXERCISE–INDUCED MUSCLE DAMAGE

Although it is known that extreme deficiencies might adversely affect athletic performance (although it is not thought to occur in athletes), there still remains the question of does antioxidant supplementation prevent exercise-induced muscle damage and consequently improve future performance? It is generally recognized that various forms of exercise results in increased markers of oxidative stress including non-damaging protocols such as a $\dot{V}O_2$max test (Ashton et al 1999), as well as damaging protocols such as downhill running (Close et al 2004). Since increased ROS production has been associated with exercise-induced muscle damage and prolonged losses of muscle function, it has been suggested that supplementation with antioxidants could increase recovery and hence improve subsequent performance. Furthermore, it has been shown in animal models that approximately 3 days following muscle-damaging exercise there is a secondary small loss of muscle force that is likely to be attributable to ROS, and therefore the use of antioxidant supplementation to prevent this has been proposed.

Studies investigating antioxidant supplementation and the recovery from exercise-induced muscle damage have given rise to equivocal findings. Many studies have demonstrated that antioxidant supplementation may attenuate some of the markers of exercise-induced oxidative stress such as increased EPR signal (Ashton et al 1999, Close et al 2004) or protein carbonyls and MDA (Goldfarb et al 2005) and even attenuated secondary losses in muscle force (McArdle et al 2001). It could therefore be concluded that antioxidant supplementation reduces post-exercise muscle damage and could improve future performance. However, such a conclusion should not be made. The mere presence of ROS at a time similar to the observed pathology (i.e. post-exercise muscle damage) should not be used to imply ROS as the cause; this conclusion should only be made following antioxidant intervention. There is some modest evidence to suggest that antioxidant supplementation may alleviate some of the symptoms of delayed onset muscle soreness, although other studies have not shown any effect (see Close et al 2005c for a review). Moreover, evidence regarding improved subsequent performance following antioxidant supplementation is lacking. We have recently shown that vitamin C supplementation may result in a delayed recovery of muscle function following muscle-damaging exercise, thus potentially impairing future performance.

It is proposed that inhibition of cellular oxidation has little effect on the scale of muscle damage that occurs and as such plays no part in improving future performance; however, ROS inhibition through antioxidant supplementation may inhibit subsequent adaptive responses. Consequently it can be concluded that whereas the role of an increased ROS production in exercise-induced damage remains equivocal, there is ever-increasing evidence that increased ROS production plays a major role as a signalling mechanism for adaptation of skeletal muscle following exercise. Therefore there does not appear to be any physiological benefits of antioxidant supplementation to increase recovery time from damaging exercise and again the use of antioxidants in this manner should be questioned.

CONCLUSIONS AND RECOMMENDATIONS

The key to the story appears to be back to cellular redox balance (Fig. 8.1). Although the body is clearly subjected to increased levels of ROS during periods of intense exercise, it is able to account for this by increasing cellular antioxidant enzymes achieved through the up-regulation of redox-sensitive transcription factors, maintaining redox balance. There is no convincing evidence that athletes are deficient in exogenous antioxidants and therefore the need for supplementation must be questioned. Although exogenous antioxidants such as vitamins C and E are important in maintaining redox balance it must be stated that these vitamins are required in relatively small amounts, and these amounts are usually consumed in a healthy diet. For example, the RDA for vitamin C is ~60 mg per day and supplementation of 1000 mg per day (a value seen in many over-the-counter vitamin supplements) is not only unnecessary but may prevent adaptation to the exercise.

Evidence regarding beneficial effects of antioxidant supplementation on performance is also lacking, although their effects on preventing exercise-induced muscle damage is somewhat equivocal. There is some evidence that following lengthening muscle contractions, secondary muscle damage occurs approximately 3 days post-exercise which may be, at least in part, attributable to reactive oxygen species. Some studies have demonstrated attenuation of this damage through antioxidant supplementation and have therefore advocated the use of antioxidants. However, the question must again be asked as to what is the role of ROS following such exercise. There is increasing evidence that the role of ROS is to act as signalling molecules, signalling the cell to adapt, preventing future damage. Furthermore, it is known that phagocytic cells produce ROS and specifically target these against micro-organisms, and that this process, known as 'the oxidative burst' is essential in host defence. ROS are produced by phagocytes to attack bacteria, viruses and, in the case of exercise-induced muscle damage, to attack degenerated cells. Consequently, as opposed to the most often cited pathological role of ROS, there is growing evidence that ROS produced following exercise may play a key physiological role, both assisting the cell to recover from the initial damage and protecting the cell from future events. With this knowledge, combined with the lack of evidence that antioxidant supplementation has any beneficial effects on athletic performance, the use of antioxidant supplementation in athletes consuming a healthy diet should not be recommended.

KEY POINTS

1. Free radicals are constantly produced by mammalian skeletal muscle. At rest this production of free radicals is usually matched by antioxidant defence systems maintaining 'redox balance'. These antioxidant defence systems include both endogenous antioxidants such as glutathione and exogenous antioxidants such as vitamin C.
2. Exercise increases the production of free radicals, largely due to increased oxygen flux through the mitochondria but also through alternative pathways including xanthine oxidase within endothelial cells, NAD(P)H oxidase, phagocytes and nitric oxide from nitric oxide synthases.
3. Free radicals are capable of attacking all major structures including proteins, lipids, carbohydrates and nucleic acids, causing irreparable damage to the cell and its genetic material.

continued

KEY POINTS — cont'd

4. However, there is growing evidence that free radicals also act as signalling molecules, controlling the activity of a number of transcription factors. This results in the up-regulation of antioxidant defence enzymes and cytoprotective proteins. Therefore, in response to exercise, the body is able to up-regulate antioxidant defences, maintaining redox balance.
5. There is no conclusive evidence to suggest that athletes should supplement antioxidants to improve performance or to increase recovery time. Conversely, there is growing evidence to suggest that large doses of antioxidants may delay recovery and/or attenuate the beneficial adaptations to training.

ACKNOWLEDGMENTS

The authors would like to thank the biological and biotechnological scientific research council (BBSRC), the food standards agency (FSA) and world cancer research fund (WCF) for their continued financial support, and Professor Malcolm J. Jackson and Dr Anne McArdle (University of Liverpool) for their scientific advice in the preparation of this chapter.

References

Ashton T, Young IS, Peters JR et al 1999 Electron spin resonance spectroscopy, exercise, and oxidative stress: an ascorbic acid intervention study. Journal of Applied Physiology 87:2032–2036

Bailey DM, Davies B, Young IS et al 2003 EPR spectroscopic detection of free radical outflow from an isolated muscle bed in exercising humans. Journal of Applied Physiology 94:1714–1718

Bunnell RH, De Ritter E, Rubin SH 1975 Effect of feeding polyunsaturated fatty acids with a low vitamin E diet on blood levels of tocopherol in men performing hard physical labor. American Journal of Clinical Nutrition 28:706–711

Cheeseman KH, Slater TF 1993 An introduction to free radical biochemistry. British Medical Bulletin 49:481–493

Close GL, Ashton T, Cable T et al 2004 Eccentric exercise, isokinetic muscle torque and delayed onset muscle soreness: the role of reactive oxygen species. European Journal of Applied Physiology 91:615–621

Close GL, Ashton T, McArdle A, Jackson M 2005a Microdialyis studies of extracellular reactive oxygen species in skeletal muscle: Factors influencing the reduction of cytcochrome c and hydroxylation of salicylate. Free Radicals in Biology and Medicine. Available online 9th August 2005

Close GL, Kayani A, Vasalaki A, McArdle A 2005b Skeletal muscle damage with exercise and aging. Sports Medicine 35:413–427

Close GL, Ashton T, McArdle A, MacLaren DPM 2005c The emerging role of free radicals in delayed onset muscle soreness and contraction induced muscle injury. Comparative Biochemistry and Physiology Part A: Molecular & Integrative Physiology 142:257–266

Coombes JS, Powers SK, Rowell B et al 2001 Effects of vitamin E and alpha-lipoic acid on skeletal muscle contractile properties. Journal of Applied Physiology 90:1424–1430

Coombes JS, Rowell B, Dodd SL et al 2002 Effects of vitamin E deficiency on fatigue and muscle contractile properties. European Journal of Applied Physiology 87:272–277

Davies KJA, Quintanilha AT, Brooks GA, Packer L 1982 Free radicals and tissue damage produced by exercise. Biochemical and Biophysical Research Communications 31:1198–2005

Goldfarb AH, Bloomer RJ, McKenzie MJ 2005 Combined antioxidant treatment effects on blood oxidative stress after eccentric exercise. Medicine and Science in Sports and Exercise 37:234–239

Halliwell B 1994 Free radicals and antioxidants: a personal view. Nutrition Reviews 52:253–265

Halliwell B, Gutteridge JMC 1999 Free radicals in biology and medicine. Oxford University Press, Oxford

Jackson MJ 1999 An overview of methods for assessment of free radical activity in biology. Proceedings of the Nutrition Society 58:1001–1006

Lawler J, Powers S 1998 Oxidative stress, antioxidant status, and the contracting diaphragm. Canadian Journal of Applied Physiology 23:23–55

McArdle A, Pattwell D, Vasilaki A et al 2001 Contractile activity-induced oxidative stress: cellular origin and adaptive responses. American Journal of Physiology and Cell Physiology 280:C621–C627

McCord JM 1985 Oxygen derived free radicals in post-ischaemic tissue injury. New England Journal of Medicine 312:159–163

Marshall RJ, Scott KC, Hill RC et al 2002 Supplemental vitamin C appears to slow racing greyhounds. Journal of Nutrition 132:1616S–1621S

Packer L 1994 Antioxidant properties of lipoic acid and its therapeutic effects in prevention of diabetes complications and cataracts. Annals of the New York Academy of Sciences 783:257–264

Packer L, Gohil K, deLumen B, Terblanche SE 1986 A comparative study on the effects of ascorbic acid deficiency and supplementation on endurance and mitochondrial oxidative capacities in various tissues of the guinea pig. Comparative Biochemistry and Physiology. B: Comparative Biochemistry 83:235–240

Powers HJ, Bates CJ, Downes R et al 1988 Running performance in Gambian children: effects of water-soluble vitamins or iron. European Journal of Clinical Nutrition 42:895–902

Powers SK, DeRuisseau KC, Quindry J, Hamilton KL 2004 Dietary antioxidants and exercise. Journal of Sports Science 22:81–94

Symons M 1978 Chemical and biochemical aspects of electron spin resonance. Van-Nosstrand-Reinhold, London

Vina J, Gomez-Cabrera M, Domenech E et al 2005 Free radicals generated in exercise act as signals to modulate mitochondrial biogenesis and the expression of antioxidant genes. Free Radical Research 39:S31

Watson TA, Callister R, Taylor R et al 2005 Antioxidant restriction and oxidative stress in short-duration exhaustive exercise. Medicine and Science in Sports and Exercise 37:63–71

Chapter 9

Dietary supplements and nutritional ergogenic aids

Ron J Maughan

LEARNING OBJECTIVES

After studying this chapter, you should be able to:

1. Appreciate the prevalence of use of supplements in sports.
2. Balance the perceived efficacy of supplements with their cost.
3. Categorize supplements according to their perceived effects.
4. Evaluate the efficacy of selected supplements from research findings.
5. Be aware of the possible adverse effects of some supplements.

INTRODUCTION

Nutritional ergogenic aids may be defined in many different ways. Taking a literal but narrow definition, that of nutrients shown to be capable of improving exercise performance, results in the identification of no more than a handful of entities that meet these criteria. If the definition is extended to include any substance ingested by mouth that may improve exercise performance, then the list embraces most of the many hundreds or even thousands of products to be found on the shelves of sports nutrition stores.

There is, or at least should be, a distinction between dietary supplements, which are substances that are added to the diet and which may or may not be normal components of foodstuffs and may or may not have a defined role in nutrition and metabolism, and nutritional supplements which are, or which contain, normal dietary components and which have a well established role in human nutrition. The vitamins, for example, can clearly be categorized as nutritional supplements, but boron, though it is normally present in foods and is widely sold as a supplement, plays no essential role in human metabolism (Bender & Bender 1997).

A full evaluation of the evidence for and against many hundreds of supplements on sale to athletes and of the contexts in which they are, or should be, used is clearly beyond the scope of this short review, and the reader is referred to some of the more extensive reviews available (Maughan 1999, Maughan et al 2004, Talbott 2003).

PREVALENCE OF SUPPLEMENT USE

There are many published surveys of reported supplement use among various groups of athletes. Although many of these can be criticized individually, the overall picture is of widespread use of supplements. It is important to recognize, however, that the overall picture of supplement use among athletes is perhaps not very different from that in the general population. A meta-analysis of 51 published surveys involving 10 274 male and female athletes suggested an overall prevalence of use of about 46% (Sobal & Marquart 1994). A survey of almost 8500 adult Americans conducted between 1998 and 2002 showed an overall prevalence of supplement use of about 19% (Kelly et al 2005). Data from the US National Health and Nutrition Examination, another survey of US adults carried out over a similar time period, however, showed that 52% of respondents in the survey reported the use of at least one dietary supplement within the preceding month (Radimer et al 2004). The discrepancy reflects the ambiguity inherent in many of the survey instruments used as to what constitutes a supplement and how usage is defined.

COSTS AND BENEFITS

It seems clear that supplements should be used only after a careful cost-benefit analysis has been conducted. On one side of the balance are the rewards, the most obvious of which is an improved performance in sport, and on the other side lie the costs and the risks. Vitamin and mineral supplements are generally perceived as being harmless, and the one-a-day multivitamin tablet is seen as an insurance policy 'just in case'. Many herbal products are also used, even though there is little or no evidence to support their claimed benefits. The fact that most of these supplements enjoy only brief periods of popularity before disappearing from the marketplace suggests that any benefits perceived by athletes are not strong enough to warrant continued use or recommendation to friends and colleagues. Although these supplements are mostly benign, this is not always the case. Routine iron supplementation, for example, can do more harm than good, and the risk of iron toxicity is very real (Eichner 2000).

Under current legislation that governs the manufacture, distribution and use of supplements in most countries there is no requirement for sellers to show that products are safe before they are offered for sale. In many cases, there have been no long-term toxicity studies; given the tendency for athletes to exceed the recommended doses of supplements and to use various combinations of different supplements, it seems unlikely that such prospective studies will ever be done. Safety should always be a primary consideration, but athletes seeking to gain a competitive advantage are reluctant to wait until safety and efficacy are proved before deciding to use a particular product. The American Food and Drugs Administration (FDA), prompted in part by a number of fatalities associated with supplement use, is now proposing to introduce legislation that will regulate the manufacture and distribution of dietary supplements (Food and Drugs Administration 2003). At present, however, dietary supplements are not evaluated by regulatory agencies and inaccurate labelling of ingredients is known to be a problem. Internet selling has also effectively removed most of the national controls that are in place to protect the consumer.

There is limited information on the efficacy of most of the dietary supplements currently on sale. The margin between success and failure in sport is often vanishingly small – usually measured in fractions of one per cent, but even with the most careful standardization of experimental conditions, the sensitivity of laboratory tests of exercise performance may not allow them to identify effects that are meaningful to the athlete (Hopkins et al 1999). Failure to show statistically significant effects of supplement use in laboratory trials of exercise performance may not mean that there is not a beneficial effect for the athlete. Most laboratory tests of supplement use do not have adequate statistical power to give confidence in the outcome, and they often also lack the precision and validity necessary to extrapolate to the athletic arena. They are usually conducted over only short timescales, and use subject populations that are not representative of the target consumer group.

Athletes who take supplements often have no clear understanding of the effects of the supplements they are using, and commonly cited sources of information include coaches, fellow athletes and lay magazines. Much of the information available to athletes and those who advise them is produced by the supplement sellers themselves, and cannot be expected to give an unbiased view. Professional help is therefore needed to inform the decisions made by athletes.

CATEGORIES OF SUPPLEMENTS

Athletes take supplements for many different reasons, but the primary driving factor is the prospect of an improved performance in competition. Supplements may be broadly categorized by their target function as follows:

1. Promoting tissue (muscle) growth and repair
2. Weight loss and fat loss
3. Enhancing energy supply and delaying fatigue
4. Promoting immune function and resistance to illness and infection
5. Central nervous system effects
6. Maintaining joint health
7. Promoting recovery after training or competition
8. Sports drinks, energy bars, etc.

Supplements may come in many different forms. Some are normal foods, taken at a specific time for a specific purpose. Many supplements are purified or concentrated food components, while others are more exotic edible compounds, often of plant origin. Although doping agents are clearly defined according to the schedules issued by the World Anti-Doping Agency and periodically updated, there is a category of supplements that has a pharmacological action, but are not prohibited (caffeine is a good example of such a compound) and there are others that can be effective in improving performance but whose use is not prohibited.

SUPPLEMENTS THAT MAY BE EFFECTIVE

As indicated above, athletes should use supplements only when there is good evidence of efficacy in their chosen sporting environment. It must be recognized, however, that such specific information is seldom available and that, at best, athletes have to work on a balance of probabilities. A single study, from one laboratory (often with a financial interest in the product), involving only a few (often less than 10) non-athletic subjects engaged in an unfamiliar and artificial test of cycling capacity may be the only information available. For many supplements, only a few in vivo data are available, and unrealistic extrapolations are made from these. This is certainly not an adequate basis on which to use a supplement. It may take many years before a sufficient body of information has been generated by a number of independent laboratories. Athletes are understandably reluctant to wait until efficacy is proved, when careers in sport may be short and may end at any time. Generation of information on safety should be a priority, but this normally takes even longer.

In assessing whether to use a supplement, the balance between evidence of efficacy and the risk of an adverse effect is not an equal one. Where the potential for harm is extremely small, an athlete may consider it worth experimenting with a supplement to see whether a performance benefit ensues.

The evidence for a beneficial effect of glucosamine on joint health, for example, is not entirely convincing, but there are no reported adverse effects, so the athlete who suffers from joint pain may feel justified in using it. There is now a considerable amount of information from clinical trials involving patients with osteoarthritis to show that regular (once or twice per day) long-term (about 2–6 months) treatment with glucosamine and chondroitin sulphate can reduce the severity of subjective symptoms and prevent further deterioration of joint function. It is less clear that athletes with joint pain of other aetiologies will also experience benefit. A meta-analysis of published studies concluded that 'some degree of efficacy appears probable for these preparations' but did express some cautions about the quality of the available data (McAlindon et al 2000). A more recent report (Braham et al 2003) of the effects of 12 weeks of supplementation in individuals with knee pain showed similar improvements in clinical and functional tests in the treatment and placebo groups, but 88% of the treatment group reported some improvement in knee pain compared with only 17% in the placebo group. Some would interpret the available evidence as suggesting that there may be 'responders' and 'non-responders', in which case a statistically significant effect on a mixed population may not be forthcoming. The absence of a well-defined mechanism of action is of no concern to the athlete who experiences subjective relief.

Only a few supplements can be considered here, but fuller details of these and of other supplements can be found in Talbott (2003) and in Maughan et al (2004).

BICARBONATE

Acute ingestion of large doses (0.3 g/kg body mass) of sodium bicarbonate induces a metabolic alkalosis that persists for some hours. This has the potential to improve performance in events where high rates of anaerobic glycolysis result in a metabolic acidosis. This would typically apply to events lasting from about 1–15 minutes. There is good evidence that performance may be substantially improved, but there is also a significant risk of intestinal distress, which can be debilitating. There are no significant acute or long-term health risks from occasional use in competition.

CAFFEINE

Caffeine has metabolic, cardiovascular and central nervous system effects that can improve exercise performance. Mechanisms of action are still under debate, but there is evidence of effects on strength, power and endurance, with clear implications for many sporting events. Caffeine is a weak diuretic, but this action is often over-emphasized. Recommendations to avoid caffeine use when hydration status may be stressed are probably counter-productive: total fluid intake may fall if these beverages are eliminated from the diet and the adverse effects of acute caffeine withdrawal may compromise performance. Use of caffeine is not restricted under current sport doping regulations, but its use is monitored by WADA. Performance effects are seen at low doses (2–3 mg/kg body mass), which can easily be achieved by drinking coffee, cola or other caffeine-containing beverages (Cox et al 2002). Caffeine is well absorbed in the mouth, and it escapes first-pass metabolism in the liver when absorbed by this route. There is evidence that athletes and others are now using caffeine-containing chewing gum and oral patches to achieve controlled intakes of caffeine.

CREATINE

Creatine use is widespread in strength and power sports and it has become one of the most popular supplements in the last decade. Creatine is normally present in meat, and the diet of the non-vegetarian supplies about 1 g per day. The daily requirement is about 2 g, so any not supplied from the diet must be synthesized from amino acid precursors. Ingestion of about 10–20 g of creatine for 4–5 days can substantially increase the total creatine content of skeletal muscles and about two-thirds of this is in the form of creatine phosphate. Increasing the availability of this high-energy source can lead to improvements in events lasting a few seconds, especially when repeated short sprints are performed with incomplete recovery. There is also evidence of significant strength gains after only a few days of supplementation. Supplementation is often accompanied by an acute gain of 1-2 kg of body mass, most of which is water (skeletal muscle is 75% water). Creatine has generated much controversy as it can be effective in improving performance (although not all studies show a positive effect, the balance of the available evidence does support this), but its use is not prohibited in sport at the present time. There are no reports of adverse effects on health or performance from long-term use, but only limited evidence is available.

CARNITINE

Carnitine is sold widely in health stores and in sports shops and is promoted as an agent for increasing fat metabolism. For athletes this would have the effect of sparing glycogen stores and thus increasing endurance: it could also help in weight-sensitive sports where athletes must compete in a specific weight category or where performance is impaired by a high body fat content. Carnitine is also sold as an obesity treatment capable of reducing body fat stores in the overweight population. L-carnitine has two important functions in muscle: it is involved in transfer of fatty acids across the mitochondrial membrane for oxidation, and it buffers any increase in mitochondrial acetyl CoA concentration, maintaining the free CoA concentration. There is therefore a potential for increasing endurance performance by increasing fat metabolism because of the key role played by carnitine in the transport of fat into mitochondria and regulating metabolism in the mitochondria. If carnitine supplementation is to be effective, it should increase the carnitine content of muscle and increase fat oxidation. At the present time, however, there is no evidence that muscle carnitine levels can be increased by carnitine supplements and there is no evidence that fat metabolism is increased by carnitine supplements. There is also no experimental evidence from properly controlled studies to show an improvement in exercise performance. On the basis of the available information, there is currently no scientific basis for advising healthy athletes to supplement their diets with L-carnitine in an attempt to improve athletic performance. In addition, the use of D-carnitine, which is present in some supplements, should be avoided as it may cause a deficiency of L-carnitine and could decrease performance. In spite of the absence of evidence, carnitine sales remain buoyant.

PROTEIN AND AMINO ACIDS

A high lean body mass, and especially a high muscle mass, confers a definite advantage in sports that require strength and power. The idea that athletes need a high-protein diet to achieve a high muscle mass is intuitively attractive, and indeed there is evidence that the requirement for protein is increased by physical activity. It is hardly surprising, therefore, that protein supplements are perhaps the most popular dietary supplement in sport. Although there is an increased need for protein, however, this can easily be met from the diet provided that energy intake is sufficient to meet energy demands, and specific protein supplementation is seldom warranted. Because of the high energy intakes of athletes in training, even a diet with a lower than normal protein content (perhaps as low as 8–10% of total energy intake, compared to the 12–15% in the diet of the 'normal' population) can meet protein needs. There is some evidence that the timing of protein intake may be important, and high-protein supplements and high-protein energy bars may be a convenient way to meet this need in athletes. There is little evidence to support beneficial effects of supplementation with individual amino acids, but free form amino acids are widely used in sport.

ADVERSE EFFECTS OF SUPPLEMENTS

Anyone purchasing a dietary supplement might feel entitled to expect that it contains the ingredients stated on the label and nothing else. There is, however, a large body of evidence to show that some supplements may not meet the standards that consumers expect. In contrast to the tight regulations that govern the manufacture of pharmaceuticals, there is no requirement for supplement manufacturers to adhere to the same degree of quality during the manufacture, storage and distribution of their products. The lack of a requirement for strict quality control in the manufacture of dietary supplements has resulted in some products failing to meet the expected standards. The American Food and Drugs Administration (FDA) has required some manufacturers to recall a number of products (Food and Drugs Administration

2003). Product recalls because of inadequate content include a folic acid product with only 34% of the stated dose. The FDA has also recently recalled
products containing excessive doses of vitamins A, D, B_6 and selenium
because of potentially toxic levels of these components. Some products have
been shown to contain potentially harmful impurities (lead, broken glass,
animal faeces, etc.) because of poor manufacturing practice.

There is a further concern regarding the use of dietary supplements that
affects mainly the elite athlete who is liable for drug testing under the regulations of the World Anti-Doping Agency (WADA). The regulations that
govern drug abuse in sport are based on the principle of strict liability and
the offence lies in the presence of a prohibited substance in the athlete's
urine sample rather than in the deliberate consumption of that substance.
A consequence of this is that an athlete is responsible for ensuring that any
supplement ingested is free from prohibited substances that could give rise
to a positive test. There is, however, no easy way for the athlete to know what
compounds may be present in any supplements they purchase.

It may seem that it should be easy to ensure that a product is free from
contamination, but this is not so. Analysis for prohibited substances requires
sophisticated equipment and is expensive. It also cannot guarantee the
absence of prohibited substances. In the case of nandrolone, for example, a
positive test may result from the ingestion of as little as 2–3 µg of nandrolone
(19-nortestosterone) or of the related compounds 19-norandrostenedione and
19-norandrostenediol: both of these latter compounds have been sold as
dietary supplements, although both are now specifically included on the
WADA list of examples of prohibited steroids. The sensitivity of the analytical
procedures for the presence of these compounds is about 1 µg per gram. A
supplement such as a protein powder, which an athlete might consume in
a dose of 20–30 g, could therefore give rise to a positive test even though it
had been analysed and no nandrolone had been found.

To assess the extent of the problem, the IOC commissioned the testing
laboratory at the German Sports University in Cologne to conduct a survey
(dopinginfo.de 2002). Between October 2000 and November 2001 a total of
634 non-hormonal nutritional supplements were purchased in 13 countries
from 215 different suppliers. Of the 634 samples analysed, 94 (14.8%) were
found to contain steroid hormones or prohormones that were not declared
on the label. Reliable data could not be obtained on a further 66 samples
(10.4%) because of analytical problems, but some these products may also
have contained steroids. Of all positive supplements, 23 samples (24.5%)
contained compounds related to nandrolone and testosterone, 64 samples
(68.1%) only contained prohormones of testosterone, seven samples (7.5%)
only contained prohormones of nandrolone. A total of 49 supplements contained one steroid, but 45 contained more than one steroid and eight products
contained five or more different steroid compounds. The positive supplements had a highly variable content of anabolic androgenic steroid (from
0.01 µg/g to 190 µg/g) and this varied between tablets or capsules within

the same container. It is important to recognize also that only steroids were tested for: other prohibited substances may well have been present.

In relation to the total number of products purchased per country most of the positive supplements were bought in the Netherlands (25.8%), in Austria (22.7%), in the UK (18.8%) and in the USA (18.8%). The labels on the products showed that all of the supplements that were found to contain steroids were produced by companies located in one of only five countries (USA, Netherlands, UK, Italy and Germany), although products purchased in other countries were also found to be contaminated; 21.1% of the nutritional supplements from prohormone selling companies contained anabolic androgenic steroids, whereas proportionally fewer (9.6%) of the supplements from companies not selling prohormones were positive.

Products that were found to include prohibited steroids included amino acids and protein powders, creatine, carnitine, ribose, guarana, zinc, pyruvate, vitamins and minerals, and a range of herbal extracts. Many of these products are in common use among athletes.

CONCLUSIONS

Dietary supplement use is a prominent part of modern society and the use of supplements in sport is widespread. For athletes eating a varied diet in amounts sufficient to meet their energy demands, most of the available supplements are probably without effect. However, for the athlete in search of performance enhancement, the prospect of even a small performance improvement is seen as a risk worth taking.

KEY POINTS

1. The use of dietary supplements in sport is widespread, but varies between sports and cultures.
2. The supplements industry is a global business and has a powerful financial motive in promoting supplement use.
3. Athletes are cautioned against the indiscriminate use of dietary supplements. A cost-benefit analysis should be conducted to assess the evidence for and against supplement use, even though many parts of the equation are unknown.
4. The absence of evidence of efficacy should not be construed as evidence of a lack of effect as most supplements have been incompletely evaluated. Safety data on most supplements are also lacking.
5. Some supplements, notably bicarbonate, caffeine and creatine, can improve performance in some situations.
6. Some supplements suffer from lack of quality control during manufacture, leading to inappropriate labelling and to the presence of extraneous materials.

References

Bender DA, Bender AE 1997 Nutrition: a reference handbook. Oxford University Press, Oxford

Braham R, Dawson B, Goodman C 2003 The effect of glucosamine supplementation on people experiencing regular knee pain. British Journal of Sports Medicine 37:45–49

Cox GR, Desbrow B, Montgomery PG et al 2002 Effects of different protocols of caffeine intake on metabolism and endurance performance. Journal of Applied Physiology 93:990–999

dopinginfo.de 2002 Analysis of non-hormonal nutritional supplements for anabolic-androgenic steroids: an international study. http://www.dshs-koeln.de/biochemie/rubriken/07_info/07_020320e.pdf

Eichner ER 2000 Minerals: iron. In: Maughan RJ (ed) Nutrition in sport. Blackwell, Oxford, p 326–338

Food and Drugs Administration 2003 FDA proposes manufacturing and labeling standards for all dietary supplements. www.fda.gov/bbs/topics/NEWS/dietarysupp/background.html. 7 March 2003

Hopkins WG, Hawley JA, Burke LM 1999 Design and analysis of research on sport performance enhancement. Medicine and Science in Sports and Exercise 31:472–485

Kelly J, Kaufman D, Kelley K 2005 Recent trends in use of herbal and other natural products. Archives of Internal Medicine 165:281–286

McAlindon TE, LaValley MP, Gulin JP, Felson DT 2000 Glucosamine and chondroitin for treatment of osteoarthritis: a systematic quality assessment and meta-analysis. JAMA 283:1469–1475

Maughan RJ 1999 Nutritional ergogenic aids and exercise performance. Nutrition Research Reviews 12:255–280

Maughan RJ, King DS, Lea T 2004 Dietary supplements. Journal of Sports Science 22: 95–113

Radimer K, Bindewald B, Hughes J et al 2004 Dietary supplement use by US adults: data from the National Health and Nutrition Examination Survey, 1999–2000. American Journal of Epidemiology 160:339–349

Sobal J, Marquart LF 1994 Vitamin/mineral supplement use among athletes: a review of the literature. International Journal of Sports Nutrition 4:320–324

Talbott SM 2003 A guide to understanding dietary supplements. Haworth Press, Binghampton NY

Chapter **10**

Nutritional concerns of female athletes

Katherine A Beals and Melinda M Manore

LEARNING OBJECTIVES

After studying this chapter, you should be able to:

1. Discuss the major nutritional concerns most common in active females.
2. Identify the three types of dietary patterns that lead to poor nutrient intakes in active females.
3. Identify the micronutrients most likely to be low in the diets of active females.
4. Discuss the role that energy intake has on macronutrient and micronutrient intakes.
5. Describe the three components of the female athlete triad and their interrelationship.
6. Discuss the health consequences that may result if a female athlete suffers from one or more components of the female athlete triad.

INTRODUCTION

For many female athletes, nutrition is a balancing act. They know they need to eat enough to meet energy and nutrient needs so as to ensure optimal performance. Yet many of these same women feel that they need to limit or restrict their energy intake in order to control their body weight. These opposing dietary concerns can place the female athlete at nutritional risk.

This chapter will examine the nutrition concerns unique to the active/ athletic female. It begins with a description of three common dietary patterns that may place a female athlete at nutritional risk (chronic dieting, disordered eating, and vegetarianism). Next, the micronutrients often found to be lacking in the diets of active women are addressed. Finally, the chapter concludes with a discussion of the female athlete triad (i.e. disordered eating, menstrual dysfunction, and low bone mineral density (BMD)), a group of disorders that not only have nutritional consequences but, also, nutritional causes.

DIETARY PATTERNS PLACING THE FEMALE ATHLETE AT NUTRITIONAL RISK

It is beyond the scope of this chapter to cover each and every dietary practice and/or pattern that could potentially place the female athlete at nutritional risk. Thus, this section will be confined to what are considered to be three of the most common nutritionally comprising dietary patterns affecting active women, including chronic dieting/energy restriction, disordered eating, and vegetarianism.

CHRONIC DIETING/ENERGY RESTRICTION

Female athletes, like their non-athletic counterparts, are often preoccupied with their body weight/shape and many are trying to control their weight (Beals 2004). However, unlike non-athletes, female athletes are hoping that weight loss will not only improve their appearance but enhance their performance; goals that can often be conflicting (Beals 2004). This is especially true for athletes competing in thin-build or weight-dependent sports in which a low body weight is thought to confer a competitive advantage. For example, athletes participating in sports that are judged (e.g. figure skating, gymnastics, diving) often feel pressure to conform to the low body weight and small body size ideals that are typically endorsed by the judges. Similarly, athletes participating in sports that require economy of movement (e.g. distance running, cycling, swimming) may feel that weight loss will improve their speed, efficiency, and ultimately their endurance. Finally, athletes participating in sports with a weight classification (e.g. rowing, martial arts, body building) are under pressure to make weight and often attempt to 'diet down' into a weight category below their natural weight for a presumed competitive advantage (Beals 2004).

For most healthy female athletes, 'going on a diet' for a discrete period of time probably poses little nutritional risk (Manore & Thompson 2000). However, serious nutritional deficiencies may arise for the athlete who severely and/or chronically restricts energy intake. It has been estimated that recreational athletes (i.e. those exercising 6–10 hours per week) need approximately 2200–2500 kcal/day for weight maintenance while competitive female athletes (i.e. those exercising 10–20 hours/week) need at least 2500–2800 kcal/week to maintain body weight (Manore & Thompson 2000). Elite female athletes and those participating in prolonged endurance events (e.g. marathons, triathlons, centuries) likely require more than 3000 kcal/day (Manore & Thompson 2000) (Box 10.1).

BOX 10.1   HOW DO YOU KNOW IF AN ACTIVE FEMALE IS NOT EATING ENOUGH?

If a female athlete is not eating enough food she may experience some of the following symptoms:

- Hungry, irritable, and may have a difficult time concentrating before or during her exercise routine. Sometimes she may even get shaky and light-headed. This may be especially true if she exercises around 3–4 p.m. in the afternoon and has not eaten since lunch, or if she exercises before eating breakfast.
- Poor growth rates for young and adolescent female athletes. The diet must provide enough fuel for growth and menstruation, building and repair of muscle tissue, as well as exercise.
- She may stop having her menstrual periods. This may be a sign that the body does not have enough energy to fuel exercise and the reproductive functions of the body. An athlete does not have to have disordered eating to stop having their period. Many female athletes stop menstruating if they are exercising hard and not eating enough food and kilocalories, even if they are making good food choices.
- She is losing weight. This means the athlete is not providing enough fuel for both exercise and weight maintenance. If the athlete is restricting energy intake and exercise intensity is high, muscle tissue as well as fat is being used for fuel.
- She is maintaining weight at the current energy intake and exercise expenditure level, but amenorrhoea or oligomenorrhoea is present, exercise-related injuries are present, and/or no improvement in exercises training despite high levels of exercise.

Energy restriction and nutrient intake

If energy requirements are not met, macronutrient (particularly protein and carbohydrate) and micronutrient intakes will likely be insufficient to support training and competition. Indeed, research indicates that female athletes with low energy intakes often have protein and carbohydrate intakes below those recommended for active individuals (Beals & Manore 1998, Coyle 1995, Tipton & Wolfe 2004). Adequate protein is essential to maintain and/or repair muscle tissue and cover the cost of any protein used for energy during exercise (Tipton & Wolfe 2004). Moreover, without enough protein the athlete may be at greater risk for sustaining injuries and/or experience prolonged healing times (Manore & Thompson 2000, Tipton & Wolfe 2004). Recovery from strenuous exercise may also be delayed (Tipton & Wolfe 2004). Finally, of particular importance to strength athletes, inadequate protein intakes will limit strength and power gains (Tipton & Wolfe 2004).

Some athletes, like their non-athletic counterparts, have been drawn to the allure of rapid weight loss claimed by low-carbohydrate diets. While carbohydrate restriction is particularly detrimental to endurance performance, it can also negatively impact strength performance (especially if body protein is being used to support glucose needs) (Burke et al 2004, Coyle 1995, Jeukendrup 2004). Inadequate carbohydrate intake (<5 g/kg/day) will compromise both muscle and liver glycogen stores (Manore & Thompson 2000). The result is more rapid glycogen depletion and an earlier onset of muscular fatigue (muscle glycogen depletion) and metal fatigue (liver glycogen depletion and subsequent low blood glucose) during exercise (Burke et al 2004).

It is not unusual for female athletes to restrict dietary fat as a method of weight loss (Beals & Manore 1998). Certainly, the health benefits of a diet low in saturated fat extend to athletes as well as sedentary individuals. However, if dietary fat intake is too low (<10–15% of total daily energy intake), the intake and absorption of the fat-soluble vitamins and the essential fatty acids may also be inadequate (Manore & Thompson 2000). In addition, research suggests that an extremely low-fat diet reduces intramuscular triglyceride concentration, resulting in lower whole body lipolysis, total fat oxidation, and nonplasma fatty acids oxidation during exercise which could negatively impact endurance performance (Coyle et al 2001). Finally, an association between very low-fat diets and menstrual dysfunction has been proposed; however, it may have been more a function of the low total energy intake that often accompanies the fat restriction (Manore & Thompson 2000).

Not only can energy restriction compromise macronutrient intakes but it can also negatively impact vitamin and mineral intakes – particularly iron, calcium, magnesium, zinc and the B complex vitamins (Beals & Manore 1998, Manore 2002, Manore & Thompson 2000). As will be described in greater detail further on in the chapter, these micronutrients are particularly important for active women as they play important roles in energy production, haemoglobin synthesis, maintenance of bone density and immune function.

Energy restriction and the timing of nutrient intake

Research indicates that it is not only what the female athlete eats that impacts performance, but when she eats it. It is generally recommended that athletes, particularly endurance athletes, consume a carbohydrate-rich meal containing approximately 200–300 g of carbohydrate 1–4 hours before exercise (American College of Sports Medicine 2000). Athletes who chronically diet tend to restrict energy intake during the day and consume most of their calories at night (Beals 2004). Such a dietary pattern is detrimental to performance of the female athlete, particularly that of the endurance athlete, as she will come to her workout with compromised carbohydrate stores and will experience more rapid glycogen depletion and muscular fatigue, thus rendering her unable to perform at an optimal level.

DISORDERED EATING

Disordered eating is a general term encompassing a spectrum of abnormal and harmful eating behaviours that are used in a misguided attempt to lose weight or maintain a lower than normal body weight (Table 10.1). Disordered eating behaviours are often depicted on a continuum. At either end of this continuum are the clinical eating disorders anorexia nervosa (characterized by self-starvation) and bulimia nervosa (characterized by regular bingeing and purging) while in between lies subclinical versions of these disorders along with a whole host of variations therein. It is important to note that athletes rarely fall neatly within one eating disorder category. Rather they often cross categories at different times during their disorder and many display symptoms of more than one disorder simultaneously (Beals 2004).

The effects of disordered eating on the nutritional status, health and performance of an athlete are a function of the severity and duration of the disordered eating behaviours as well as the physiological demands of the sport (Beals 2004). For example, an individual who engages in severe energy restriction or who has been bingeing and purging for a long time will probably experience a greater decrement in performance than one who has engaged in milder weight-control behaviours for a shorter period of time. Likewise, endurance sports and other physical activities with high energy demands (e.g. distance running, swimming, cycling, basketball, and field and ice hockey) are likely to be more negatively affected than sports with lower energy demands (e.g. diving, gymnastics, weightlifting). Finally, athletes who train at a high intensity (e.g. elite athletes) are apt to have greater performance decrements than those who engage in lower-intensity exercise (e.g. recreational athletes).

Athletes suffering from anorexia nervosa or subclinical anorexia are at risk for nutritional deficiencies similar to those previously described for athletes who severely and/or chronically restrict energy intake. The degree of nutritional risk is directly related to the severity and duration of the energy restriction and corresponding energy deficit, such that the more severe the energy restriction the greater the nutritional risk. Additional health effects associated with

Table 10.1   Disordered eating classifications

Anorexia nervosa	A clinical eating disorder characterized by a refusal to maintain body weight at or above a minimally normal weight for age and height (e.g. weight loss leading to maintenance of body weight less than 85% of that expected; or failure to make expected weight gain during period of growth, leading to body weight less than 85% of that expected). The individual exhibits an intense fear of gaining weight or becoming fat even though underweight and severe body image disturbance.
Bulimia nervosa	A clinical eating disorder characterized by recurrent episodes of binge eating (out of control eating of a large amount of food in a discrete period of time) followed by compensatory purging behaviours including self-induced vomiting, misuse of laxatives, diuretics, enemas, or other medications, fasting or excessive exercise occurring on average, at least twice a week for 3 months. Self-evaluation is unduly influenced by body shape and weight.
Binge eating disorder	A recently recognized eating disorder that resembles bulimia nervosa and is characterized by episodes of uncontrolled eating (or bingeing). It differs from bulimia, however, because its sufferers do not purge their bodies of the excess food, via vomiting, laxative abuse or diuretic abuse.
Eating disorders not otherwise specified	A clinical eating disorder category recently added to the DSM-IV to describe a condition that meets some but not all of the criteria for anorexia nervosa and bulimia nervosa. 1. Nervosa are met except that, despite substantial weight loss, the individual's current weight is in the normal range. 2. All of the criteria for bulimia nervosa are met except binges occur at a frequency of less than twice a week or for a duration of less than 3 months. 3. An individual of normal body weight who regularly engages in inappropriate compensatory behaviour after eating small amounts of food (e.g. self-induced vomiting after the consumption of two cookies). 4. An individual who repeatedly chews and spits out, but does not swallow, large amounts of food.
Subclinical eating disorders	The term *subclinical eating disorder* has since been frequently used by researchers to describe considerable eating pathology and body weight concerns in both athletes and non-athletes who do not demonstrate significant psychopathology or who fail to meet all the DSM-IV criteria for anorexia nervosa, bulimia nervosa or EDNOS. Indeed, many athletes do not meet the technical criteria for a clinical eating disorder, despite severely restricting energy intake, engaging in self-induced vomiting, or using laxatives, diuretics and excessive exercise in an effort to lose weight. Conversely, athletes may use none of these methods but still suffer from an obvious eating disturbance

chronic or severe energy restriction and the resulting weight loss (or maintenance of a dangerously low body weight) include decreased basal metabolic rate, cardiovascular and gastrointestinal disorders, depression, menstrual dysfunction and the resulting decrease in bone mineral density (Eichner 1992) (Table 10.2).

Table 10.2 Health consequences of disordered eating behaviours

Weight control behaviour	Physiological effects and health consequences
Fasting or starvation	Promotes loss of lean body mass, a decrease in metabolic rate, and a reduction in bone mineral density. Increases the risk of nutrient deficiencies. Promotes glycogen depletion, resulting in poor exercise performance.
Diet pills	Typically function by suppressing appetite and may cause a slight increase in metabolic rate (if they contain ephedrine or caffeine). May induce rapid heart rate, anxiety, inability to concentrate, nervousness, inability to sleep, and dehydration. Any weight lost is quickly regained once use is discontinued.
Diuretics	Weight loss is primarily water, and any weight lost is quickly regained once use is discontinued. Dehydration and electrolyte imbalances are common and may disrupt thermoregulatory function and induce cardiac arrhythmia.
Laxatives or enemas	Weight loss is primarily water, and any weight lost is quickly regained once use is discontinued. Dehydration and electrolyte imbalances, constipation, cathartic colon (a condition in which the colon becomes unable to function properly on its own) and steatorrhoea (excessive fat in the faeces) are common. May be addictive, and athlete can develop resistance, thus requiring larger and larger doses to produce the same effect (or even to induce a normal bowel movement).
Self-induced vomiting	Largely ineffective in promoting weight (body fat) loss. Large body water losses can lead to dehydration and electrolyte imbalances. Gastrointestinal problems, including oesophagitis, oesophageal perforation, and oesophageal and stomach ulcers, are common. May promote erosion of tooth enamel and increase the risk for dental caries. Finger calluses and abrasions are often present.
Fat-free diets	May be lacking in essential nutrients, especially fat-soluble vitamins and essential fatty acids. Total energy intake must still be reduced to produce weight loss. Many fat-free convenience foods are highly processed, with high sugar contents and few micronutrients unless the foods are fortified. The diet is often difficult to follow and may promote binge eating.

continued

Table 10.2   Health consequences of disordered eating behaviours — *cont'd*

Weight control behaviour	Physiological effects and health consequences
Saunas	Weight loss is primarily water, and any weight lost is quickly regained once fluids are replaced. Dehydration and electrolyte imbalances are common and may disrupt thermoregulatory function and induce cardiac arrhythmia.
Excessive exercise	Increases risk of staleness, chronic fatigue, illness, overuse injuries and menstrual dysfunction.

Reprinted, with permission, from K A Beals, Disordered eating among athletes: a comprehensive guide for health professionals, 2004, pages 84–85, Table 6.1. Human Kinetics, Champaign IL. Originally adapted with permission from ACSM's Health and Fitness Journal. Lippincott, Williams & Wilkins.

Athletes with bulimia nervosa or subclinical bulimia are at risk for many of the same nutritional and health complications as those with anorexia nervosa (e.g. nutrient deficiencies, chronic fatigue, endocrine abnormalities and bone mineral density reductions). In addition, the bingeing and purging behaviours add some unique nutritional, cardiovascular and gastrointestinal complications.

Bingeing frequently causes gastric distension that, in rare cases, can result in gastric necrosis and even rupture (Pomeroy & Mitchell 1992). Oesophageal reflux and subsequent chronic throat irritation are also common and may increase the risk for oesophageal cancer (Carney & Andersen 1996).

Purging (via diuretics, laxatives, enemas or self-induced vomiting) significantly increases an athlete's risk for dehydration (Carney & Andersen 1996). Electrolyte imbalances, particularly hypokalaemia (i.e. low blood potassium levels), are also common in individuals who engage in purging behaviours and can have debilitating effects on health) (Carney & Andersen 1996). Purging can also lead to dangerous disruptions in the body's acid–base balance and life-threatening alterations in the body's pH. Self-induced vomiting typically results in an increase in serum bicarbonate levels and thus leads to metabolic alkalosis (increase in blood pH). On the other hand, individuals who abuse laxatives are more likely to develop metabolic acidosis (decrease in blood pH) secondary to loss of bicarbonate in the stool (Carney & Andersen 1996). Purging via excessive exercise increases the athlete's risk for overtraining syndrome and overuse injuries (Beals 2004).

Cardiovascular complications associated with bingeing and purging are usually secondary to the electrolyte imbalances induced by purging. As described earlier, hypokalaemia can result in potentially life-threatening cardiac arrhythmias. In addition, individuals who abuse ipecac may have myocarditis (inflammation of the middle layer of the heart muscle) and various cardiomyopathies (Carney & Andersen 1996). The gastrointestinal complications associated with purging depend on the purging methods used and can include throat and mouth ulcers, dental caries, abdominal cramping, diarrhoea and haemorroids (Pomeroy & Mitchel 1992) (Table 10.2).

Surprisingly, anecdotal evidence (i.e. reports from coaches and personal accounts by athletes with disordered eating) suggests that athletes practising disordered eating behaviours often experience an initial, albeit transient, increase in performance (Beals 2004). The reasons for this temporary increase in performance are not completely understood but may be related to the initial physiological and psychological effects of starvation and purging (Beals 2004). Starvation and purging are physiological stressors and, as such, produce an up-regulation of the hypothalamic-pituitary-adrenal axis (i.e. 'the fight-or-flight response') and an increase in the adrenal hormones: cortisol, adrenaline (epinephrine) and noradrenaline (norepinephrine). These hormones have a stimulatory effect on the central nervous system that can mask fatigue and evoke feelings of euphoria in the eating disordered athlete. In addition, the initial decrease in body weight (particularly before there is a significant decrease in muscle mass) may induce a transient increase in relative maximal oxygen uptake per kilogram of body weight ($\dot{V}O_2$max) (Ingjer & Sundgot-Borgen 1991). Moreover, with weight loss, athletes may feel lighter, which may afford them a psychological boost, particularly if they believe that lighter is always better in terms of performance. Nonetheless, it should be emphasized that any initial improvements in performance are transient. Eventually, the lack of sufficient calories, macro- and micronutrients will cause the body to break down and performance to suffer.

VEGETARIANISM

Vegetarianism as a dietary practice has increased steadily over the past two decades. It has been estimated that approximately 5.4% of the United Kingdom population are vegetarians while 2.5% of Americans and 4.5% of Canadian adults report following a vegetarian diet (Barr & Rideout 2004). The number of athletes or active individuals who ascribe to vegetarian diets is currently unknown. However, given that vegetarians often report other healthy behaviours, including higher levels of physical activity (Barr & Rideout 2004, Nieman 1999), it could be speculated that it represents a substantial percentage.

A number of health benefits have been associated with vegetarian diets including reduced risks for obesity, type 2 diabetes, hypertension, cardiovascular disease and some cancers (Fraser 1999, Key et al 1999). Whether a vegetarian diet is associated with beneficial or detrimental effects on athletic performance remains questionable. Of greatest concern is whether a vegetarian diet can meet the nutritional requirements of athletes. A recent review of the scientific literature concluded that a well-planned and varied vegetarian diet can meet the needs of athletes (Barr & Rideout 2004). In addition, observational studies of vegetarian and non-vegetarian athletes have found no differences in performance or fitness associated with the amount of animal protein consumed (Barr & Rideout 2004). Similarly, short-term intervention studies, in which subjects consumed vegetarian and non-vegetarian diets for periods of 2–6 weeks, observed no differences in performance parameters

(Barr & Rideout 2004). Despite this research, it should be noted that following a vegetarian diet, particularly one that contains no animal products (i.e. a vegan diet), requires diligence on the part of the athlete to ensure that nutrient needs are met, most notably protein, iron and vitamin B_{12}.

Protein. It has been hypothesized that vegetarian athletes may be at risk for inadequate protein intakes. While it is true that the protein content as well as protein quality of many plant-based foods is lower than that of animal products and research consistently shows that vegetarians, on average, consume less protein than their omnivorous counterparts, protein intakes for both groups are generally well above the Recommended Dietary Allowance (RDA) (American Dietetic Association 2003). Moreover, since athletes typically have higher energy requirements (and, consequently, higher energy intakes), even a diet with a relatively low percentage of energy from protein will provide sufficient absolute amounts of protein (Barr & Rideout 2004). The possible exception would be athletes who are following a vegetarian diet and also engaging in severe/chronic dieting and/or disordered eating behaviours (Barr & Rideout 2004, Barr & Broughton 2000).

Iron. Studies consistently show that the total iron intake is similar between vegetarians and non-vegetarians (Barr & Rideout 2004). Nonetheless, the lower bioavailability of non-haem iron (the only form of iron in plant foods) relative to haem iron (only found in foods of animal origin), the low iron intake among the female population in general, and the potential for increased iron losses with intense physical activity (e.g. gastrointestinal blood losses, haematuria from footstrike haemolysis in runners), renders iron a nutrient of concern for the female vegetarian athlete. Very few studies have examined the iron status of vegetarian athletes. Research among non-athletes indicates that prevalence of iron deficiency is similar among vegetarians and omnivores while the iron depletion (low iron stores as evidenced by low serum ferritin) is significantly more prevalent (Barr & Rideout 2004). One could assume that similar results would be found among vegetarian athletes.

As indicated in Chapter 6, iron deficiency (anaemia) will certainly impair endurance performance. The impact of iron depletion (without anaemia) on athletic performance is currently controversial (Sinclair & Hinton 2005). Regardless, since iron depletion can progress to anaemia, intervention at the iron depleted stage is prudent and warranted.

Vitamin B_{12}. As indicated in Chapter 6, vitamin B_{12} is found naturally only in foods of animal origin; thus, vegetarians who exclude all animal products from their diet (i.e. vegans) are at risk for inadequate intakes. It should be noted, however, that increasing numbers of vegan foods and beverages are being fortified with B_{12}, making deficiencies rare. There are currently few studies examining vitamin B_{12} intakes among vegetarian athletes; thus, it is difficult to make specific intake recommendations. To be safe, vegetarians, particularly vegans, should be mindful of consuming B_{12} fortified foods and/or a dietary supplement providing 2 µg/day.

MICRONUTRIENTS OFTEN LACKING IN THE DIETS OF FEMALE ATHLETES

The most common nutrition issues that contribute to low micronutrient intakes in active women are inadequate energy intake and/or poor food selection. As previously mentioned, any time energy intake is chronically and/or severely restricted, intakes of almost all micronutrients will be low and status can be compromised. In addition, it is not uncommon for active females to eliminate foods or food groups from the diet, especially meat and dairy foods, which decreases micronutrients found in these foods (Manore 2005). For example, if dairy foods are eliminated then the intake of bone-building nutrients can be low. However, even under circumstances of adequate energy intake, female athletes can have low micronutrient intakes. The most common micronutrients found to be low in the diets of active females include bone-building nutrients (calcium, magnesium, vitamin D), iron, zinc, and the B vitamins, especially folate and vitamin B_6. All of these nutrients are discussed in detail in Chapter 6 of this text; thus, we will present a brief overview of these micronutrients as they apply to the female athlete.

BONE-BUILDING NUTRIENTS

CALCIUM AND VITAMIN D

Female athletes often have low intakes of the bone-building nutrients, especially if they have eliminated dairy foods from their diet. Manore (2002) reviewed the research assessing calcium intake in female high school and collegiate athletes and found that mean intakes ranged from 500–1623 mg/day, with most studies reporting mean intakes <1000 mg/day. The lowest intakes of calcium are typically reported in athletes who participate in sports where body weight and/or image are important (ballet, gymnastics, and track and field events). These individuals also have the greatest risk for amenorrhoea, which can lead to poor bone mineral density and increased risk of stress fracture. The Dietary Reference Intake (DRI) for calcium is 1300 mg/day for young females between the ages of 9 and 18 years, and 1000 mg/day for adult females 19–50 years of age (IOM 1997).

All female athletes, especially those who report menstrual disturbances, need to be encouraged to consume adequate calcium in either dairy foods, calcium fortified products or supplements. For those athletes with lactose intolerance, care should be taken to assure adequate calcium is consumed using other calcium-rich foods (e.g. calcium fortified soy milk or orange juice) and/or calcium supplements. However, optimal calcium absorption and good bone health cannot occur without adequate intakes of vitamin D and normal blood oestrogen concentrations. Athletes need to be reminded that all the bone-building nutrients are required. Calcium intake alone will not assure an athlete of adequate bone density. For athletes that live in northern climates, where winter light is limited, and who exercise primarily indoors, vitamin D status may be poor. For these athletes, a calcium supplement fortified with other bone-building nutrients, including vitamin K, magnesium and vitamin D, may be necessary. Adequate energy and protein intake are also important for bone health.

MAGNESIUM

Magnesium is an important component of bone, but also important for energy metabolism, protein synthesis and neuromuscular transmission (Manore & Thompson, 2000). In the United States, the typical magnesium density of the diet is 120 mg/1000 kcal (4184 kJ) and the RDA is set at 310–320 mg/day (IOM 1997). Thus, it is easy to see that active women who restrict energy intake will have low magnesium intakes, especially if energy intakes are less than 2000 kcal/day (8368 kJ). For example, Beals & Manore (1998) reported that 54% of their female athletes with subclinical eating disorders (mean energy intake = 1989 kcal/day (8322 kJ)), consumed <100% of the RDA for magnesium and 8% consumed <66% of RDA. Like calcium, athletes in thin-build sport are most likely to report less than optimal intake of dietary magnesium. Foods high in magnesium include whole grains and cereals, beans and legumes, meat, fish, milk and yogurt, and some nuts (almonds and sunflowers), vegetables (broccoli, green beans, carrots and potatoes) and fruits (bananas).

TRACE MINERALS

IRON

Iron deficiency (low ferritin concentrations <20 μg/L) is one of the most prevalent nutrient deficiencies in the world. According to the World Health Organization (2003), ~4–5 billion people, or 66 to 80% of the world's population, are iron deficient without anaemia and 2 billion people – over 30% of the world's population – have iron deficiency anaemia. In the United States, iron deficiency anaemia is ~3–5% in women overall, while iron deficiency without anaemia is 12–15%. However, based on recent reports, the prevalence of iron deficiency without anaemia is 25–35% in active women (Sinclair & Hinton 2005). This higher incidence of iron deficiency without anaemia in female athletes is usually attributed to four primary factors: (1) poor intakes of meat, fish and poultry products that contain, in haem iron, the most absorbable form of iron in the diet, (2) decreased bioavailability of the iron in the diet, which means that the iron being consumed is not being absorbed due to high fibre intakes and other food compounds that decrease iron absorption, (3) increased losses of iron in sweat, blood, urine and faeces, and (4) low energy intakes. Thus, there are a number of factors that may be contributing to why iron status is low in a particular athlete.

The consequences of iron deficiency without anaemia on exercise and work performance have recently been examined. Research shows that iron supplementation in women with low ferritin concentrations, even when serum iron levels are normal, significantly decreased 15-km running times compared to controls who were not supplementing (Hinton et al 2000). For this reason, all active females should be encouraged to have their iron status checked yearly. If poor status is indicated, recommend that they see their doctor and a dietitian that can help them identify why iron status may be poor and work to correct the problem. If poor iron intake is indicated, then eating haem sources of iron, using iron fortified foods, and/or taking iron supplements will help reverse the deficiency. Because iron supplements may cause gastrointestinal distress, finding alternatives to supplements may be necessary.

For women 19–50 years, the RDA for iron is 18 mg/day (IOM 2001). Based on survey data in the USA, pre- and post-menopausal women consume ~12 mg/day of iron. In addition, the US diet has an iron density of ~6 mg/1000 kcal (4184 kJ/day), so unless good food choices are made the diet will be low in iron. Although active women may appear to be getting adequate amounts of iron in their diet, much of this iron is from non-haem fortified foods such as breakfast cereal, energy and breakfast bars, and fat-free or low-fat snacks, which have low bioavailability.

ZINC

Zinc has multiple functions within the body, but is especially important as a component of various enzymes, maintains the structural integrity of proteins and assists in the regulation of gene expression (IOM 2001). Without zinc the body cannot grow and develop properly, or build and repair muscle tissue. Currently there are over 100 different enzymes within the body that require zinc (IOM 2001). Manore (2002) reviewed the mean dietary zinc intakes of active female athletes and found that most have zinc intakes below the RDA of 8 mg/day (IOM 2001). At the present time there are no good assessment measures for zinc, so we do not know the number of active females with low zinc status. Thus, assessing zinc intake is one of the best ways of determining if status might be low. Like iron, the lower zinc intakes of active women are usually attributed to low energy intakes and lower intakes of animal products, which are good sources of zinc. Female athletes who avoid animal products and limit intakes of whole or fortified cereals and grains may need zinc supplements.

B VITAMINS

The B vitamins (e.g. riboflavin, niacin, vitamin B_6, folate and vitamin B_{12}) are especially important for energy metabolism and the regeneration of new cells, including new red blood cells. For active women who eat a highly processed diet and/or restricted energy intake, intakes of these nutrients may be low. The B-complex vitamins most commonly assessed in cross-sectional studies of female athletes are riboflavin, vitamin B_6, vitamin B_{12} and folate. A review of the literature shows that the intake of B vitamins varies dramatically, with ~10–60% of female athletes consuming <100% of the recommended levels for these nutrients (Manore 2002). Of the B-complex vitamins, vitamin B_6 and folate are frequently low in the diets of female athletes (Manore 2000), especially those with restricted energy intakes or with disordered eating behaviours (Beals & Manore 1998). This brief overview will focus on vitamin B_6 and folate. See Chapter 6 for an in-depth review of B vitamins and exercise.

VITAMIN B_6

Vitamin B_6 (pyridoxine) has a number of functions related to energy metabolism and, thus, to exercise and exercise performance. As one would expect, the dietary intakes of vitamin B_6 are generally lower in active females with poor energy intakes. Hansen & Manore (2005) reviewed the metabolic studies done with active and/or sedentary individuals consuming known amounts of vitamin B_6 and found that ~1.5–2.3 mg/day of vitamin B_6 are required to maintain plasma levels of pyridoxal 5' phosphate (PLP) concentrations above the cutoff value of 30 nmol/L. PLP is the active form of vitamin B_6 in the blood. In 1989 RDA for vitamin B_6 was 1.6 mg/day for women, but was decreased to 1.3 mg/day for women (19–50 years of age) in 1998 (IOM 1998). Thus, the current RDA for vitamin B_6 may not be high enough for active females to maintain good vitamin B_6 status. Again, vitamin B_6 is also low in individuals who report consuming <1900 kcal/day (Hansen & Manore 2005).

FOLATE

Folate is the one of the B vitamins that appears to be consistently low in the diets of female athletes. A review of the literature by Manore (2002) found no studies reporting mean folate intakes ≥400 µg/day in female athletes, with mean folate intakes ranging from 126 to 364 µg/day (Manore 2002). The RDA for folate is 400 µg/day (IOM 1998). Beals & Manore (1998) report one of the few studies examining both dietary folate intake and blood levels in active women. They found that 53% of their female athletes consumed <400 µg/day of folate based on 7-day weighed food records. Those athletes with the lower energy intakes (<1900 kcal/day) had the lowest folate intakes. Overall they found 4% of their athletes to be in negative folate balance (plasma folate ≤3 ng/mL); however, nearly 50% of their athletes reported supplementing. Thus, the assumption is that folate status would be lower had the athletes not been supplementing with folate.

Active females need to increase their daily intake of folate to the current RDA of 400 µg/day. Folate is especially high in leafy green vegetables, fortified cereals and grains, nuts, legumes, liver and brewer's yeast. If these types of foods are not consumed in the diet, supplementation may be necessary.

THE FEMALE ATHLETE TRIAD

The female athlete triad (Triad) refers to three distinct yet interrelated disorders: (a) disordered eating, (b) menstrual dysfunction, and (c) low BMD (Otis et al 1997). Although any of these disorders can, and do, occur in isolation, they often follow a typical developmental pattern. In an attempt to improve performance and/or meet the aesthetic demands of her sport, the female athlete begins to diet. For any number of reasons, the dieting becomes increasingly severe and eventually progresses to disordered eating. The energy imbalance and hormonal alterations resulting from the disordered eating leads to menstrual dysfunction, which eventually results in decreased bone mineral density and possibly premature osteoporosis (Otis et al 1997).

Not only is the Triad born out of nutritional deficiencies as illustrated by the etiological pattern above, but it carries significant nutritional implications for the female athlete. Since disordered eating was previously covered in this chapter, the following section will focus on menstrual dysfunction and low BMD.

MENSTRUAL DYSFUNCTION

While menstrual dysfunction afflicts only approximately 2–5% the general female population it has been shown to be as high as 79% among female athletes participating in certain sports (e.g. gymnastics, distance running, swimming, dance) (Warren & Perlroth 2001). A number of theories have been proposed for the significantly higher prevalence among female athletes. In the early 1970s a low body weight and/or body fat were thought to be the primary cause of amenorrhoea seen in physically active women; however, research conducted in the mid 1980s demonstrated neither body weight nor body composition varies significantly between amenorrhoeic and eumenorrhoeic athletes (Beals & Warner 2005). Subsequent research has focused on the impact of exercise on menstrual dysfunction. The so-called *exercise-stress* hypothesis purports that the stress of exercise training, like other chronic stressors, activates the hypothalamic-pituitary-adrenal (HPA) axis, which disrupts the GnRH pulse generator and results in menstrual dysfunction (Warren & Perlroth 2001). More recently, however, research has shown that it is not exercise per se that induces menstrual dysfunction but, rather, the energy deficit that often results from exercise (Loucks et al 1998). This energy drain theory holds that failure to provide sufficient calories to meet energy requirements and support the carbohydrate needs of the brain causes an alteration in brain function that disrupts the GnRH pulse generator through an as yet undetermined mechanism (Beals & Warner 2005). In a series of studies, Anne Loucks and her colleagues clearly demonstrated that low energy availability is at the root of hypothalamic menstrual dysfunction (Beals & Warner 2005). The threshold of energy availability needed to maintain normal menstrual function has been estimated to be approximately 30 kcal/kg lean body mass per day (Loucks & Thuma 2003).

Interestingly, female athletes who experience menstrual dysfunction, particularly amenorrhoea, often demonstrate little concern for the disruption in their cycles; in fact, they often express relief at the 'break' (Otis & Goldingay 2000). Similarly, some coaches simply dismiss menstrual dysfunction, believing it is a natural result of hard training. Despite these attitudes, it should be emphasized that menstrual dysfunction is not a normal response to training; rather, it is a clear indication that health is being compromised. The health consequences of menstrual dysfunction are well documented and include infertility and other reproductive problems, decreased immune function, and an increase in cardiovascular risk factors. Perhaps most importantly, menstrual dysfunction is directly and positively associated with decreases in BMD (Otis et al 1997).

LOW BMD

Low BMD is independently linked to both disordered eating and menstrual dysfunction and has the potential to negatively impact both the athlete's health and performance (Beals & Warner 2005). Research indicates that lumbar BMD can be reduced by as much as 20% in amenorrhoeic athletes compared with their eumenorrhoeic counterparts (Wolman et al 1990). Of greatest immediate concern is the increased risk for stress fractures. Research indicates that amenorrhoeic athletes (24–61%) are at a greater risk than their eumenorrhoeic counterparts (9–29%) (Beals & Warner 2005). In addition, bone formation rates (measured by serum osteocalcin, which is a common blood marker used to assess bone formation) are reduced in those with amenorrhoea and are associated with lower BMD in the hip and spine (Beals & Warner 2005).

It is important to note that even brief interruptions in normal menstrual function can negatively impact BMD. For example, Drinkwater and colleagues (1984) found that spinal BMD of athletes varied by level of menstrual irregularity; eumenorrhoeic athletes had higher BMDs than oligomenorrhoeic athletes, who had higher BMDs than amenorrhoeic athletes. Other studies have shown that luteal suppression and anovulation can also produce reductions in BMD (Beals & Warner 2005).

Spinal BMD appears to be the most negatively affected by Triad-related bone loss, whereas total body BMD, and more specifically hip BMD (weight-bearing bones), appear to be protected by weight-bearing exercise (Beals & Warner 2005). Moreover, research indicates that bone density lost as a result of menstrual dysfunction may never be completely regained, even given a return to normal menses. Drinkwater and colleagues (1986) followed 16 female athletes (nine amenorrhoeic and seven eumenorrhoeic) for a total of

3 years, during which time seven of the amenorrhoeic athletes regained menses. The mean BMD for the two athletes who remained amenorrhoeic continued to decline (–3.4%), while the BMD for the eumenorrhoeic athletes remained relatively unchanged. The average BMD for the amenorrhoeic athletes who regained menses increased significantly (about 6%) during the first year; however, the increase slowed to only 3% the following year and then ceased altogether the year after that. Thus, victims of the Triad likely will not achieve peak BMD in youth and they will be at increased risk for fractures for the rest of their lives.

As previously described, female athletes with menstrual dysfunction and/or low BMD need to pay particular attention to consuming adequate amounts of energy (to correct the negative energy balance), protein, and bone-building nutrients, such as calcium, vitamin D and vitamin K. Other important nutrients for bone health include magnesium and potassium (New et al 2000, Weaver 2001).

CONCLUSION

There is increasing pressure on women to be thin or thinner. This pressure may be particularly pronounced for female athletes who strive to meet the predominant sociocultural body weight/shape ideals, but also meet the weight requirements of their particular sport. This pressure may lead to potentially harmful patterns of chronic dieting or disordered eating that not only increase the athletes' risk for nutritional deficiencies but also menstrual dysfunction and subsequently low BMD.

Female athletes need to be educated regarding the adverse nutritional, health and performance effects of severe and/or chronic energy restriction. In addition, they need to understand the far-reaching consequences of menstrual dysfunction, particularly with respect to BMD. Strategies to help the female athlete optimize health and performance include the identification of an appropriate and healthy body weight, good eating habits and techniques for maintaining these habits for a lifetime.

KEY POINTS

1. Two of the most common nutritional issues that arise in the active female are energy restriction for weight loss and disordered eating behaviours, which can contribute to inadequate nutrient intakes.
2. Three common dietary patterns that can lead to poor nutrient intakes are chronic dieting, disordered eating and vegetarianism.
3. The most common micronutrients found to be low in the diets of active females are calcium, magnesium, iron, zinc and selected B vitamins (vitamin B_6, folate).

continued

> **KEY POINTS — cont'd**
>
> 4. Energy intakes below that required to maintain weight can lead to poor intakes of protein and carbohydrate necessary to sustain physical activity and maintain lean tissue, and micronutrients, such as iron, zinc, folate and calcium.
> 5. Disordered eating, menstrual dysfunction and osteoporosis are the three components of the female athlete triad. If left untreated, individuals diagnosed with the female athlete triad can have severe bone loss and increased fracture rates.

References

American College of Sports Medicine, American Dietetic Association and Dietitians of Canada 2000 Nutrition and athletic performance. Medicine and Science in Sports and Exercise 32:2130–2145

American Dietetic Association, Dietitians of Canada 2003 Vegetarian diets. Journal of the American Dietetic Association 103:748–765

Barr SI, Broughton TM 2000 Relative weight, weight loss efforts and nutrient intakes among health-conscious vegetarian, past vegetarian and nonvegetarian women ages 18–50. Journal of the American College of Nutrition 19:781–788

Barr SI, Rideout CA 2004 Nutritional considerations for vegetarian athletes. Nutrition 20(7–8):696–703

Beals KA 2004 Disordered eating among athletes: a comprehensive guide for health professionals. Human Kinetics, Champaign IL

Beals KA, Manore MM 1998 Nutritional status of female athletes with subclinical eating disorders. Journal of the American Dietetic Association 98:419–425

Beals KA, Warner SE 2005 The female athlete triad. In: Ransdell L, Petlichkoff L (eds) Ensuring the health of active and athletic girls and women. National Association for Girls and Women, Reston VA, p 205–232

Burke LM, Kiens B, Ivy JL 2004 Carbohydrates and fat for training and recovery. Journal of Sports Science 22:15–30

Carney CP, Andersen AE 1996 Eating disorders: guide to medical evaluation and complications. Psychiatric Clinics of North America 19:657–679

Coyle EF 1995 Substrate utilization during exercise in active people. American Journal of Clinical Nutrition 61(suppl):968S–979S

Coyle EF, Jeukendrup AE, Oseto MC et al 2001 Low-fat diet alters intramuscular substrates and reduces lipolysis and fat oxidation during exercise. American Journal of Physiology, Endocrinology and Metabolism 280:E391–398

Drinkwater BL, Nilson K, Chesnut CH III et al 1984 Bone mineral content of amenorrheic and eumenorrheic athletes. New England Journal of Medicine 311:277–281

Drinkwater BL, Nilson K, Ott S, Chesnut CH 3rd 1986 Bone mineral density after resumption of menses in amenorrheic athletes. JAMA 256:380–382

Eichner ER 1992 General health issues of low body weight and undereating in athletes. In: Brownell KD, Rodin J, Wilmore JH (eds) Eating, body weight and performance in athletes: disorders of modern society. Lea & Febiger, Philadelphia, p 191–201

Fraser GE 1999 Association between diet and cancer, ischemic heart disease, and all-cause mortality in non-Hispanic white Californian Seventh-Day Adventists. American Journal of Clinical Nutrition 70(suppl):532S–538S

Frisch RE 1987 Body fat, menarche, fitness, and fertility. Human Reprod 2:521–533

Hansen CM, Manore MM 2005 Vitamin B_6. In: Wolinsky I et al (eds) Sports nutrition. Vitamins and trace elements. 2nd edn. CRC Press, Boca Raton FL, 81–91

Hinton PA, Giordano C, Brownlie T, Haas JD 2000 Iron supplementation improves endurance after training in iron-depleted, nonanemic women. Journal of Applied Physiology 88:1103–1111

Ingjer F, Sundgot-Borgen J 1991 Influence of body weight reduction on maximal oxygen uptake in female elite athletes. Scandinavian Journal of Medical Science in Sport 1:141–146

IOM (Institute of Medicine, Food and Nutrition Board) 1997 Dietary reference intakes for calcium, phosphorus, magnesium, vitamin D, and fluoride. National Academy Press, Washington DC

IOM (Institute of Medicine, Food and Nutrition Board) 1998 Dietary reference intakes for thiamin, riboflavin, niacin, vitamin B6, folate, vitamin B12, pantothenic acid, biotin, and choline. National Academy Press, Washington DC

IOM (Institute of Medicine, Food and Nutrition Board) 2001 Dietary reference intakes: vitamin A, vitamin K, arsenic, boron, chromium, copper, iodine, iron, manganese, molybdenum, nickel, silicon, vanadium, and zinc. National Academy Press, Washington DC

Jeukendrup AE 2004 Carbohydrate intake during exercise and performance. Nutrition 20:669–77

Johnson MD 1994 Disordered eating in active and athletic women. Clinical Sports Medicine13:355–369

Key TJ, Davey GK, Appleby PN 1999 Health benefits of a vegetarian diet. Proceedings of the Nutrition Society 58:271–275

Loucks AB, Thuma, JR 2003 Luteinizing hormone pulsatility is disrupted at a threshold of energy availability in regularly menstruating women. Journal of Clinical Endocrinology and Metabolism 88:297–311

Loucks AB, Verdun M, Heath EM 1998 Low energy availability, not stress of exercise, alters LH pulsatility in exercising women. Journal of Applied Physiology 84(1):37–46

Manore MM 2000 The effect of physical activity on thiamin, riboflavin, and vitamin B-6 requirements. American Journal of Clinical Nutrition 72:598S–606S

Manore MM 2002 Dietary recommendations and athletic menstrual dysfunction. Sports Medicine 32:887–901

Manore MM 2005 Feeding the active female: Part 1. ACSMs Health and Fitness Journal 9:26–28

Manore MM, Thompson J 2000 Sport nutrition for health and performance. Human Kinetics, Chicago

Nieman DC 1999 Physical fitness and vegetarian diets: Is there a relation? American Journal of Clinical Nutrition 70(suppl):570S–575S

O'Keefe KA, Keith RE, Wilson GD, Blessing DL 1989 Dietary carbohydrate intake and endurance exercise in trained female cyclists. Nutrition Research 5:25–36

Otis CL, Goldingay R 2000 The athletic woman's survival guide: how to win the battle against eating disorders, amenorrhea, and osteoporosis. Human Kinetics, Champaign IL

Otis CL, Drinkwater B, Johnson M et al 1997 American College of Sports Medicine position stand. The female athlete triad: disordered eating, amenorrhea, and osteoporosis. Medicine and Science in Sports and Exercise 29:i–ix

Pomeroy C, Mitchell JE 1992 Medical issues in the eating disorders. In: Brownell KD, Rodin J, Wilmore JH (eds) Eating, body weight and performance in athletes: disorders of modern society. Lea & Febiger, Philadelphia, p 202–221

Sinclair LM, Hinton PS 2005 Prevalence of iron deficiency with and without anaemia in recreationally active men and women. Journal of the American Dietetics Association 105:975–978

Tipton KD, Wolfe RR 2004 Protein and amino acids for athletes. Journal of Sports Science 22:65–79

Warren MP, Perlroth NE 2001 The effects of intense exercise on the female reproductive system. Journal of Endocrinology170:3–11

Weaver C 2000 Calcium requirements of physically active people. American Journal of Clinical Nutrition 72(2 suppl):579S–584S

Wolman RL 1990 Bone mineral density levels in elite female athletes. Annals of the Rheumatic Diseases 49:1013–1016

World Health Organization 2003 Nutrition. Micronutrient deficiencies. Battling iron deficiency anaemia. http://www.who.int/nut/ida.htm. Accessed August 2005

Chapter **11**

Chronobiology and nutrition

Jim Waterhouse

LEARNING OBJECTIVES

After studying this chapter, you should be able to:

1. Understand the basic principles of chronobiology, namely: the similarities and differences between homeostasis and chronobiology; the distinction between the endogenous and exogenous component of a circadian rhythm; the principles underlying constant routine and forced desynchronization protocols; the structure and function of the 'body clock'; the need for zeitgebers and their mechanism of action.
2. Relate the above concepts to food intake, the digestion of food and the metabolism of absorbed foodstuffs.
3. Be aware of the differences from young adults that exist in these rhythmic processes in babies and in old people, as well as be able to explain how

and why rhythms of food intake and metabolism change after time-zone transitions, during night work and when fasting.

4. Outline the extent to which mealtimes might act as a zeitgeber.

CHRONOBIOLOGY

The concept of homeostasis is a key one in physiology and biochemistry. It refers to the control of physiological functions at a 'steady state', to which they return when perturbed. Thus, body (core) temperature is maintained within narrow limits in spite of changes in the heat load to which the individual is exposed, and blood glucose levels are controlled despite discontinuous food intake.

Technological developments have enabled an increasing range of variables to be monitored, for example, gut temperature and its intra-luminal pressure, while developments in biochemical assays now enable very small volumes of blood, saliva or other body fluids to be collected at frequent intervals and assayed for a whole range of substances. Such developments have not called into question the viability of the concept of homeostasis but they have shown that the limits within which a variable is controlled homeostatically show a daily periodicity (Reilly et al 1997, Waterhouse et al 2002). Chronobiology is the study of what causes these rhythms and the implications they have for the individuals concerned.

Rhythms of gastrointestinal function have not been studied much in a chronobiological context. Instead, much work in humans has been performed using core (rectal) temperature, and this rhythm will be used to illustrate the principles of chronobiology. It will then be possible to apply these principles to investigations of food intake, gut function and the metabolism of food. Insofar as such rhythms are not wholly due to lifestyle, there will be implications for those whose sleep–wake cycle is changed, after a time-zone transition or during night work, for example. Further, do such rhythms exist in the newborn, and are they modified with ageing?

ORIGIN OF THE DAILY RHYTHM OF CORE TEMPERATURE

If the daily rhythm of core temperature were wholly due to an individual's lifestyle and environment, then changing these, as after a time-zone transition or during night work, for example, would result in an immediate and appropriate change in the timing of these rhythms. In practice, it has long been known that this is not the case. Time-zone transitions and night work are associated with a whole group of symptoms, called 'jet lag' and 'shift workers' malaise', respectively. These symptoms include: loss of sleep and fatigue, falls in motivation and concentration, decreased appetite and enjoyment of food, and changed bowel function.

Moreover, the rhythm of core temperature is abnormal and, until it has adjusted to the time-zone transition or night work, the symptoms persist.

This is indirect evidence that 'something else' in addition to lifestyle and the environment is involved.

There are two methods that are widely used for investigating whether an observed daily rhythm is due wholly to the individual's lifestyle and environment. They are the constant routine and forced desynchronization protocols.

Constant routines

When subjects living normally (daytime activity and night-time sleep) are studied, core temperature shows higher values in the daytime and lower values at night (Fig. 11.1). *A priori*, this rhythm might reflect the body's response to a day-orientated lifestyle, with daytime activities in a dynamic environment and nocturnal sleep and recuperation in a quiet one. This is not the case, however, as can be deduced from studies of individuals during a 'constant routine'. In this protocol, the subject is required: (1) to stay awake and sedentary for at least 24 hours in an environment of constant temperature, humidity and lighting; (2) to engage in similar activities throughout this time, generally reading or listening to music; and (3) to take identical meals at regularly-spaced intervals. Even though this protocol removes any rhythmicity due to the environment and lifestyle, the rhythm of core temperature persists, even though its amplitude is decreased (Fig. 11.1). Three deductions can be made from this result:

1. The rhythm that remains must arise from a source within the body; it is described as an endogenous component of the rhythm, and its generation is attributed to a 'body clock'.

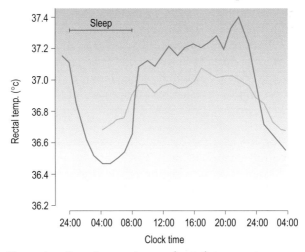

Figure 11.1   Mean circadian changes in core (rectal) temperature measured hourly in eight subjects: living normally and sleeping from 24:00 to 08:00 hours (solid line); and then woken at 04:00 hours and spending the next 24 hours on a 'constant routine' (dashed line). From Minors & Waterhouse (1981) with permission.

2. Some effect of the environment and lifestyle is present, since the amplitude of the rhythm has decreased. This component of the rhythm is termed 'exogenous'; body temperature is raised by ambient light and mental and physical activities during daytime waking, and decreased by darkness, sleep and inactivity during the night.

3. In subjects living a conventional lifestyle, these two components are in phase. This means that, during the daytime, the body temperature is raised by the body clock acting in synchrony with the environment and activity and, during the night, the clock, environment and inactivity all act to reduce core temperature.

Forced desynchronization protocol

This approach (Boivin et al 1997) is based on the observation that the body clock is not able to adjust to an imposed lifestyle whose period differs substantially from 24 hours (see later). For example, if a subject lives on 27-hour 'days' (with 9 hours of sleep and 18 hours of activity each 'day'), the endogenous component of the circadian rhythm retains a period close to 24 hours, as a result of which, 8×27-hour imposed 'days' equal 9×24-hour endogenous cycles. This length of time is called a 'beat cycle'. One result of such a protocol is that the endogenous component of the rhythm moves continually out of phase with the sleep–wake cycle and then back into phase. If core temperature is measured throughout a beat cycle, then it can be averaged in one of two ways. First, if the results from nine 24-hour cycles are averaged into a single 24-hour rhythm, any phase of this average rhythm is mixed with all phases of the imposed (27-hour) sleep–wake cycle. That is, provided that the sleep-wake cycle is similar day-by-day, any effects directly or indirectly due to the exogenous component will be cancelled out, and the average rhythm observed will represent the endogenous component of the measured rhythm. Alternatively, if the temperatures from eight 27-hour cycles are averaged into a single 27-hour rhythm, any phase of this average rhythm is mixed with all phases of the endogenous (24-hour) cycle. That is, any effects directly or indirectly due to the body clock will be cancelled out, and the average rhythm observed will represent the exogenous component of the measured rhythm.

BODY CLOCK

Humans have paired groups of cells, the suprachiasmatic nuclei (SCN), in the base of the hypothalamus, a region of the brain closely associated with the regulation of body temperature, the release of hormones, and the control of appetite and sleep (Moore 1992). One of the many pieces of evidence that the SCN is the site of the clock is that slices of brain containing this area show rhythmicity in nerve activity when the slices are cultured in vitro in constant conditions; no other region of the brain shows autonomous activity in such circumstances. The genetic and molecular mechanisms responsible for generating the activity of the clock have now been described (Clayton et al 2001).

When humans are studied in an environment in which there are no time cues – in an underground cave, for example – the daily rhythms of sleep and waking, body temperature, hormone release, and so on, continue. This fact confirms their endogenous origin, but it is observed that the period of such rhythms is closer to 25 than 24 hours and the subject becomes progressively more delayed with respect to the outside environment (Fig. 11.2). The clock-driven rhythms measured in such circumstances are called circadian (from the Latin for 'about a day').

Such circadian rhythmicity implies that the body clock needs to be adjusted continually for it to remain synchronized to a solar (24-hour) day, and this is what normally happens. Synchronization is achieved by zeitgebers (German for 'time-givers'), rhythms resulting, directly or indirectly, from the environment (Reilly et al 1997, Waterhouse et al 2002). In humans, the most important zeitgebers are the regular alternation of the light-dark cycle and the regular secretion at night of the pineal hormone, melatonin.

The effect of light depends on the time of exposure (Czeisler et al 1989, Minors et al 1991). Pulses of light that are centred in the 6-hour 'window' immediately after the trough of the body temperature rhythm (the trough normally being 03:00–05:00 hours, see Fig. 11.1) produce a phase advance; those centred in the 6-hour window before the temperature minimum, a phase delay; and pulses centred away from the trough by more than a few hours have little effect and are said to be in the 'dead phase' (Fig. 11.3). Bright light such as is found outdoors or indoors near windows produces larger phase shifts than does domestic lighting although, in practice, most humans normally have little exposure to natural daylight. Therefore, exposure to light on waking in the morning, and even to light passing through our eyelids when asleep at this time, will cause a small advance of the body clock. This

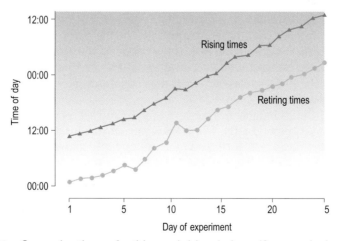

Figure 11.2   Successive times of retiring and rising during a 'free-running' experiment performed upon a single subject in temporal isolation. From Waterhouse et al (2002) with permission.

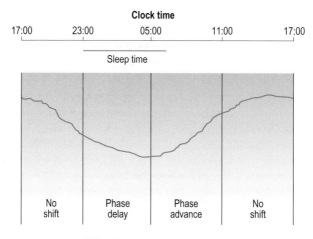

Figure 11.3   Diagrammatic illustration of a phase response curve to light. The circadian rhythm of core temperature is shown (as a marker of the body clock) and, relative to this, are shown the times when light would cause a phase advance, a phase delay, or no phase shift ('dead zone') of the body clock. The normal sleep time is shown as a horizontal line.

will result in the clock showing a period of 24 hours, synchronized to the solar day.

Ingestion of melatonin, in the form of pills, can also advance or delay the body clock according to the time at which ingestion takes place. The shifts produced tend to be in the opposite direction to those produced by light exposure at the same time. Thus, the ingestion of melatonin in the afternoon and evening tends to advance the body clock, and in the morning tends to delay it. Receptors for melatonin are present in the SCN. Since bright light also inhibits the secretion of melatonin, the phase-shifting effects of light and melatonin reinforce each other. Bright light in the early morning, just after the temperature minimum, advances the phase of the body clock – not only directly but also indirectly, since it suppresses the secretion of melatonin and so prevents the phase-delaying effect that melatonin would have exerted at this time (Lewy & Sack 1996).

These rhythmic changes in exposure to light and secretion of melatonin are normally underpinned by the whole social structure of individuals' lifestyles, including mealtimes and social, mental and physical activities. That is, it is in the daytime that we tend to eat and to be active, and at night that we fast and are inactive. Even so, these other putative zeitgebers have been found to be comparatively unimportant (see, for example, Mrosovsky 1999). The potential role of meals as a zeitgeber will be considered in more detail later.

Role of the body clock
The body clock produces daily rhythms in core temperature, plasma hormone concentrations, the outflow of the sympathetic nervous system, and

activity in the sleep centres of the brain. All of these rhythms exert effects throughout the body.

The general effects of the body clock are twofold. First, those actions involving physical and mental activity and their associated biochemical and cardiovascular changes, including the metabolism of glucose and the storage of lipid, are promoted in the daytime; those involving recovery and restitution during a period of inactivity, including the sparing of glucose and metabolism of lipid, are promoted at night. The second role is to enable preparations to be made for the switches from the active to the sleeping state, and vice versa; individuals have to prepare biologically for going to sleep and for waking up (Moore-Ede 1986). Such changes require an ordered reduction or increase in activity of a whole series of biochemical and physiological functions – and this has to be set in motion before the actual events of falling asleep or waking up take place.

To achieve the above aims, the body clock needs to be stable and robust, and not to respond to transient changes in the environment or lifestyle of the individual. For example, a clock that rapidly adjusted would compromise the phasing of the circadian rhythms of an individual who woke transiently in the night and switched on the light, or who took a nap in the daytime. The fact that the body clock is slow to adjust to changes in lifestyle makes sound ecological sense, therefore. Such stability means that, for those who undergo time-zone transitions or have to work at night, the normal synchrony between the endogenous and exogenous components of the circadian rhythms, including that of core temperature, will be lost. It is now known that it is this lack of synchrony between the body clock and the outside world that causes these individuals to suffer the symptoms of 'jet lag' (Waterhouse et al 1997) and 'shift workers' malaise' (Waterhouse et al 1992).

DIFFERENCES IN THE NATURE AND STRENGTH OF THE EXOGENOUS COMPONENT

The above principle, that a measured rhythm consists of an endogenous, clock-driven component and an exogenous component driven by the individual's lifestyle and environment, applies to all variables. In practice, however, differences exist between variables. The first difference is in those aspects of the subject's sleep–wake cycle and environment that contribute to the exogenous component of a measured rhythm. Blood pressure, heart rate and airway calibre are affected similarly to core temperature, being raised by physical and mental activity and lowered by sleep; melatonin secretion is suppressed by bright light; the levels of gut muscular and secretory activity and several hormones are modified by ingestion of food; and antidiuretic hormone (ADH) release is affected by fluid intake and posture.

The second difference between variables is in the relative size of the endogenous and exogenous components of a rhythm. Some variables appear to have large exogenous and only small endogenous components – for example, heart rate, blood pressure, the excretion of water by the kidneys, the muscular and secretory activity of the gut, and the secretion of growth hormone by the pituitary gland (which is promoted by sleep). By contrast, the excretion of potassium in the urine and the secretion of melatonin and cortisol (together with the metabolic effects of this latter hormone) have more marked endogenous components. Core temperature has components of similar magnitude (compare the amplitudes of the two curves in Fig. 11.1).

CHRONOBIOLOGY TO FOOD INTAKE, GASTROINTESTINAL FUNCTION AND METABOLISM

There is clear evidence that subjects living normally show daily rhythms of food intake, of gastrointestinal activity, and of dealing with the absorbed foodstuffs. It is less clear if all these rhythms have an endogenous component; each will be considered in turn. For a review of the field, see Waterhouse et al (1999).

DAILY PROFILES OF FOOD INTAKE AND THE ENJOYMENT OF EATING

Most humans distribute food intake unevenly over the course of the waking day; there are generally two or three main meals, conventionally described as 'breakfast', 'lunch' and 'dinner', interspersed with several snacks. The timing of the main meals has a large cultural component and is also influenced by lifestyle (including hours of work), social events and religious practice (fasting during Ramadan, for example, Khashoggi et al 1993).

Even though many of these rhythmic patterns can be seen as having a strong exogenous component, indicating integration between waking activities and food intake, there is also some evidence that an endogenous component might be present also. For example, appetite and enjoyment of food decrease transiently after a time-zone transition (Waterhouse et al 2000) and food intake is changed quite markedly during night work, the individual often 'snacking' throughout the night shift rather than eating a full meal ('lunch') in the middle of it (Krauchi et al 1990, Lennernas et al 1995, Reinberg et al 1979). These results might arise because food is being offered at what is the wrong time by the biological clock. The question is, 'How strong is the evidence that such changes indicate that the body clock plays an important role?'.

After a journey to Australia from the UK, for example (Australia is 10 time zones ahead of the UK), 'breakfast' is at about 22:00 hours, 'lunch' at about 03:00 hours, and 'dinner' at about 09:00 hours on 'body time' while it is still adjusted to UK time. Waterhouse et al (2000) found that food intake and its enjoyment recovered sooner than did other symptoms of jet lag, and before the rhythm of core temperature had become adjusted to the new time zone. Moreover, in this and another study (Waterhouse et al 2003b), the correlation between loss of appetite and the assessment of the amount of 'jet lag' was low and often non-significant. These results indicate that the link between jet lag and loss of appetite and enjoyment of food is weak. It seems likely that they are partly the result of the general fatigue and malaise associated with jet lag and due to the loss of sleep. Eating different food (or food prepared in a different way) in new surroundings might contribute to these changes.

Also, in a laboratory-based simulation of an 8-hour eastward time-zone transition, the daily pattern of meal intake adjusted almost immediately to the new local time (Fig. 11.4). As this figure shows, the pattern of intake of hot meals on control days indicated it was most common at times that could be considered to be 'lunchtime' and 'dinnertime'. On the day immediately after the time-zone shift, this pattern was altered, with hot meals most frequent at the beginning and end of the waking day, and least frequent in the middle of it. This result can be interpreted in terms of effect upon food intake of an unadjusted body clock. Thus, the increased frequency of eating a hot meal after rising might be considered to be a late evening meal (by UK time and by an unadjusted body clock); the increased frequency of eating a hot meal just before retiring can be considered as 'lunch'; and the lower frequency of eating hot meals during the daytime coincides with night on UK time. However, the pattern was essentially normal by the third post-shift day, even though the body clock, as assessed by the circadian rhythm of core temperature, had not adjusted by the third post-shift day. That is, once again, the link between the phase of the body clock and food intake has been shown to be weak.

With night work, altered eating habits might be due to several reasons, including inadequate facilities for buying or preparing food, lack of surroundings conducive to eating a meal, or the body clock (since it adjusts poorly to the schedule of night work and daytime sleep). In addition, it might be felt the 'wrong time' to eat a full meal and/or eating a full meal might not fit in with domestic arrangements, where meals would be available soon before or

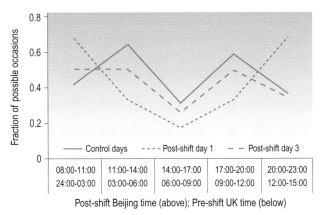

Figure 11.4 The mean fraction of possible occasions when a hot meal was eaten before (control days) and on the first and third day after (post-shift days) a simulated eastward time-zone shift of 8 hours, equivalent to flying from the UK to Beijing, China. Beijing and UK clock times are shown. (Unpublished data.)

after the night shift (dinner and breakfast, respectively, for those members of the household not working night shifts).

We investigated some of these possibilities in hospital nurses working at night using our Food Intake Questionnaire (Waterhouse et al 2003a). Taken as a whole, the questionnaire gave information about how intake of food was affected by habits, social factors, the work schedule, availability of food and by hunger; it also gave information about the type of meal chosen and subjective responses to that meal. The questionnaire was answered every 3 hours for a 'typical week', including work days and rest days.

Results (Waterhouse et al 2003a) confirmed that, compared with rest days, there was an increased frequency of eating snacks rather than larger meals during the night shifts. Also, one of the main factors affecting food intake in the night shift was the work schedule; food intake had to be fitted around this schedule. This last result was found also in a group of daytime workers who were studied in the same way, but there were differences between the two groups during their work days: the constraints imposed by the work schedule were considered by the night worker to be more severe; snacks were more common during night than day work; and meals were generally enjoyed less by the night workers, in part because snacks in general were enjoyed least. These differences tended to disappear during rest days, and both groups of subjects were more likely to eat because they felt hungry, they enjoyed their food more, and they ate hot meals more frequently.

The differences between the night and day workers during their work days indicate that the night shift imposes more restrictions upon the freedom to eat a meal when hungry. In addition, these differences might also be due to the body clock (the night worker eating near to the circadian trough of the unadjusted core temperature rhythm but the day worker eating nearer to the peak of this rhythm) and to domestic factors.

As described above, a forced desynchronization schedule is one way to separate the endogenous and exogenous components of a daily rhythm. A group of 14 students was subjected to such a protocol, living on 28-hour 'days', with 9.33 hours allocated to sleep and 18.67 hours to waking (Waterhouse et al 2004). During the waking period, subjects had some tasks to perform, but they were free to choose what they ate during breaks that would conventionally be regarded as times for breakfast, elevenses, lunch, tea, dinner and supper. During this protocol, they answered the questionnaire about food intake. By far the main reason for eating/not eating was hunger/lack of hunger rather than factors such as food availability and time-pressure. There were statistically significant effects of time within the imposed waking periods upon the type of meal eaten – 'breakfast' tending to be a snack, 'lunch' a small hot meal, and the 'evening meal' a large hot meal. Hot meals (whether small or large) were associated with more hunger before the meal, more enjoyment of the meal, and a greater degree of satiety afterwards than were cold meals.

These effects suggest that, as was the case after a time-zone transition, individuals adjust their eating habits to fit in with the imposed wake times (the exogenous component of a rhythm). By contrast, the effect of 'body time' (the endogenous component) upon food intake, the type of meal eaten, and subjective responses to the meal was much weaker and rarely reached statistical significance. That is, a large hot meal was chosen as readily for a 'dinner', and subjective responses to it were the same, whether it was eaten at a time coincident with the trough or the peak of the core temperature rhythm.

This importance of exogenous rather than endogenous factors in determining food intake has also been seen in 'spontaneous internal desynchronization'. This is a poorly-understood phenomenon that is observed in some subjects during free-running experiments (see Fig. 11.2). With it, the subject's core temperature rhythm continues with a period of about 24.5 hours, but the sleep–wake cycle adopts a period of about 16 or 33 hours. In both cases, the normal synchrony between endogenous and exogenous components is lost. It was found that meals continued to be taken at the 'normal' time with regard to the sleep–wake cycle. Thus, breakfast was taken soon after waking up (at whatever phase of the core temperature rhythm this coincided with), and so on. Moreover, the time interval between breakfast and lunch lengthened in proportion to the increase in the waking period (Aschoff et al 1986).

In summary, the evidence from altered sleep–wake schedules indicates that the endogenous component of the intake and enjoyment of food intake is rather weak.

Food intake in babies and aged individuals

Compared with the adult (18–60 years) population, babies and aged subjects have different feeding patterns. Can these sub-groups provide relevant information about the relative roles of exogenous and endogenous components of a rhythm?

In babies, adult feeding patterns have not been laid down (Honnebier et al 1989, Reppert 1989). Instead, feeding is determined by the baby and/or the carer. Often, babies are fed on demand, and this means feeding them every 4 hours or so (Weinert et al 1997). Does the baby's desire for food reflect the activity of some internal oscillator with a period of about 4 hours or does it, instead, reflect the accumulation of a drive for energy replacement? Means to distinguish between such possibilities (by altering meal times and/or the energy content of the food given) present ethical difficulties and have not been tested. Nevertheless, in principle, if the drive for food intake were wholly due to energy replacement, then changing the energy value of the food eaten would produce a proportional change in the interval between feeds; alternatively, if the drive were due only to an oscillator, then the timing of food intake would be unchanged, even though the amount taken would vary inversely with its energy content.

During infancy, the number of nocturnal feeds decreases. This reduction might indicate the increasing importance of a circadian control of food intake, but it might arise also because neurological and behavioural development lead to more attention during the daytime and more consolidated sleep at night, so preventing the desire for food from being sensed.

In subjects aged 55 years or more, there is the general finding of a decrease in day-to-day variability of many activities, including the frequency, timing and content of meals (Minors et al 1998, Sidenvall et al 1996). This change occurs in spite of decreasing commitments such as employment (which tend to limit the variability in mealtimes, as described above), and takes place in subjects who are still active and independent enough to be unrestricted in their activities. This increased freedom of choice was stressed by a recent study (Waterhouse et al 2005) comparing responses to the Food Intake Questionnaire in elderly (55+ years) subjects who were not involved in full-time work with those in younger subjects (20–48 years) who worked full time. During the weekend, the food intake pattern of neither group was influenced by 'schedule'; during the weekdays, this lack of influence persisted in the older group, but 'schedule' became an important factor for the working group. It was also found that 'habit' was recorded more frequently in older than younger subjects as a reason for eating or not eating at a particular time.

In summary, the results from older subjects indicate that the role of routine in determining their meals and activities increases, in spite of greater freedom to spend time as they wish. One effect of this increased adherence to a routine will be to strengthen the exogenous component of circadian rhythms, and this might offset the decline in strength of the endogenous component, due to atrophy of cells in the SCN, that generally accompanies ageing. For neonates, there is some evidence that a regular routine of feeding, accompanied by the regular exposure to light and to general activities by the carer that will normally accompany feeding, promotes the development of circadian rhythms and even of more general areas of development. Whether, with either group, such regular mealtimes are also acting as a zeitgeber, that is, are stabilizing the body clock to a 24-hour period, is another issue that will be addressed later.

GASTROINTESTINAL FUNCTION

In adults living on conventional sleep–wake cycles, there are daily patterns in gastrointestinal motility and the secretion of digestive juices, in the absorption of digested food products, and in the concentrations of carbohydrates, amino acids and lipids in the bloodstream. Superimposed upon these daily changes are changes occurring about every 4 hours during the daytime. These rhythms have been reviewed on several occasions (for example: Mejean et al 1988, Waterhouse et al 1999) and they are obviously closely related to the individuals' patterns of food intake; that is, they are exogenous. From a chronobiological viewpoint, the issue is whether these rhythms possess also an endogenous component that can be linked to the body clock.

To investigate this issue, baseline muscular activity and intra-luminal pH during the fasting state have been measured, as well as the responses to similar meals eaten at different times of the day. In many studies, only a few time-points have been compared, these having been obtained during the waking day and during the night when the subject is, or has been, asleep. Such studies do not enable a detailed description of any circadian rhythm to be obtained, and they suffer from the interpretive problem that day-night differences might reflect effects due to sleep as well as the endogenous body clock. Even so, there is some evidence to indicate that there is a weak circadian rhythm in the responses to food intake. Examples of this include the response to a glucose load, gastric acidity (both during fasting and after a meal), cell proliferation of the gastrointestinal mucosa, the rate of gastric emptying, gut muscle activity, the secretion of gut hormones and digestive juices, motility of the small intestine, rectal motor complexes, and the absorption of drugs and foodstuffs from the gastrointestinal tract (see reviews cited above and Auwerda et al 2001, Bjarnason & Jordan 2002, Keller et al 2001). In most cases, differences between day and night are rather small and show less activity in the night. The exception to this is gastric acidity, which is higher at night, thereby accounting for the pain associated with ulcers being worse at this time.

The observation that there is a daily rhythm in proliferation of mucosal cells of the gut has implications for cancer treatment. When cytostatic drugs (that prevent cell division) are used, their effectiveness depends in part upon the rate at which the cells are dividing. The cancerous cells (which tend to divide rapidly at all times of the day) can be targeted preferentially if the drug is administered at a time when the rate of division of the healthy cells is at its daily minimum (Bjarnason & Jordan 2002). Similarly, the finding that the absorption of drugs from the gut varies with the time of day has implications for their most efficacious time of administration (Lemmer 2004).

A rhythm in uptake of materials from the gut is one explanation of subjective reports from some subjects during constant routines; even though an identical snack is taken each hour, some subjects reported that this intake did not satisfy them during the daytime but was too much and made them feel uncomfortably bloated during the night. This has been investigated formally, using subjects on a constant routine (starting 1 hour after a normal 8-hour sleep) and eating an identical snack every 3 hours. Subjects' hunger and indigestion were assessed hourly, and just before eating on those occasions when they were required to take a snack. Over the course of the constant routine (Fig. 11.5), hunger was about normal during the daytime, but fell at the end of the constant routine, which coincided with the night. Indigestion remained low during the daytime and then rose during the night. Whether this result indicates an effect of increasing fatigue in addition to circadian influences cannot be inferred from this observation. Nevertheless, these changes could contribute to the decreased intake of food during a night shift, with meals during the night being taken not only when individuals are feeling tired but also when their temperature rhythm is close to its minimum.

Since the requirement of a 'constant routine' is to minimize the exogenous component of a rhythm experimentally, staying awake with constant activity is adequate when the measurement of core temperature is considered, because the exogenous components of this rhythm are sleep and activity. By contrast, if gut function does show circadian rhythmicity, then it is clear that such a protocol is inappropriate for studies of food uptake and the hormones

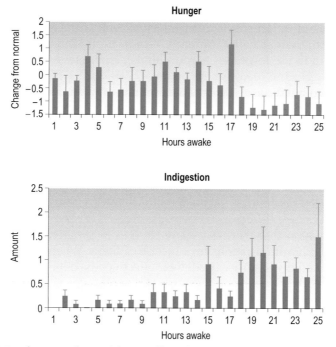

Figure 11.5   A group of 12 subjects, adjusted to a normal sleep–wake cycle and undergoing a constant routine protocol. Top, the mean (+ SE) difference in change of hunger from 'normal'; bottom, the mean (+ SE) amount of indigestion.

associated with metabolism of absorbed carbohydrate and fat. Van Cauter and co-workers (Van Cauter et al 1989, 1991) have used a constant intra-venous infusion of glucose in place of eating identical meals at equi-spaced intervals. The rationale for this procedure is that eating identical meals does not guarantee a constant uptake of nutrients into the bloodstream, depending as it does upon digestion and absorption from the gut, both of which them-selves might show circadian variation. (It will be noted that this would be a plausible inference from the study of indigestion, Fig. 11.5.) Intravenous infusion of a glucose solution overcomes this problem, and has provided valuable information about metabolic function. However, the protocol does nothing to control circadian changes in sequestration or metabolism of absorbed foodstuffs.

DEALING WITH THE PRODUCTS OF DIGESTION

During the daytime, particularly in the morning, the sensitivity of the tissues to the hormone insulin is high (La Fleur 2003, Van Cauter et al 1989). Later in the daytime and at night, the body is less able to deal with a glucose load. The increased sensitivity of the body to insulin in the earlier part of the day, coupled with the fact that eating generally takes place only in the daytime, means that most daytime energy comes from the metabolism of glucose, with the extra energy being stored in the muscles and liver as glycogen. Insulin is also lipogenic, that is, it has the property of causing the fats that are eaten to be laid down in adipose tissue. At night, by contrast, the sensitivity of the body tissues to insulin is reduced and growth hormone, whose secretion is associated with the early part of sleep (when so-called 'slow wave sleep' predominates), further reduces the effectiveness of insulin. As a result, fatty acids are released from the adipose tissue stores during the night and they, rather than glucose, are metabolized preferentially then. Also, there is an increased release of cortisol towards the end of the night, and this conserves glucose by promoting gluconeogenesis.

Since the rises in plasma glucose concentration and its uptake by the tissues begin before waking in the morning and are independent of food intake, they appear to have an endogenous component (La Fleur 2003). It is also known that cortisol has a marked endogenous component. By contrast, growth hormone has a much weaker endogenous component, its secretion being dominated by sleep onset and slow wave sleep. The result of these factors is that, after a change in the sleep–wake schedule of an individual (after a time-zone transition or during night work, for example), the hormonal rhythms will shift at rates that differ both from each other and from the sleep–wake and food intake cycles. The normal balance between glucose and lipid metabolism will be altered. This perturbation has been observed in laboratory studies (Morgan et al 1998), and a link between nocturnal glucose intake and raised LDL cholesterol has been reported (Lennernas et al 1994). The potential importance of these findings is that they might provide a link with the increased incidence of cardiovascular morbidity that is associated with night work (Waterhouse et al 1992). They are of interest to the sports participant also, since exercise is known to alter the secretion of both growth hormone and cortisol, but the position is complicated by the fact that the size and time-courses of the changes depend upon the time of exercise (Kanalev et al 2001).

Concentrations of carbohydrates, lipids and amino acids in the plasma are affected by the size and composition of meals, and so the circadian rhythms of these variables have a marked exogenous component, as do the many metabolic processes and release of hormones initiated by the uptake of these foodstuffs. The metabolic responses to a meal can depend also on the timing (Wolever & Bolognesi 1996) and combination of foods ingested. For example, the simultaneous ingestion of a meal containing carbohydrate and protein will, through the action of insulin (which is released due to the uptake of glucose and which promotes the selective clearance from the plasma of some amino acids), cause the ratio [plasma tyrosine]:[plasma tryptophan] to be lower than when the meal contains only protein (Leathwood 1989). The possible implication of this result is described in the next section.

Sports participants are interested in nutritional interventions (e.g. high-fat, high-carbohydrate diets, caffeine, etc.) that are thought to improve performance. However, their efficacy when taken at different times of the day has not been investigated; generally, these experiments are performed in the morning, following an overnight fast. Bearing in mind the metabolic consequences of these interventions, and that circadian rhythms are associated with metabolism of the food that is taken up from the gut, it is theoretically possible that the timing of the intervention will affect its efficacy.

SOME IMPLICATIONS OF CHRONOBIOLOGY AND NUTRITION

Brief mention has already been made of some of the uses to which a knowledge of the chronobiology of nutrition has been put. These include knowledge that the kinetics of uptake of a drug from the gut will depend upon its time of administration and that the timing of cell proliferation of the gut mucosa can influence the time of administration of cytostatic drugs aimed at the gut. Mention has been made also of the problem with food intake experienced by night workers, but the difficulties are so widespread that they deserve some elaboration. Other implications include the time of day of food intake and weight loss, and the effects of changed food and fluid intakes during the fast of Ramadan. Finally, it is appropriate to consider if the timing of meals and their nature act upon the body clock as a zeitgeber.

NIGHT WORK

One reason why a solution to the difficulties associated with food intake during night work is so important is that between 10–20% of the workforce of industrialized societies is involved in night work at some stage. Gastric ulcers are more common in night workers than in their day-working colleagues, and indigestion and irregularity of bowel movements are common enough to be regarded almost as 'routine' (Waterhouse et al 1992). The incentive to improve the situation stems also from two other pieces of epidemiological evidence. First, nurses working night shifts are more likely to be obese than their day-working colleagues (Niedhammer et al 1996). Second, as already described, metabolic changes produced by a meal at night differ from those produced by the same meal eaten in the daytime, there being a rise in LDL cholesterol, a predictor of cardiovascular morbidity.

When these factors are combined with the observations that eating habits are generally altered in night workers, it is clear that there is a challenge to improve the general food hygiene of night workers. This is a complex issue, because both endogenous and exogenous causes for changed eating habits seem to exist. To the extent that the body clock exerts some role in food intake, some advantage would be gained by promoting adjustment of the body clock to the night shift. Such an adjustment would also relieve sleep loss and fatigue, and so provide a further advantage to the night worker.

When exogenous factors are considered, it seems that the demands of work schedules and the problems encountered in attempting to eat with the rest of the household and family are important. A solution to these difficulties requires changes to work patterns and to lifestyle. At work, the advent of the microwave oven and the increasing awareness of a healthy diet, with more fibre and fresh produce and less fried food and cholesterol-rich foodstuffs, should both help in meeting this challenge. This would particularly be the case if these changes were coupled with improved facilities for sitting down to relax and enjoy a meal (De Castro 2002). Nevertheless, the problem of a decline in appetite and decreased enjoyment of food when tired would remain.

Changing eating habits in the home is difficult and inconvenient and raises a broader issue. Many of the difficulties encountered by night workers result from the clash between the demands of working abnormal hours on the one hand and trying to live with individuals who, like the body clock, adhere to normally phased sleep–wake schedules on the other. This problem is fundamental and currently remains rather intractable.

WEIGHT LOSS

There have been several reports which indicate that a single meal taken in the morning is associated with a better control of body mass than the same meal taken later in the day (see Keim et al 1997, for example). The mechanism involved is unclear, though changed metabolic processes during the course of the day are one possibility. There is also the possibility that energy expenditure in the daytime during routine activities is slightly greater after a meal eaten soon after rising than after one later in the day, since the early meal 'sets up' the individual for the day. This theory does not seem to have been tested; the metabolic difference that would account for the observed effect is small and would not be easy to measure. There are better ways in which to lose weight!

RAMADAN

The required practice of adherents to Ramadan is to eschew food and fluid intake between sunrise and sunset. Observance of this religious tenet by Muslims displaces energy intake and hydration to the hours of darkness and reverses the normal circadian pattern of eating and drinking. In this regard, there is some similarity with the night worker, therefore. Also, the natural tendency for humans to eat about every 3–4 hours when awake is overridden (Khashoggi et al 1993).

The long duration of diurnal fasting means that hunger, energy levels and subjective fatigue are increased above those habitually experienced at other times of the year. Furthermore, if the period of daytime fasting is fractured by spells of sleeping, the normal sleep–wakefulness cycle associated with the solar day is disrupted. Effects upon mental and physical performance are likely, and participation in physical training is likely to be impaired, even if the period of training is displaced to after darkness has fallen.

Fluid intake is also eschewed during daylight hours. A gradual dehydration therefore occurs until body water status can be restored after darkness. Since hypohydration can lead to impairments in physical performance, the lack of fluid intake compounds the effects of energy losses during the day. There are likely to be knock-on consequences for renal function during the daytime, as well as endocrine function, particularly the secretion of antidiuretic hormone and aldosterone (Reilly et al 2000).

Clearly, religious requirements during Ramadan create a profound change in the circadian profile of food and fluid intake, and of the metabolic responses produced by these actions. Detailed accounts of any changes to mental and physical performance are not currently available.

MEALTIMES AS A ZEITGEBER

The possible role of regular mealtimes both in promoting daily rhythmicity in babies and old subjects has already been mentioned. Since melatonin is to be found in breast milk (Reppert 1989), and melatonin can affect the timing of the body clock, it is possible that the mother might be able to influence her baby's rhythms by this route. This does not seem to have been investigated. However, regular breast feeding per se is likely to act as a zeitgeber, if only through the social activities and care-giving that are associated with it.

Another mechanism by which food intake might act as a zeitgeber has been suggested (summarized by Leathwood 1989). The mechanism is based on changes in the balance of amino acids in the plasma following the intake of protein-rich or carbohydrate-rich meals. Carbohydrate-rich meals, through their action upon insulin secretion and the selective uptake of certain amino acids into the cells of the body that this hormone produces, lower plasma tyrosine levels in preference to plasma tryptophan; protein-rich meals have the opposite effect. These amino acids pass into the brain in proportion to their relative concentrations in the plasma. The argument continues, therefore, that there could then be a selective increase in the uptake into the brain of tryptophan or tyrosine following a carbohydrate-rich or protein-rich meal, respectively. This would promote the synthesis of serotonin or catecholamines from their precursor amino acids (tryptophan and tyrosine), and this could, in turn, promote sleepiness (through the release of serotonin) or alertness (through the release of catecholamines).

Work with rodents has not supported the hypothesis (Leathwood 1989). It has not been shown that uptake of the amino acid into the brain is the rate-limiting step for serotonin or catecholamine synthesis and release, or that sleep and alertness can be controlled by this mechanism. Even so, reports of the value of a diet to combat jet lag that is based upon these mechanisms (with a protein-rich breakfast to promote alertness and a carbohydrate-rich evening meal to promote sleep) continue to appear, and the diet has been recommended in the past as part of a strategy for athletes going to competitions in distant time zones. Any effect of such a dietary intervention seems to be rather small, and appropriate times of exposure to, and avoidance of, bright light would seem to be a better alternative.

SUMMARY

Chronobiology deals with the effects of time upon body functions, and this chapter deals with the daily intake of food and its metabolism. The first section deals with some of the evidence for possession of a 'body clock' and some of its effects upon the physiology and biochemistry of the body.

There is a clear rhythm of food intake, due mainly to our habits and lifestyle. This pattern of intake is reflected in gut function and the metabolism of digested materials. One of the key issues is whether the observed rhythms contain an endogenous component, that is, part of the rhythm is mediated by the body clock. The evidence indicates that the endogenous component is weak for food intake, but that it is more pronounced for the metabolism of food.

One implication of the existence of an endogenous component is that the rhythm of food intake and metabolism will not adjust fully and immediately to changes in the sleep–wake pattern because the body clock is slow to adjust to such changes. As a result, problems are to be expected during the feast of Ramadan, after time-zone transitions, and during night work, for example. Each of these is considered, and recommendations made where possible.

The evidence that food intake might be used to promote adjustment of the body clock after time-zone transitions is outlined. It is concluded that the effect, if present, is weak.

KEY POINTS

1. Chronobiology deals with temporal changes in body functions.
2. There is clear evidence for a 'body clock' which affects many aspects of physiology and biochemistry.
3. Food intake is determined mainly by our habits and lifestyle, and this is reflected in gut function and the metabolism of digested materials. However, there is evidence that these processes are influenced also by the body clock, particularly when the hormonal control of metabolism is considered.
4. Since the body clock adjusts to changes in the sleep–wake cycle only slowly, the rhythms of food intake and metabolism will not adjust fully and immediately to time-zone transitions and night work.
5. Current knowledge provides a rationale for reducing these difficulties.

ACKNOWLEDGMENT

The author wishes to acknowledge the significant contributions of Professor Greg Atkinson, Dr Ben Edwards, Dr Barry Drust and Professor Tom Reilly in the writing of this chapter.

References

Aschoff J, von Goetz C, Wildgruber C, Wever R 1986 Meal timing in humans during isolation without time cues. Journal of Biological Rhythms 1:151–162

Auwerda J, Bac D, Schouten W 2001 Circadian rhythm of rectal motor complexes. Diseases of the Colon and Rectum 44:1328–1332

Bjarnason G, Jordan R 2002 Rhythms in human gastrointestinal mucosa and skin. Chronobiology International 19:129–140

Boivin D, Czeisler C, Dijk D-J et al 1997 Complex interaction of the sleep–wake cycle and circadian phase modulates mood in healthy subjects. Archives of General Psychiatry 54:145–152

Clayton J, Kyriacou C, Reppert S 2001 Keeping time with the human genome. Nature 409:829–831

Czeisler C, Kronauer R, Duffy J et al 1989 Bright light induction of strong (Type 0) resetting of the human circadian pacemaker. Science 244:1328–1333

DeCastro J 2002 Age-related changes in the social, psychological, and temporal influences on food intake in free-living, healthy, adult humans. Journal of Gerontology, Series A – Biological Science and Medical Science 57:M368–M377

Honnebier M, Swaab D, Mirmiran M 1989 Diurnal rhythmicity during early human development. In: Reppert S (ed.) Development of circadian rhythmicity and photoperiodism in mammals. Perinatology Press, New York, p 221–244

Kanaley J, Weltman J, Pieper K et al 2001 Cortisol and growth hormone responses to exercise at different times of day. Journal of Clinical Endocrinology and Metabolism 86:2881–2889

Keim N, VanLoan M, Horn W et al 1997 Weight loss is greater with consumption of large morning meals and fat-free mass is preserved with large evening meals in women on a controlled weight reduction regimen. Journal of Nutrition 127:75–82

Keller J, Groger G, Cherian L et al 2001 Circadian coupling between pancreatic secretion and intestinal activity in humans. American Journal of Physiology – Gastrointestinal and Liver Physiology 280:G273–G278

Khashoggi R, Madani K, Ghaznawi H, Ali M 1993 The effects of Ramadan fasting on body weight. Journal of Islamic Medical Association of North America 25:44–45

Krauchi K, Nussbaum P, Wirz-Justice A 1990 Consumption of sweets and caffeine in the night shift:relation to fatigue. In: Horne J (ed.) Sleep '90. Pontenagel Press, Bochum, p 62–64

La Fleur S 2003 Daily rhythms in glucose metabolism: suprachiasmatic nucleus output to peripheral tissues. Journal of Neuroendocrinology 15:315–322

Leathwood P 1989 Circadian rhythms of plasma amino acids, brain neurotransmitters and behaviour. In: Arendt J et al (eds) Biological rhythms in clinical practice. John Wright, London, p 136–159

Lemmer B 2004 Chronopharmakologie. Tagesrhythmen und Arzneimittelwirkung. Wissenschaftliche Verlagsgesellschaft mbH, Stuttgart

Lennernas M, Akerstedt T, Hambraeus L 1994 Nocturnal eating and serum cholesterol of three-shift workers. Scandinavian Journal of Work and Environmental Health 20:401–406

Lennernas M, Hambraeus L, Akerstedt T 1995 Shift related dietary intake in day and shift workers. Appetite 25:253–265

Lewy A, Sack R 1996 The role of melatonin and light in the human circadian system. Progress in Brain Research 111:205–216

Mejean L, Bicakova-Rocher A, Kolopp M et al 1988 Circadian and ultradian rhythms in blood glucose and plasma insulin of healthy adults. Chronobiology International 5:227–236

Minors D, Waterhouse J 1981 Circadian rhythms and the human. Wright PSG, Bristol

Minors D, Waterhouse J, Wirz-Justice A 1991 A human phase-response curve to light. Neuroscience Letters 133:36–40

Minors D, Atkinson G, Bent N et al 1998 The effects of age upon some aspects of lifestyle and implications for studies on circadian rhythmicity. Age and Ageing 27:67–72

Moore R 1992 The organisation of the human timing system. Progress in Brain Research 93:101–117

Moore-Ede M 1986 Physiology of the cireadian timing system: predictive versus reactive homeostasis. American Journal of Physiology – Regulatory and Integrative Physiology 250:R737–R752

Morgan L, Arendt J, Owens D et al 1998 Effects of the endogenous clock and sleep time on melatonin, insulin, glucose and lipid metabolism. Journal of Endocrinology 157:443–451

Mrosovsky N 1999 Critical assessment of methods and concepts in nonphotic phase shifting. Biological Rhythm Research 30:135–148

Niedhammer I, Lert F, Marne M 1996 Prevalence of overweight and weight gain in relation to night work in a nurses cohort. International Journal of Obesity 20:625–633

Reilly T, Atkinson G, Waterhouse J 1997 Biological rhythms and exercise. Oxford University Press, Oxford

Reilly T, Atkinson G, Waterhouse J 2000 Exercise, circadian rhythms and hormones. In: Warren M, Constantine N (eds) Sports endocrinology. Humana Press, Totowa NJ, p 391–420

Reinberg A, Migraine C, Apfelbaum M 1979 Circadian and ultradian rhythms in the eating behaviour and nutrient intake of oil refinery operators (Study 2). Chronobiologia (suppl 1):89–102

Reppert S (ed.) 1989 Development of circadian rhythmicity and photoperiodism in mammals. Perinatology Press, New York

Sidenvall B, Lennernas M, Anna-Christina E 1996 Elderly patients' meal patterns – a retrospective study. Journal of Human Nutrition and Dietetics 9:262–272

Van Cauter E, Desir D, Decoster C et al 1989 Nocturnal decrease in glucose tolerance during constant glucose infusion. Journal of Clinical Endocrinology and Metabolism 69:604–611

Van Cauter E, Blackman I, Roland D et al 1991 Modulation of glucose regulation and insulin secretion by circadian rhythmicity and sleep. Journal of Clinical Investigation 88:934–942

Waterhouse J, Folkard S, Minors D 1992 Shiftwork, health and safety. An overview of the scientific literature 1978–1990. HSE contract research report. Her Majesty's Stationery Office, London

Waterhouse J, Atkinson G, Reilly T 1997 Jet lag. Lancet 350:1611–1616

Waterhouse J, Akerstedt T, Lennernas M, Arendt J 1999 Chronobiology and nutrition: internal and external factors. Canadian Journal of Diabetes Care 23 (suppl 2):82–88

Waterhouse J, Edwards B, Nevill A et al 2000 Do subjective symptoms predict our perception of jet lag? Ergonomics 43:1514–1527

Waterhouse J, Minors D, Waterhouse M et al 2002 Keeping in step with your body clock. OUP, Oxford

Waterhouse J, Buckley P, Edwards B, Reilly T 2003a Measurement of, and some reasons for, differences in eating habits between night and day workers. Chronobiology International 20:1075–1092

Waterhouse J, Nevill A, Edwards B et al 2003b The relationship between assessments of jet lag and some of its symptoms. Chronobiology International 20:1061–1073

Waterhouse J, Jones K, Edwards B et al 2004 Lack of evidence for a marked endogenous component determining food intake in humans during forced desynchronisation. Chronobiology International 21:443–466

Waterhouse J, Edwards B, Reilly T 2005 A comparison of eating habits between retired or semi-retired aged subjects and younger subjects in full-time work. Biological Rhythms Research 36:195–218

Weinert D, Sitka U, Minors D et al 1997 Twenty-four-hour and ultradian rhythmicities in healthy full-term neonates: exogenous and endogenous influences. Biological Rhythm Research 28:441–452

Wolever T, Bolognesi C 1996 Time of day influences relative glycaemic effect of foods. Nutrition Research 16:381–384

Chapter **12**

The practical aspects of sports nutrition

Jeanette Crosland

LEARNING OBJECTIVES

After studying this chapter, you should be able to:

1. Describe which foods are the major sources of carbohydrate and protein.
2. Appreciate the steps necessary to provide information which is appropriate to match the requirements of the individual.
3. Appreciate the complexity of using glycaemic index in a mixed diet.
4. Describe simple methods of assessing hydration status available to athletes.
5. Describe some simple strategies which will help the travelling athlete.
6. Appreciate the need for athletes to be able to shop and cook adequately in order to be able to comply with nutritional strategies for sport.
7. Describe some simple hygiene rules which will help to ensure the safety of athletes.
8. Appreciate the extra nutritional issues which may be present for athletes with disabilities.

INTRODUCTION

This chapter is designed to be very different to the other chapters of the book. Its aim is to encourage the sports scientist to look at the available facts and translate them into practical information that informs the athlete. Some examples are presented which give an insight to quantities, choices, practical skills, and potential barriers to compliance with nutrition recommendations which can enhance performance.

FOOD

Athletes do not eat carbohydrate, protein and fat. Athletes eat food. Research might indicate ideal intakes of carbohydrate and protein for a 24-hour period, or for specific times during the athlete's day – prior to training, post-training, etc. However, few athletes have the knowledge and/or time to work out what these numbers mean in terms of real food. A printed dietary analysis indicating an average carbohydrate intake of 2.5 grams per kg body weight and suggesting that a minimum of 6 grams per kg body weight is needed to ensure sufficient energy stores for training, might be factually correct, but it will not help the athlete to achieve this goal. Practical advice is needed too.

Calculating dietary intake is the first step to helping the athlete, but it should be borne in mind that the results of dietary analysis can be inaccurate for a number of reasons:

- athletes changing eating habits to simplify recording
- athletes failing to record those foods which might 'embarrass' them
- athletes failing to record accurate description such as type of milk, size of portion, description of cooking method
- analysers failing to translate portion sizes correctly
- use of cheap imported programmes for analysis which contain inappropriate foods and quantities
- analysers failing to find the most appropriate food when identical items are not in the data base
- inappropriate conclusions being made on the basis of the number of days food analysis used.

The next step is to translate the calculations into foods and dietary strategies. Sports dietitians and sports nutritionists are practitioners who work with such numbers all the time and can readily translate nutrition into food. Ideally these professionals should be used to provide the practical information to athletes, but all sports scientists should have some appreciation of how to equate the theoretical requirements to real food portions. The following example takes one set of theoretical requirements and translates them into foods.

Example one

It is suggested that an ideal carbohydrate intake to ensure glycogen stores are maximized for endurance training can be as high as 10 grams of carbohydrate per kg body weight. A 55-kg female long-distance runner aiming to achieve this while maintaining a healthy well balanced diet based on complex carbohydrates (the popular advice available to the nation) might find herself eating:

- 90 g breakfast cereal (three times national average portion) plus 200 mL milk
- 2 slices of bread
- 3 apples
- 2 bananas
- 4 slices of bread as sandwiches
- 120 grams of rice (cooked weight) as rice salad – quite a large portion as a side salad
- 300 grams (cooked weight) pasta (a LARGE plate when cooked)
- 2 fruit scones
- 2 pots of yogurt
- ½ can of beans on two slices toast
- 4 Jaffa cakes.

In this plan no account has been taken of protein such as meat/fish/chicken, etc. which need to be added plus perhaps a low-fat sauce and maybe vegetables or salad. Can such an athlete actually eat all this? Would some refined sugary foods help to reduce the quantities of food eaten? What is the individual's current intake? Is a compromise needed? While some lighter weight females may have no problem with these quantities, a blanket presumption that because the theory dictates this is the amount needed could lead to problems of compliance. Familiarity with food portions and the nutritional content of food is an advantage if not a necessity when working in this situation.

An ability to calculate the actual nutritional content of a food is useful, but at least an appreciation of portion sizes and the carbohydrate and protein content of those portions can help. A useful way to begin to understand food portions is to read labels. They can sometimes be difficult to follow – an indication of the problems encountered by athletes. Questions to consider are as follows. How much of different foods make a portion? What does 150 grams of pasta look like? How much carbohydrate and protein does this contain? If an athlete draws the amount of rice on the plate with their hand – what does this equate to?

As a rough guide, Tables 12.1 and 12.2 indicate approximately how much food is needed to provide 50 grams of carbohydrate and 10 grams of protein. These are based on averages for a selection of foods only, but they do provide a rough guide to portions and numbers. Some athletes may consider these portions large, others may eat two or three times these quantities at one meal.

Table 12.1   Examples of food portions containing 50 g of carbohydrate

Amount of food in grams providing 50 grams of carbohydrate	Household description
Bagel with honey	1 bagel 1 teaspoon honey
150 g pasta – cooked weight	5 heaped tablespoons
160 g rice – cooked weight	4 heaped tablespoons
135 g baked beans + 2 slices toast	$\frac{1}{3}$ can beans with two slices bread
30 g corn flakes 200 mL milk, apple	
2 slices bread sandwich with ham/tuna/chicken plus 200 mL fruit juice	
75 g quick-cook porridge	1 mug full
60 g cornflakes	10 tablespoons
65 g Weetabix	3–4 biscuits
100 g bread	3 slices
100 g malt loaf	3 slices
Jacket potato	1 medium
Bananas	2 large
Apples	4 medium
70 g sultanas	2 heaped tablespoons
140 g dried apricots	18 apricots
410 g tinned fruit in fruit juice	1 tin
Majority of cereal/breakfast bars	2 bars
800 mL isotonic sports drink	

Note: These are approximate values. Checking individual brands may give slightly different values.

GLYCAEMIC INDEX

The glycaemic index of foods is a factor which is thought to be a useful consideration in some aspects of sports nutrition. The glycaemic index of a food is a ranking based on the immediate effect of the food on blood sugar levels, when compared with a reference food such as pure glucose. The use of high glycaemic index foods post-exercise may assist the body in restoring its glycogen stores more rapidly, aiding refuelling prior to future training/competition bouts. There is some evidence that lower GI foods may be beneficial prior to exercise and that our general diet, in terms of good health, should be based on carbohydrate foods with a low to medium GI. This principle works relatively easily when single foods are considered. For example some higher

Table 12.2 Examples of food portions containing 10 g of protein

Amount of food in grams providing 10 grams of protein	Household description
30 g meat	1 small slice
30 g chicken	
45 g fish	
45 g tuna canned in brine – when drained	½ small tin
200 g baked beans	Small tin
80 g egg	1½ eggs (1 egg contains 6 g protein)
30 g skimmed milk powder	
300 ml lower fat milk	
320 ml sweetened soya milk	
40 g cheese	
125 g tofu (steamed)	
40 g peanuts	
50 g cashew nuts	
200–250 g low-fat fruit yogurt	1½ to 2 pots
140 g red kidney beans caned and drained	3 heaped tablespoons
Bread	3½ slices
150 g pasta – cooked weight	5 heaped tablespoons
380 g boiled rice	2 bowls

GI foods include sports drinks, bread, jelly sweets, cornflakes and rice cakes. Most of these would make quite acceptable post-training snacks. Some lower GI foods which might usefully be included in the general day-to-day diet of athletes might include jam, carrots, peas, pasta, milk and yogurt and fruits such as peaches, apples, grapes. However, if the athlete decides to add milk to their cornflakes, the GI of the resulting snack is affected.

The GI of a meal is a weighted average of the GI factors of the carbohydrate containing foods within the meal. The actual weighting is based on the proportion of the total carbohydrate for the meal which is contributed by the carbohydrate containing foods in that meal. For example, if a meal contains two slices of bread providing 30 g carbohydrate and three teaspoons jam also providing 30 g carbohydrate, the GI of the meal will be the GI value for bread plus the GI for jam divided by 2. However, the proportion of the total carbohydrate provided by each food must be considered and with more complicated examples there is a fair amount of maths involved. Consequently, at a practical level, many practitioners find that with the majority of athletes a simple use of high GI foods for post-training snacks may be the easiest option.

PERSONALIZING NUTRITION INFORMATION

Within any sport and even within the same team, each individual athlete will have different requirements based on their body weight, position in team, periodization of training and body weight targets. It is important for each athlete to be given specific targets and advice to meet their own personal demands. For example, using similar food patterns and approximated figures, the intakes shown in Table 12.3 may be calculated from basic estimations of need.

The variation in the quantities of food needed by each athlete can be seen from the table. On a practical note it can be seen from the following examples that it is possible for even strength-based athletes to ensure sufficient protein to meet requirements by consuming foods as opposed to supplements.

These examples could vary considerably. The endurance runner may need to increase his carbohydrate to 10 g per kg body weight prior to a marathon, or decrease his intake during periods of lesser activity or injury. The intake of the rugby player could change during a phase of intensive power training. Other players within the same team may be aiming to lose body weight/body fat and require a different intake – others may be attempting to bulk up and need much higher requirements.

Athletes may also have ethnic backgrounds that make these particular food choices totally unacceptable and the same nutritional requirements may have to be met with Afro-Caribbean, Asian, Indian or vegetarian foods.

A key feature throughout this process is that the athlete understands what he or she is doing and why. It is important to understand which are the foods rich in carbohydrate and those rich in protein, while remembering the cross over, i.e. rich sources of carbohydrate which also provide protein. With practice the athlete will then be able to formulate their own daily food plans based on the theoretical requirements for their sport.

The issue of fat is one which often confuses athletes. Reducing fat to minimize weight gain or to make room for sufficient carbohydrate is sensible, but does the athlete understand that message. Do they believe they are on a no-fat diet? There is a misconception that this is an aim of the ideal diet for sport among some athletes.

Fat should not be avoided and indeed a certain amount of fat in the diet is essential. It is important to encourage athletes to look at using healthier types of fat such as those high in monounsaturated fat (olive oil, rapeseed oil) and polyunsaturated fats (sunflower seed oil and soya oil). It is vital for athletes to include some fat to ensure an adequate intake of essential fatty acids, as well as fat soluble vitamins. Some athletes may need advice on how to avoid excess intakes of fat and how to avoid saturated fat which does not confer health

Table 12.3   Examples of food intakes for two different athletes

Example one: 60-kg endurance runner – male (Estimated requirements)	Example two: 90-kg rugby player, forward – male (Estimated requirements)
480 g carbohydrate (8 g per kg body weight – middle point of endurance requirements)	720 g carbohydrate (8 g per kg body weight – middle point of power/strength requirements)
78 g protein (1.3 g per kg body weight – middle point of endurance requirements)	144 g protein (1.6 g per kg body weight – middle point of power/strength requirements)
Approximate food intake	Approximate food intake
Breakfast	Breakfast
200 mL orange juice	200 mL orange juice
30 g cereal plus 100 mL milk	90 g cereal plus 200 mL milk
2 slices bread plus jam	4 slices bread plus jam
Mid-morning	Mid-morning
1 cereal bar	1 cereal bar
200 mL apple juice	200 mL apple juice
apple	apple and yogurt
Lunch	Lunch
2 slices bread plus 30 g meat (1 slice)	4 slices bread plus 90 g tuna ($^1/_2$ can drained)
Salad	Salad, including 1 egg
Large banana	Large banana
Malt loaf 2 slices	Malt loaf 3 slices
Evening meal	Evening meal
90 g chicken breast plus tomato-based sauce	120 g chicken breast plus tomato-based sauce
300 g cooked pasta	300 g cooked pasta
Cooked vegetables	Cooked vegetables
Large banana	Large banana Coffee plus 2 spoons sugar
During/after training	During/after training
1 L isotonic sports drink	1.5 L isotonic sports drink
1 cereal bar	1 cereal bar
50 g jelly sweets	50 g jelly sweets 300 mL milk shake

benefits in the way that monounsaturated and polyunsaturated fats do. These might include:

- swapping butter for an olive oil or sunflower oil based spread – using a lower fat version if weight is an issue
- using olive oil in cooking in small amounts
- avoiding processed take-away meals with high-fat contents
- avoiding pastry based foods such as pies, sausage rolls, etc.
- ensuring that snacks for sport are high carbohydrate and low fat, rather than buying crisps from vending machines at sports venues
- planning appropriate post-training food rather than relying on the fast food outlets passed on the way home
- using a lower fat milk rather than avoiding milk.

FLUIDS

Sports science is crucial in enabling athletes to know their own hydration status and to establish strategies for maintaining hydration. The use of osmometry and hydrometers has become commonplace in testing and training environments. The weighing of individuals before and after training to establish fluid loss and hence sweat rate is also common practice. During this process it is important to remember the simple practical implications such as removing as much clothing as possible to avoid weighing sweat, removing sweaty trainers and socks, drying hair for water sports, passing urine before initial weighing but not passing urine before the final weight (unless urine is to be collected) and taking account of any fluid drunk during the exercise – preferably with a small weight scale to aid calculation. Good practice will give good results.

But what happens to the athlete when no support services are available? A number of quick indicators of hydration status can be useful reminders to the athlete to ensure good and appropriate hydration:

- Colour of urine – which should be pale straw coloured. Dark urine indicates dehydration and clear urine may indicate over-hydration or rapid passing of consumed fluid.
- Frequency of passing urine. Failure to pass urine for long periods should remind athletes of the need to drink. Similarly, having to get up in the night several times may indicate too much fluid has been consumed!
- Amount of urine passed.
- Smell of urine – strong urine indicates dehydration.

The need for athletes to practise drinking is important. Despite accurate calculations of requirements, many people find drinking before, during and after sport very difficult, and need to spend time learning how to do it.

In terms of the fluid used, athletes must be comfortable with their choice of drink in advance of competition. There is an obvious advantage to using the drink provided by sponsors in some events such as marathons. However, athletes should purchase samples and test the drink in advance. Sponsored drinks are common in team sports; however, in some teams the consensus might be that drinks are too strong. Therefore the solution is provided in a more dilute form. This has implications for energy content and sodium content, which may have varying levels of importance in different sports and different environmental conditions.

Sponsored drinks usually mean free bottles – an excellent idea, but bottles should be named and athletes should only drink from their own bottle. Sharing of bottles means sharing of germs. Where 'sports' bottles are used regularly it is also important that the bottles are sterilized regularly. Bottles which regularly contain sweet drinks are an ideal breeding ground for germs. The sterilizing solution used for babies' bottles, available in tablet or liquid form, is an ideal way to sterilize sports bottles.

TRAVEL

Once good nutritional habits have been established it is important that athletes maintain these habits, which can be particularly difficult during periods of travel.

JOURNEYS

It is important to take account of the whole journey time, from door to door, not just flight time. Sufficient food and drinks for the whole period are needed. The time spent in cars or sitting in airports can be used as eating time. Normal habits and quantities should be taken into account and the food and drinks planned to match as closely as possible the quantities and timing of normal meals. This may mean using packed food rather than airline meals which are often inadequate and not popular. Contacting the airline in advance with special dietary requirements can sometimes help.

It is wiser to carry more food than is needed to allow for the unexpected delays to flights, delays receiving baggage, long transfer times, etc. Even when travelling just within one country, it is possible to encounter delays on the road or railway. Carrying snacks that will not perish, such as cereal bars, dried fruit, low fat biscuits and lower fat savoury snacks, as well as the planned meals, will ensure that any unforeseen gaps are filled. Extra fluid should be carried, particularly on aeroplanes, which have a tendency to cause dehydration. Alcohol should be avoided during flights for the same reason.

EATING OUT

When travelling to training or competition, carrying sufficient food for post-exercise eating is a good idea but it may be necessary to find a restaurant in order to eat a full meal during long journeys. The meal should be low in fat and replace the carbohydrate and protein needed by the athlete. Food eaten during travelling must provide sufficient and adequate nutrition to allow training or competition to occur as soon as is needed. In restaurants it may be necessary to ask for extra potato; rice or pasta and bread can also be requested as an extra. Choosing main dishes without rich sauces, asking for pizzas that do not contain too many toppings, avoiding chips, opting for jacket potatoes, selecting undressed salads, and avoiding creamy deserts will all help to ensure that the next training session is well fuelled.

PLANNING

The principles of eating the best foods to ensure that nutrition optimizes performance may look relatively simple to the sports scientist. However, for the athlete who has to cope with training, possibly work or college, sleeping, perhaps having a family and social life – cooking and preparing food can be a major issue. Athletes often need help with planning and organizing food in such a way as to make sure that they eat what they know is the best food for them rather than what is fastest and easiest to obtain.

Planning begins with the theory – what are the requirements for the athlete? What does this mean in food terms? The practical application of this involves ensuring that the appropriate food is available at the right time. This can be further broken down into: shopping, storing and cooking appropriate foods.

The first step is a shopping list that ensures that the correct foods are purchased. Those foods then need to be stored. A store cupboard and freezer that can hold appropriate dried and frozen foods to make food preparation easier are essential time savers. Tins of tuna, low-fat custard, cooked red kidney beans, chopped tomatoes, sweetcorn, are good examples of tinned foods that can be made into a variety of dishes. Other basics such as stock cubes, dried milk, dried pasta and rice, cous cous, jars of lower fat sauce are useful additions to a store cupboard. A freezer, even a small one, is useful for keen athletes. They can be used to store bread, pizza bases, meat, fish, chicken portions and frozen vegetables which all form the basics of a meal and with careful choice can help the athlete to make a fast and appropriate meal.

Another useful store is a supply of appropriate snack foods which can be picked up quickly on the way to work or training. The snacks must be appropriate for the type of sport. Some kit bags contain a lot more kit than others, which can make perishable foods such as bananas a distinct problem.

COOKING

As previously mentioned, time is exceedingly tight for many athletes. Cooking may not be the first priority. There should also be no presumption made that the athlete (or their other household members) have the ability to cook what may seem simple food. In line with much of the population cooking skills may be limited to following the microwave instructions on a ready meal pack. A few guidelines for successful cooking are:

- Food must be fast. Recipes must be simple and not time consuming.
- Good food can be prepared faster than the time it takes to visit a take-away!
- Ingredients may need to be familiar and easy to purchase at local shops.
- Recipes should have been designed or adapted to meet the needs of the athlete – high in carbohydrate, with an appropriate amount of protein and low in fat. Most athletes will not want to spend time adapting inappropriate recipes themselves.
- Equipment which speeds up cooking can be useful such as a microwave, pressure cooker, and small portable 'grilling machines'.
- Equipment which cooks food slowly with minimal preparation can also be useful, such as slow cookers and bread making machines.
- Good cooking needs good shopping and food storage – see previous section on planning.

FOOD HYGIENE – THE FORGOTTEN SCIENCE OF SPORTS NUTRITION

Food hygiene is based on our knowledge of microbes and the potentially devastating effect they can have on our health and well-being. While food poisoning is never pleasant and is not conducive to good training, even worse is the scenario of being smitten just before a major competition. A few rules of basic hygiene should be observed by all.

STORE FOOD APPROPRIATELY

Perishable food should be kept in a refrigerator which is maintained at 0°C to 5°C. Left-over food should be removed from cans and stored in a dish with a lid, foil or cling film covering – but not stored too long. Foods in jars usually need to be stored in the fridge after opening. Meat should be stored at the bottom of the fridge to ensure that blood does not drip onto other foods. The fridge should not be overloaded or it will not work efficiently.

Foods in the freezer should be maintained at −18°C. After removing food from the freezer it should be thoroughly defrosted before using. Never refreeze food.

Root vegetables should be stored separately from other vegetables because of the risk of contamination from soil. If you are eating fruit and vegetables without cooking them, make sure that they are thoroughly washed.

SENSIBLE HYGIENE

- Check use-by dates on food, do not use out-of-date food.
- Do not use cracked eggs.
- Wash hands before handling food.
- Keep work surfaces clean – disinfect them regularly.
- Bleach or replace dish cloths regularly, as they harbour germs.
- Food should always be appropriately well cooked. Cook food thoroughly and serve it piping hot.
- When travelling and eating in hotels make sure that the water is safe, avoid shellfish, avoid scoop ice creams as the temperature at the surface is always too high and make sure that drinks bottles are sterilized regularly if they are re-used.

ATHLETES WITH DISABILITIES

Athletes with disabilities may need to consider a number of issues which will affect their nutritional requirements or the provision of those requirements.

Energy, carbohydrate and protein requirements may be different for athletes who use wheelchairs. This will be based on the functionality of their limbs and how mobile they are at times of the day when they are not taking part in sport.

Good hydration is vital. Adequate fluid intake is vital for sport and a poor fluid intake may also result in urine infections in athletes who use catheters. Dehydration also increases the risk of epilepsy, causing fits in people who are prone. Athletes with spinal cord injures will not sweat below the lesion in their spine. However, their sweat rate above the lesion can increase many fold and dehydration is still an issue. Good monitoring will help individuals to determine what their own sweat rate is. Some wheelchair users suffer from a problem called autonomic dysreflexia. Any athlete reporting this problem should establish their hydration strategies in conjunction with their medic and sports dietitian as bowel, bladder and drinking habits can influence the occurrence of autonomic dysreflexia which can cause sudden and massive increases in blood pressure.

Access to toilets may be an issue at some venues and this may affect the athlete's desire to drink the amount of fluid needed for good hydration. Some athletes may also need assistance in accessing drinks while using a wheel-chair. This may be physical assistance or the setting up of the drinks container in such a way as to allow free access. Access to food at eating venues, in shops and when cooking may have to be taken into account.

Visually impaired athletes may prefer information in an audio form or pre-sented as an email which can be accessed and 'read' using a voice synthesis system. Traditional methods of recognizing dehydration may not work for the visually impaired but indicators such as frequency of passing urine, how much urine is passed and the smell of urine can work very well.

CONCLUSION

Sports nutrition is a science, but it is a science with a very practical application. Those working at the interface with athletes need to be aware of the practical issues that affect compliance with nutritional guidelines. An appreciation of these issues and some suggestions for coping with them will help the athlete to maximize their performance through good nutrition.

KEY POINTS

1. Food or nutrition. The principles of nutrition are well documented and good guidelines are available. However, these principles must be translated into foods for the athlete.
2. Every athlete is individual and their nutrition plans and strategies should reflect this.
3. A number of life situations will impact on the nutritional intake of athletes and it is important to have plans in place to cope with these situations. These would include such issues as training times, competition days, travelling and eating out.
4. Basic shopping and cooking skills are important to an individual's ability to follow sound nutritional advice. A basic grasp of food hygiene will help to protect athletes from illness.
5. Athletes in wheelchairs may have different nutritional requirements to able-bodied counterparts. Other disabilities may merit consideration in the practicalities of information and food provision.

Further reading

Griffin J 2001 Food for sport – eat well, perform better. J Crowood, London

Leeds A, Brand Miller J, Foster-Powell K, Colagiuri S 1996 The glucose revolution. Hodder & Stoughton, London

O'Connor H, Brand Miller J, Colagiuri S, Foster Powell K 2000 The glucose revolution. In: The pocket guide to sports nutrition. Hodder & Stoughton, London

Stear S 2004 Fuelling fitness for sports performance. The British Olympic Association, London

Glossary

Activity-induced energy expenditure Energy expenditure due to physical activity.

Anaplerosis The replenishment of metabolites that have been removed from a metabolic pathway. In the case of the TCA cycle anaplerosis refers to the entry of carbon into the TCA cycle, by routes other than acetyl CoA entry via the citrate synthase reaction.

Antioxidant A chemical that reduces the rate of particular oxidation reactions, where oxidation reactions are chemical reactions that involve the transfer of electrons from a substance to an oxidizing agent.

Basal metabolic rate Rate of energy expenditure necessary for maintaining the basal functions of the body.

Biomarkers A measurable biological parameter which varies simply and quickly in response to changes in nutrient intake. Thus in dietary surveys there should be concordance between estimates of dietary intake and level of biomarker, e.g. urine nitrogen and protein intake.

Body clock Paired groups of cells in the suprachiasmatic nuclei that generate a circadian rhythmic output.

Chronobiology The study of the effects of time upon biological processes.

Circadian Having a period of about a day, generally in the region 24–25 h.

Cofactor Any substance that needs to be present in addition to an enzyme to catalyze a certain reaction. Some cofactors are inorganic, such as the metal atoms zinc, magnesium, iron, and copper in certain forms. Others, such as vitamins, are organic, and are known as coenzymes. Some cofactors undergo chemical changes during the course of a reaction (i.e. being reduced or oxidized).

Constant routine A protocol that minimizes the exogenous component of a circadian rhythm, thereby enabling the endogenous component to be investigated in more detail.

Cytoskeleton The network of proteins that contributes to the structure and organization of a cell.

Dehydration The process of losing water. In the case of exercise, essentially by the process of sweating.

Desynchronized A state in which the endogenous and exogenous components of a circadian rhythm are out of phase.

Diet-induced energy expenditure Energy cost of processing food.

Dietary counselling Giving advice to individuals which should take into account the person's whole lifestyle.

Direct calorimetry Determination of energy expenditure by measuring heat production of the body.

Endogenous rhythm The component of a *circadian* rhythm that is generated by the *body clock.*

Entrainment The process by which the body clock is adjusted to be in phase with a *zeitgeber.*

Euhydration Being in water balance.

Exogenous rhythm The component of a circadian rhythm that is generated by factors other than the body clock, the sleep–wake or light–dark cycles, for example.

Fat-free mass Mass of the body minus total mass of fat.

Fat mass Total of ether-extractable substances in the body; the mass of the body minus fat-free mass.

Fatty acid A simple lipid consisting of carbon, hydrogen and oxygen only, and the building block of a triglyceride. It is the useable source of energy from fats in which it is oxidized via β-oxidation and then the TCA cycle.

Fatty acid binding protein (FABP) A group of fatty acid transporters found both in the plasma membrane ($FABP_{pm}$) and cytosplasm ($FABP_c$).

Fatty acid translocase (FAT) A fatty acid transporter found in the membrane of skeletal muscle cells.

Fatty acid transport protein (FATP) A fatty acid transporter found in the membrane of skeletal muscle cells.

Ferritin A primary storage form of iron found in the mucosal cells, spleen, bone marrow and liver.

Food atlas A book of photographs of varied portion sizes of common foods. It enables individuals to indicate the amount of food eaten but may not be very precise and may induce bias.

Food composition tables A catalogue of the chemical (nutrient) composition of common foods. Such tables are normally essential parts of any appraisal of dietary intake but can introduce large errors (especially if used inexpertly).

Forced desynchronization A protocol which separates the endogenous and exogenous components of a circadian rhythm.

Free radical Atomic or molecular species with unpaired electrons on an otherwise open shell configuration. These unpaired electrons are usually highly reactive, so radicals are likely to take part in chemical reactions.

Gluconeogenesis The process by which glucose is synthesized from non-carbohydrate precursors such as amino acids, e.g. alanine and glutamine.

Glycaemic index A ranking system for carbohydrates based on their immediate effect on blood glucose concentrations. It compares carbohydrates (gram for gram) in individual foods, providing a numerical, evidence-based index of postprandial glycaemia.

Glycaemic load Is a ranking system for carbohydrate content in food portions based on their glycaemic index and the portion size.

Glycogenolysis   The breakdown of glycogen by removal of a glucose molecule and addition of phosphate to produce glucose-1-phosphate. The glucose-1-phosphate is then converted to glucose-6-phosphate and enters glycolysis.

Glycolysis   A biochemical pathway by which a molecule of glucose is oxidized to two molecules of pyruvic acid.

Haem   The iron-containing molecule found in haemoglobin.

Haem iron   Iron that is part of haemoglobin and myoglobin and found only in animal-based foods such as meat, fish and poultry.

Homocysteine   An intermediate metabolite in the metabolism of the amino acid methionine. High blood levels of homocysteine are associated with increased risk for cardiovascular disease.

Hyperhydration   The steady state of increased water in the body – usually as a result of imbibing fluids.

Hypernatraemia   The state where there is a high plasma sodium concentration in the blood.

Hypohydration   The steady state of reduced water in the body – usually as a consequence of sweat loss or lack of sufficient fluid intake.

Hyponatraemia   The state where there is a low plasma sodium concentration in the blood.

Indirect calorimetry   Determination of energy expenditure by measuring oxygen consumption and possibly carbon dioxide production and converting it to heat production.

Iron-deficiency anaemia   The last stage of iron deficiency in which red blood cell production has declined and there is a decreased ability to transport oxygen.

Iron-deficiency erythropoiesis   The second state of iron deficiency that is characterized by a decrease in serum iron and the iron transported on transferrin, which can lead to the decreased ability to synthesize new red blood cells.

Iron depletion   The first stage of iron deficiency, when low serum ferritin concentrations are low due to depletion of stored iron.

Jet lag   The symptoms that appear transiently after a time-zone transition across 3 or more time zones; it is due to desynchronization.

Lipid peroxidation   The oxidative degradation of lipids. It is the process whereby free radicals remove electrons from the lipids in cell membranes, resulting in cell damage.

Lipolysis   The breakdown of triglycerides stored in fat cells to free fatty acids and glycerol.

Nitrogen balance   A proxy measure for protein balance, as proteins are the main nitrogen-containing substances in the body, and is used by researchers to establish protein requirements. Nitrogen balance exists when nitrogen intake from the diet is equal to nitrogen excretion via urine, faeces and sweat. Negative nitrogen balance occurs when nitrogen intake is less than nitrogen excretion; and positive nitrogen balance occurs when nitrogen intake is greater than nitrogen excretion.

Non-haem iron   The form of iron that is not part of haemoglobin or myoglobin and found in animal and plant foods.

Nutritional epidemiology The application of the principles of epidemiology to the study of food intake and nutritional status.

Oxidative burst The rapid release of reactive oxygen species from different types of cells. Usually denoting the release of these ROS from immune cells, e.g. neutrophils and macrophages, as they come into contact with their targets.

Oxidative stress An imbalance between pro-oxidants and anti-oxidants, with the former prevailing. Oxidative stress is a term used for damage to cells individually, thus the organs and tissues composed of those cells and ultimately the organism. Oxidative stress is caused by reactive species. These include (but are not limited to) superoxide, singlet oxygen, peroxynitrite or hydrogen peroxide.

Oxidize The loss of an electron by a molecule, atom or ion.

Physical activity index Ratio of total energy expenditure and basal metabolic rate.

Placebo An inactive substance (pill, liquid, etc.), which is administered as if it were a therapy, but which has no therapeutic value other than the placebo effect.

Reactive oxygen species (ROS) Include oxygen ions, free radicals and peroxides both inorganic and organic. They are generally very small molecules and are highly reactive. ROSs form as a natural byproduct of the normal metabolism of oxygen and have important roles in cell signalling.

However, during times of stress, ROS levels can increase dramatically which can result in significant damage to cell structures.

Reduce The gain of an electron by a molecule, atom or ion.

Rehydration The process of regaining water.

Reliability The extent to which a measurement can be repeated (assuming no real change has occurred). Food intake is constantly changing and what an individual eats for a particular day, week, month may not be a good (reliable) reflection of what they normally would eat – thus compromising the ability to give advice or draw useful conclusions.

Shiftworkers' malaise The symptoms that appear during night work; it is due to desynchronization.

Transamination The process by which an amino group (NH_2) is transferred from a donor compound, usually an amino acid, to another chemical compound, usually an oxo acid.

Transferrin The transport protein for iron found in the blood.

Triglyceride (Also known as triacylglycerol) is the storage form of lipids in adipose tissue and skeletal muscle composed of a glycerol molecule esterified with three fatty acids.

Validity The extent to which any measurement measures what it is intended to do. With any sort of dietary survey there is a common tendency to under-report food intake, especially of less desirable food items, thus compromising the validity of the assessment.

Zeitgeber   A rhythm in the external environment with a period equal to, or close to, 24 h that entrains the body clock.

Index